Natural Energy

Natural*Energy*

A CONSUMER'S GUIDE

TO LEGAL, MIND-ALTERING,

AND MOOD-BRIGHTENING

HERBS AND SUPPLEMENTS

Mark Mayell

Three Rivers Press | *New York*

Copyright © 1998 by Mark Mayell

All rights reserved. No part of this book may be reproduced or transmitted in
any form or by any means, electronic or mechanical, including photocopying,
recording, or by any information storage and retrieval system, without
permission in writing from the publisher.

Published by Three Rivers Press, a division of Crown Publishers, Inc., 201 East
50th Street, New York, New York 10022. Member of the Crown Publishing Group.

Random House, Inc. New York, Toronto, London, Sydney, Auckland
www.randomhouse.com

THREE RIVERS PRESS and colophon are trademarks of Crown Publishers, Inc.

Printed in the United States of America

DESIGN BY LYNNE AMFT

Library of Congress Cataloging-in-Publication Data
Mayell, Mark
Natural energy : a consumer's guide to legal, mind-altering, and
mood-brightening herbs and supplements / by Mark Mayell. — 1st pbk. ed.
p.   cm.
Includes bibliographical references and index.
1. Psychotropic plants.   2. Psychotropic drugs.   3. Nootropic agents.
4. Herbs—Therapeutic use.   5. Dietary supplements.
I. Title.
RM315.M357   1998
615'.788—DC21   97-24045
                                        CIP

ISBN 0-517-88812-2 (pbk.)

10   9   8   7   6   5   4   3   2   1

First Edition

This book is a reference guide. The tools, techniques, and suggestions here are not intended to substitute for medical advice or treatment. Any application of the ideas or recommendations in this book is at the reader's discretion and risk.

Contents

◉

Acknowledgments

Editors Leslie Meredith, Sherri Rifkin, and Joanna Burgess of Harmony Books supported the project and offered many valuable suggestions. Agent Nat Sobel of Sobel Weber Associates ably assisted my efforts from proposal to finished manuscript. Bob Bonanno, M.D., Alan R. Hirsch, M.D., Christopher Hobbs, Bill Thomson, and Laurel Vukovich deserve thanks for various types of help and guidance. I'd also like to thank the folks at Healthy.Net, the producers of Health-World Online (www.healthy.net), for their service that provides free access to Medline, and the staff at the College of Pharmacy, University of Illinois at Chicago, for their invaluable Napralert natural products and medicinal plants database. Family members and friends who have been supportive throughout this project include Hillary Mayell White, Dick White, Kathryn Grammer, Bob Bruce, and especially my wife, Jeanne Mayell.

Author's Note

◉

This book is a consumer's guide to natural mind-altering substances. It is the author's intent neither to endorse the taking of these herbs and supplements nor to proscribe their use. Rather, the purpose of this book is to offer definitive, up-to-date information about mind-altering herbs and supplements, and to encourage a more enlightened and realistic discussion of their effects, their relative benefits and risks, and why people take them. The goal is to allow individuals to make educated choices about what they want—and don't want—to put in their bodies and minds.

By definition, substances that can alter mind or mood and affect behavior or performance can impact personal health. While an attempt has been made to provide thorough information on the relative safety and the potential side effects of every substance, it is impossible to cover all contingencies. Nor is it possible to take into consideration every individual's unique physical makeup and situation. Readers are encouraged to seek the advice of their doctors or natural health practitioners if they have medical conditions or have any reservations at all about taking the substances described in this book.

Ultimately, the choice to use any substance lies with the individual, who must be ready to accept full responsibility for his or her actions.

Preface

Recently my seven-year-old son came to me with a strange complaint. "Everything seems like it's going too fast," he said. In what way, I asked, doubtful that at his tender age he was ready to voice a philosophical reservation about the hurried nature of modern society. He wasn't. "Last night when I slept over at Billy's house," he said, "I couldn't fall asleep. And now this morning I can't sit still and when I do things it's like I'm rushing."

"Well, did you drink some Coca-Cola over at Billy's?"

"No."

"What about Pepsi?"

"Oh yeah, I had some of that."

Welcome to the world of mind-altering substances, little guy. Since he isn't provided caffeinated beverages at home, when he does consume a cola the effects are clear to him: he feels juiced, hyped-up, speedy. It's the same feeling experienced by the eight out of ten Americans over the age of twelve who use caffeine regularly. Yet, at seven, my son now is aware of something that millions of other kids, and even plenty of adults, don't know or refuse to recognize: caffeine is a drug. The fact that it is rarely packaged and promoted as a drug—NoDoz, Vivarin, and the like account for only a fraction of caffeine consumption—and that producers freely market it to children does not alter its status as a psychoactive substance.

By the same token, three out of five adult Americans regularly consume alcohol and one out of four smoke or chew tobacco. Alcohol and nicotine happen to be two of the most potent, toxic, and addictive mind-altering drugs ever identified. Yet in the United States and throughout most of the rest of the world, they're legal, socially accepted, and widely advertised. People use them much as they have for centuries: to be stimulated or relaxed, to promote conversation and friendship, to celebrate or just to escape.

Americans may be loath to admit it, but they take mind-altering and mood-boosting substances with remarkable alacrity. What they don't do, unfortunately, is give much thought to why they use these substances, what the long-term health implications are, and whether less-toxic alternatives with similar properties might exist. Clearly, the wide range of social and cultural factors that surround, for example, alcoholic beverages and their use—what's been called Western society's "drinking complex"—outweigh the specific actions alcohol has on the mind and body for the vast majority of people who drink. But it's also true that when people drink at home alone to relax after a day at work, or consume alcohol late at night in an attempt to promote sleep, they are overlooking other, equally effective mind-alterants available to them no farther away than the nearest natural foods store.

Knowing and acknowledging that you're taking a mind-altering drug, as my son recently discovered, is the first step toward responsible use. Equally important is to make informed choices, based not on social pressures and marketing hype but on a realistic understanding of substances' relative risks and benefits.

PART ONE

Introduction to Mind~Altering Substances

Types of Mind ~ Alterants

◉

FROM STIMULANTS TO APHRODISIACS

A few years ago I put together a somewhat tongue-in-cheek birthday present for my wife. It was a jewelry box that contained not necklaces and earrings but what I labeled "nature's little helpers," after the "mother's little helpers" of the Rolling Stones' song from the 1960s. Each of the box's compartments held a different category of natural mind-alterant: a few capsules of ginseng and the amino acid phenylalanine in the stimulant section; some melatonin and valerian in the relaxant section; ginkgo for boosting the brain and some essential oil of Rose for brightening the mood. On tiny cards I briefly described what each substance was, what it did, how to use it, and how much to take.

The gift was an immediate success with my wife, and friends and family who heard about the gift box put in requests. Those tiny cards gradually accumulated more and more information, and I soon realized that the topic of natural mind-alterants was curiously overlooked in the crowded personal health market.

Any number of books and magazine articles have been devoted to natural ways to lose weight, decrease your risk of cancer or heart disease, regulate your digestive system, and cure your backache. But information about the effects that herbs, amino acids, nutritional supplements, essential oils, and other natural substances have on mind, mood, and behavior is harder to come by.

I'm convinced that a large part of the reason for the apparent reluctance of writers and publishers to explore this field has to do with certain cultural biases that are still prevalent in North America, if not much of the rest of Western society. Both elements of the term "natural mind-alterant" cause confusion and even outright resistance among a part of the public, though there is evidence of an increased openness in recent years. The word *natural* has, admittedly, been used in so many euphemistic and variable ways in popular books and products that its meaning has become dangerously thin. For some it means little more than an empty promotional promise, akin to "new and improved." For others it is high praise, denoting safety, effectiveness, and environmental appropriateness.

Mind-alterant shares a pejorative context with a whole host of related words with nevertheless distinct meanings, including drug, narcotic, and high. People often react negatively and unthinkingly to the whole concept of mind-alterants, even (often especially) those who take these substances many times every day. When I mentioned I was writing a book on natural mind-altering substances to an acquaintance a few months ago, her first response was, "You're going to warn people away from these, right?" I mildly replied not necessarily, and alluded to the tens of millions of people whose everyday abuse of conventional mind-alterants, from alcohol to cigarettes to sleeping pills, was hardly reason to endorse the status quo. Might an examination of potential alternatives be useful?

The terms used to frame the discussion are crucial for moving beyond the level of cliché and sound-bite. To promote useful dialogue, before looking at the individual mind-alterants it is worthwhile to address the issue of what is meant by such words as natural, mind-altering, stimulant, relaxant, inebriant, and so forth.

NATURAL VERSUS SYNTHETIC

The definition of *natural* used here will be a utilitarian and relativistic one that falls some-where between the most loose (anything that appears in a natural foods store) and the most strict (the unchanged products of nature). That is, natural products are herbs, nutrients, and compounds derived from nature or based upon substances found in nature without added extraneous ingredients or unnecessary processing. Note that, by this definition, most of the conventional mind-alterants in Western societies, including coffee, tobacco, and alcohol, are natural. By the same token, various mind-alterants currently considered illicit, from cocaine to marijuana, are natural. Neither the conventional nor the illicit mind-alterants are covered in detail for a number of reasons, including the fact that a vast amount of information has already been collected in other books. Here the primary concern is with legal, readily available alternatives to these substances, many of which have similar actions on the mind and body.

Any useful definition of natural must be relative, because even obvious distinctions may blur under closer examination. One of the most potent natural mind-alterants is kava. Kava is a plant—what could be more natural? Well, many researchers say that for thousands of years humanity has selectively bred kava for certain properties. The plants are basically no longer found in the wild. They propagate only with the help of humans, who cut off a stem of an existing plant and stick it in the ground, not exactly a reproductive technique found in pre-humanity nature. If humanity were to disappear from the earth tomorrow, within a short time in all likelihood kava would also become extinct. So, is this substance "natural"? Yes, because it is possible to distinguish between certain types of human actions on a natural product and still consider it natural.

Most people would also agree that the ground-up, powdered root of a kava plant is natural. But herbal producers often take herbs such as kava and select certain compounds for extraction and/or standardization, sometimes at the expense of other compounds that also naturally occur in the plant. Other ingredients may be added to the resulting powder, which is then encapsulated and bottled. Is the kava product you pick up off the natural foods store's shelf natural, or not? Again, yes, relative to the vast majority of synthetic pharmaceutical drugs, whether over-the-counter or prescription-only. At this point, however, questions about the degree of processing of a natural product begin to become important. Many synthetic drugs are concentrated forms of a single isolated compound, unlike plants that may have many active ingredients with synergistic or counterbalancing effects.

In a number of cases (particularly the nutrients, some hormones, and a few substances that act much like certain brain chemicals known as neurotransmitters, all described in this chapter), natural can even encompass laboratory synthesis. For example, melatonin is a natural bodily hormone. Supplement producers can obtain it either by isolating it from animals' pineal glands or by synthesizing it in the laboratory. Either way, melatonin is the same molecule. Obtaining it synthetically is easier, cheaper, and cleaner than laboriously pulling only the melatonin out of ground-up organs, and the vast majority of the melatonin on the market today is synthetic. Nevertheless, for our purposes it is considered natural because the original substance is based upon a naturally occurring compound. On the other hand, synthetic or so-called nature-identical essential oils don't deserve the term natural. Chemists cannot match the exquisite balance and identity of the hundreds of compounds found in many essential oils, and the resulting synthetic products are clearly inferior to natural essential oils.

It is also worth noting that even conventional pharmaceutical drugs often have a basis in the natural world. Pharmacologists estimate that one-quarter of the prescriptions written in North America today are for drugs whose origins can be traced to plants and herbs. These include the drug digitalis (from components of the leaves of the purple foxglove plant) for heart conditions; reserpine (from Indian snakeroot) for hypertension; and of course all of the potent pain-killing morphine-based drugs (from the opium poppy). Even aspirin is seminatural, since a close relative (salicin) of one of its compounds was originally identified in white willow bark and the meadowsweet plant. Modern medicine's natural pharmacopoeia is actually much larger than most people recognize.

Strictly from a utilitarian standpoint, the natural mind-alterants examined in this book include many substances familiar to anyone who has ever shopped in a natural foods store:

■ Herbs: green tea, ginseng, Siberian ginseng/ eleuthero, ephedra/ma huang, guarana, maté, kola nut, St. John's wort, ginkgo, valerian, California poppy, kava, yohimbé

- Amino acids: phenylalanine, tyrosine, tryptophan, 5-hydroxytryptophan, GABA, and pyroglutamate
- Essential oils: Rose, Jasmine, Neroli, Peppermint, Basil, Rosemary
- Nutritional substances: choline and DMAE

An additional category includes compounds that are modeled, sometimes exactly and sometimes not, on substances normally found in the human body, including:

- Hormones: melatonin and vasopressin

A final category also straddles the line between natural and synthetic:

- Semisynthetic substances with analogs in the plant world: Hydergine, piracetam, and deprenyl

---

A W A R O F W O R D S

The thirty-two natural mind-alterants just mentioned represent a wide range of substances with considerable variations in their actions on body and mind. All too often, discussions about these substances and their actions take place without sufficient regard to important distinctions. For example, a certain percentage of the population can be expected to react to a book on natural mind-alterants along the lines of "this is a book about drugs, drugs are bad, ban this book." Another percentage may well react quite differently, along the lines of "cool, natural ways to get high!"

Quite possibly, this book will disappoint both camps. Those who think that "just say no" is an effective idea for influencing people's use of mind-altering substances will not accept the underlying reality recognized and acknowledged here: for vast numbers of people mind-alterants serve a purpose and individuals choose to use them. On the other hand, though it is certainly possible to use some of the substances covered in this book to get high (and a short section of the book is devoted to inebriants), such "nonmedical" or "recreational" applications don't fairly represent the range of substances and their actions considered here. Indeed, few of the substances here are merely recreational highs, but rather are substances that people take with specific purposes in mind, those purposes being to alter the mind in a way that allows for greater stimulation, relaxation, concentration, sexual pleasure, and so forth.

The best general terms for the group of substances included here are *mind-altering* and *psychoactive,* referring to the whole range of possible changes in consciousness, from mild stimulation to vivid hallucinations, from slight relaxation to stupefaction. A lesser-used term with a similar meaning is *psychotropic,* from the Greek roots *psyche* for life, soul, or breath, and *tropein* for turning, thus acting on or affecting the spirit or mind. A similar construction, coined even more recently, in 1973, is *nootropic,* from the Greek *noos* for mind. Its popular usage, however, has been restricted to refer to smart drugs (see Brain Boosters, pages 9–10).

These words to describe substances that alter mind and mood are all preferable to a general term such as *drugs,* especially when it is used in a phrase like "the war on drugs." Admittedly, whether natural or synthetic in origin, substances that affect the function of mind and body can legitimately be considered drugs. That includes all of the substances in this book. Yet the label *drug* has been politicized to the degree that it obscures as much as it reveals. Young people have begun to refer to the war on drugs as "the war on *some* drugs," noting that Americans take vast quantities of legal drugs for medical, disease-curing reasons; vast quantities of legal drugs for questionably medical, mind-altering purposes (from mood enhancers like Prozac to anxiety reducers like Valium); and vast quantities of legal drugs for totally nonmedical reasons (such as virtually all consumption of caffeine, alcohol, and tobacco). For many Americans who live outside mainstream culture, the war on drugs is simply shorthand for "the war on *someone else's* drugs." A clearer definition of terms would be a first step toward reconciling conflicting points of view.

- -
THE MAIN MIND-ALTERING ACTIONS
- -

Numerous attempts have been made to classify the diverse actions of mind-altering substances. Most of the more recent ones are variations on a model proposed by the German writer Louis Lewin in his classic 1924 book *Phantastica.* Lewin devised five primary categories for mind-alterants: euphorica, such as opium; excitantia, such as tobacco and caffeine; hypnotica, such as sleep-inducing kava; inebrianta, for which alcohol is the prototype; and phantastica, such as vision-inducing peyote.

Modern writers have adapted and expanded Lewin's categories, based on new research and increased knowledge about substances' actions. For example, in his important 1972 book *Narcotic Plants,* William Emboden slightly modified Lewin by grouping most central nervous system depressants into one category. In 1979, an influential group of scholars and botanists proposed a new word for Lewin's phantastica and Emboden's hallucinogens: *entheogen,* from the Greek root *theos* for god, thus "becoming god within." In his 1995 book *Pharmako/Poeia,* poet and ethnobotanist Dale Pendell utilizes four of Lewin's original categories but replaces hypnotica with *thanatopathia*–plants that offer "a taste of death," as tobacco.

For the purposes of this book, it is not important to organize all the relevant herbs and other natural substances into rigid categories. Within any model that might be adopted, one would expect much crossing over among categories, such that substances would be an inebriant to one person, a stimulant to another, and a euphoric to a third. Rather, a discussion of the categories themselves helps to identify the wide range of potential properties exhibited by mind-altering substances. The categories and properties most prominent in succeeding chapters are the following:

Stimulants

These are what Lewin categorizes as excitants, substances that increase the action of the central nervous system and lead to improved alertness, greater ability to concentrate, and enhanced physical and mental endurance. Stimulants range from relatively mild ones such as caffeine to super-potent ones, including synthetic amphetamine derivatives (and even LSD) that are classified as controlled substances and have drastic effects on mental function that can go quite a bit beyond what is usually considered stimulation.

Part two, which groups all of the natural stimulants, includes a discussion of four herbs that contain caffeine, the predominant conventional stimulant in modern society. One of these herbs is green tea (see chapter 2), which, although it has the same amount of caffeine as black tea, when prepared in the traditional method can have a lower caffeine content. The other three are exotic caffeinated herbs, guarana, maté, and kola nut (see chapter 5), which are increasing in popularity outside their origins in South America and Africa. While caffeine is definitely a prominent active compound in these herbs, it may not be the only one. A few of these caffeinated herbs, particularly green tea, may also have additional compounds that suggest it is a more healthful source of caffeine than coffee.

Other chapters in this section explore diverse alternatives to caffeinated herbs. Ephedra, or ma huang as the Chinese refer to it (see chapter 4), is not caffeinated, though its principal active compound, ephedrine, has similar effects on the mind. Ephedrine is more potent than caffeine and as a result ephedra has become one of the most controversial herbs on the market today. Certain amino acids, particularly phenylalanine and tyrosine, can also provide an energy lift, and in chapter 6 we look at what they offer and how they work.

Another prominent class of natural stimulants is strengthening or tonic herbs. Ginseng and Siberian ginseng/eleuthero (see chapter 3) do not contain central nervous system stimulants as potent as caffeine and ephedrine. Rather, these ancient herbs work in the body in slightly different ways to increase energy levels, prevent fatigue, improve mood, and possibly even increase libido.

Quite a few of the mind-altering substances covered in the other sections of the book can be mildly stimulating, especially the brain boosters covered in part four and yohimbé, covered in part six.

Mood Brighteners

These are substances that elevate the spirits, dispel the blues, reduce anxiety, and increase feelings of cheerfulness and optimism. Since the development of Prozac in 1974 by researchers at Eli Lilly, conventional pharmaceutical mood brighteners like it have become best-selling drugs with markets measured in the billions of dollars. Many of the most successful are, like Prozac, classified as selective serotonin reuptake inhibitors (SSRIs), though an even newer category is selective noradrenaline reuptake inhibitors (SNRIs). These work by promoting the activity in the brain of serotonin and noradrenaline, neurotransmitters with potential mood-elevating effects, among others.

Mood brighteners are generally considered to be less potent and less toxic than antidepressants, though both classes of drugs may benefit certain types of depression. Major mood disorders include clinical depression, manic depression, schizophrenia, and other conditions. These are serious illnesses, not the kind of condition you want to try to address merely by taking some herb or nutrient (though these may play a beneficial role in a broader treatment plan). Doctors define clinical depression as a continuing, whole-body illness characterized by a variety of symptoms, such as decreased energy or fatigue, thoughts of suicide, sleep problems, and changes in appetite and weight. An estimated ten million Americans each year suffer from major depression.

Temporary low moods and feelings of anxiety are much more common, affecting almost everybody every now and then. Natural mood brighteners are perfectly appropriate for such conditions, and in some cases their actions on the mind can be attributed to the same types of effects on neurotransmitters as the more toxic conventional mood brighteners. Substances such as St. John's wort (see chapter 7) and three exquisite essential oils, Rose, Jasmine, and Neroli (see chapter 8; to distinguish essential oils from herbs, we'll follow the convention of capitalizing the names of essential oils), rarely promote euphoria but can frequently alleviate mild depression and enhance an overall sense of well-being.

Many of the stimulants described in part two tend also to have minor mood-brightening effects. In addition, a number of natural mind-alterants in other sections of the book have mood-elevation as a "side effect" of their main function. For example, the brain boosters in part four, especially ginkgo, can often alleviate the age-related depression associated with decreased circulation of blood and oxygen to the brain. Relaxants, too, can have important effects on serotonin and other neurochemicals that affect mood, such as melatonin. These natural substances include melatonin, 5-hydroxytryptophan, and kava.

Brain Boosters

Brain boosters constitute a relatively recent category of potentially mind-altering substance. People take brain-boosting herbs, nutrients, and smart drugs primarily to enhance brain function and prevent age-related declines in mental performance. They are also frequently taken to increase short- and long-term memory, enhance certain types of learning, boost creativity and motivation, and improve other aspects of thinking and intelligence.

The classic brain boosters are the smart drugs, but the term has also come to encompass nutritional substances (such as choline, DMAE, and pyroglutamate; see chapter 10) and herbs (such as ginkgo; see chapter 11) with smart-drug effects. The term *smart drug* is generally reserved to refer to synthetic or semisynthetic drugs that may be available in

North America only by prescription. Even this simple classification, however, is not clear-cut. At high doses, some nutrients can have drug-like effects, and some of the smart drugs appear to be as safe as certain nutrients.

The mechanisms by which brain boosters act vary from one substance to another. Among the common actions are brain boosters' ability to protect the brain from free radical damage; increase blood flow to or circulation within the brain and thus its supply of oxygen; and boost the levels or the activity of certain neurotransmitters, such as dopamine, noradrenaline, and acetylcholine, that have positive effects on aspects of mental functioning. Many brain boosters may slow the aging of the brain in a way that promotes its full and efficient functioning.

An improvement in recall or an apparent increase in intelligence is usually thought to be more "brain-altering" than to have "mind-altering" effects. Yet because many of the brain boosters have varied actions, quite a few do have important mind-altering effects. There is significant crossover with the effects of the stimulants. Brain boosters may cause increases in alertness, concentration, and endurance; stimulants frequently (though not uniformly) have positive effects on the ability to perform mental tasks and other aspects of mental performance. Many people also experience an elevation of mood and noted prosexual effects from taking certain brain boosters.

The medical establishment in North America does not generally recognize any brain-boosting substances as useful for normal, healthy people. A few of the smart drugs, such as deprenyl and Hydergine, do have approved uses in the treatment of certain conditions that cause elderly people to develop problems with memory, attention, and mood. Use of smart drugs among normal, healthy persons has gained wider acceptance in Europe, where dozens of products are now promoted as brain boosters. Among the many pharmaceutical smart drugs, in chapter 9 we take a close look at four (vasopressin, deprenyl, piracetam, and Hydergine) that are among the more established and safest of the category. Though they're not typically considered brain boosters per se, the essential oils that promote clearheadedness (Peppermint, Basil, and Rosemary) discussed in chapter 12 share a few of the same properties.

Relaxants

Relaxants of one kind or another are among the most popular mind-altering substances worldwide. Partly this is because stimulants are also widely consumed—relaxants may be necessary to unwind or induce sleep after a day of drinking coffee and smoking cigarettes. Americans consume thirty million sleeping pills a day; the national appetite for benzodiazepines such as Valium to reduce anxiety is almost as voracious. Prescription relaxants are typically potent substances, with a high potential for abuse and numerous side effects. Alcohol, which has been used by humanity for thousands of years, is basically a relaxant.

A slew of alternative terms with meanings similar to *relaxant* are used to describe substances' ability to reduce the activity of the central nervous system, calm muscles, and promote sleep. These terms include *sleep aid, hypnotic,* and *soporific,* which all refer primarily to an ability to promote sleep, and the more generic *downer, sedative,* and *depressant,* connoting an overall reduction in vital bodily functions, such as circulation and nervous system activity. Dose can be crucial—a low level of a relaxant might mainly promote calmness and reduce anxiety, a slightly higher dose induce sleep, higher still act as an inebriant, and yet more act as a general anesthetic. The effect may also be slightly different over time, as is often noted with alcohol. A drink or two may seem mainly stimulating, yet after an hour or two the depressant effects on the nervous system win out, making the person relaxed or even sleepy.

The most potent of the conventional relaxants are the *tranquilizers,* used both to induce sleep and calm psychotic patients, and the *narcotics. Narcotic* is another word that has lost some of its usefulness as a result of lack of agreement on the exact meaning. In the nineteenth century narcotic was used in much the same manner we now use mind-altering and psychoactive. This use continued as recently as the early 1970s, if the title of Emboden's book *Narcotic Plants* is an indication. Gradually, however, narcotic has taken on another, equally misleading meaning. In the United States politicians and the police often use it as a synonym for "illegal drug," a usage that has even made it into the judicial system. Substances regulated by the Harrison Narcotic Act, including the stimulant cocaine, are legally considered narcotics.

The word's original meaning remains the most useful. Narcotic is from the Greek *narkoun* for "to benumb." Its earliest use in En-glish has been traced back six hundred years to Chaucer, who referred specifically to opium and other drugs with similar effects. Narcotics in the original sense are opium and similar drugs that induce sleep, lethargy, and eventually stupor. Initially they may induce euphoria, often they are useful for reducing pain, and ultimately they may be addictive over the long term. The true narcotics now include the potent alkaloids isolated from opium (such as morphine and codeine) and semisynthetic opium derivatives (such as heroin).

None of the substances described in parts two through six are true narcotics. California poppy (see chapter 14), though it is in the same plant family as the opium poppy, a true narcotic, does not derive its actions from the same potent, and addictive, compounds. Nor do any of the herbal relaxants in part five have the addictive properties of the true narcotics. The natural relaxants described here, including the herb valerian (see chapter 13); the hormone melatonin (see chapter 15); and the amino acids tryptophan, 5-hydroxytryptophan, and GABA (see chapter 16) are generally milder in their effects than the prescription sedatives or tranquilizers. The natural relaxants tend to be safer, too, and they can be just as useful as more potent prescription drugs for the effects most people desire: occasional relief from nervous tension or temporary sleeplessness.

Inebriants

Of course, the principal mainstream inebriant in modern society is alcohol. The word *inebriate* is from the Latin *ebriare,* to make drunk, to excite or exhilarate as with alcohol. A closely related term, also widely associated with the drug alcohol, is *intoxicant*. A slight but important distinction exists. *Intoxicate* is derived from the Latin *toxicum,* for poison. To be intoxicated is literally to be poisoned in a way that causes loss of control, physically and mentally. In Western societies both inebriation and intoxication are almost always associated with drunkenness from alcohol, or from even more injurious substances. To become intoxicated, however, is more pejorative, with its connotations of self-induced poisoning. Inebriation at least leaves open the possibility that the experience is not mere drunkenness but a losing of the normal constraints on the self to experience rapture or ecstasy, a return, as author Jonathan Ott notes, to inebriation's first use in English in 1526 as "heavenly drunkenness of the spirit." (See Ott's extraordinary and encyclopedic *Pharmacotheon* for a much more thorough examination of what is meant by inebriation and many of the other terms described here.)

Inebriants can also usefully be described as agents that induce euphoria or ecstasy. *Euphoria* is from the Greek *euphoros,* for "healthy, bearing well," thus a feeling of well-being or elation, the buoyancy of being carried along in one's endeavors. *Ecstasy* is from the Greek *ek* for out and *histanai,* for "to set, stand." It sometimes gets translated as "to derange" but a more literal meaning is to be put outside of oneself, to experience a state of such overwhelming rapture or delight or feeling that the mind or soul withdraws from the body and soars into another, higher, realm.

In comparison, the term *deliriant* has more

in common with intoxicant than euphoriant. The word is from the Latin *de* for "away" and *lira* for "furrow"; thus to plow outside the furrow—to go nuts, to be crazy. Deliriants cause disordered, disturbed, sometimes violent and self-destructive behavior. They may also cause hallucinations. Substances capable of causing such extreme states are highly toxic.

Given these distinctions, kava (see chapter 17) is more legitimately an inebriant or euphoriant. In lower doses, of course, kava is primarily a relaxant, just as a few drinks of an alcoholic beverage can be relaxing while a few more can be inebriating. The other relaxants grouped in part five, however, tend to be milder than kava, and are either ineffective as inebriants or not generally taken in doses high enough to cause that effect.

Aphrodisiacs

Substances that tend to increase libido (sexual desire) and boost sexual performance may be the most controversial category from the perspective of medical scientists, most of whom contend that aphrodisia is all in the mind. According to the *American Medical Association Encyclopedia of Medicine,* "In fact, no substance has a proven aphrodisiac effect, although virtually anything may produce the desired results if the person taking it believes strongly enough that it will work." The mind can indeed be a potent aphrodisiac (the placebo effect is as high as 50 percent for aphrodisiac properties), but there are also a number of potential mechanisms for natural substances to boost aspects of sexuality: by diminishing sexual inhibition while intensifying sensory feelings (kava, for example); by affecting bodily levels of male and female sex hormones (ginseng, possibly); by increasing or decreasing brain levels of neurotransmitters associated with sexual desire (various substances); and by improving blood supply to erectile tissue such as the penis (yohimbé, ginkgo). Natural substances can not only increase short-term sexual desire but can nourish and support the sex glands and the entire hormonal and reproductive systems, thereby increasing overall sexual vigor and possibly fertility.

Given the skepticism that the term aphrodisiac generates, a useful substitute that is frequently used is *prosexual,* popularized recently in *Better Sex Through Chemistry* by John Morgenthaler and Dan Joy. They define a prosexual drug or nutrient as "any substance that can improve sex or sexual health."

Chief among the prosexual substances is yohimbé (see chapter 18). In fact, it is the source for a compound that is approved by the FDA as a treatment for male impotence. It is one of the few compounds, natural or synthetic, that does have medical acceptance as a promoter of male erections, if not male sexual response.

Substances covered in other sections that are also taken by some for prosexual effects include kava, the smart drug deprenyl, and even ginseng. Ginkgo's positive effects on circulation can in some cases promote better sexual function. The floral essential oils just mentioned as mood boosting are also often the same ones that people find useful for increasing sexual desire.

Humanity's use of mind-altering and mood-boosting substances is virtually universal. As far back in time as records go, the evidence indicates that people have sought out and used drugs to alter consciousness, primarily though not exclusively in spiritual contexts. As widely afield as anthropologists search, they've found that societies also include various types of mind-alterants in their cultural, social, and medical practices. One estimate is that some 4,000 plants yield mind-altering compounds. Only a very few cultures, such as the Inuit, who live in the severe climate of the far north with a very limited selection of plants to use, appear to have no traditional mind-altering substances.

Indeed, anthropologists and psychopharmacologists who have researched humanity's use of inebriating substances have found mind-alterants tightly, even ineradicably, interwoven into the pattern of human history. Recent scholarly books on the topic have referred to mind-alterants as "essential substances" and humanity's pursuit of them as "the fourth drive" (after hunger, thirst, and sex). From this perspective, the use of stimulants, relaxants, inebriants, and other mind-alterants, for reasons that may range from the divine (to achieve an ecstatic communion with nature or one's gods or goddesses) to the mundane (to promote sleep, increase alertness, or reduce anxiety), is seen to be a basic human activity. Taking mind-altering drugs is evidently so ingrained in public behavior and individual psyche that we ignore it at the peril of not fully knowing ourselves.

Certainly, mind-alterants are deeply ingrained in modern American society. Virtually the entire adult population of the United States makes regular use of mind-altering or mood-boosting substances. Each day the average American drinks three-and-one-half cups of coffee (one estimate is that 80 percent of coffee drinkers are addicted to the drug) and more than 20 ounces of (usually caffeinated) soft drinks. Americans consume more than 22 billion gallons of beer and another two billion gallons of other alcoholic beverages. An estimated forty million Americans are addicted to tobacco; at least thirteen million are considered heavy drinkers. Eighty million have tried marijuana or some other illicit drug in their lifetimes; about twelve million used illicit drugs last year alone. Prescription drugs to reduce anxiety and improve mood are taken by tens of millions. All this drug taking doesn't occur in a vacuum, of course—coffee, alcohol, and soft drinks, in that order, are the three foods most often consumed or mentioned on prime-time television. U.S. alcoholic beverage producers spend billions of dollars each year to promote their drug.

Two of the psychoactive drugs, opium and alcohol, with the longest histories of human use, plus a third, coca, with a shorter but still significant history, now play crucial roles in modern societies' approaches to mind-altering substances in general. Opium has important medicinal merits and a high potential for abuse; its nonmedical use is illegal and

tightly controlled. Coca has very limited medicinal uses and is also tightly controlled. Alcohol has no medicinal uses but is a prominent social drug, advertised, promoted, and accepted from the lowest to the highest strata of society. The respective histories of these three drugs reveal a number of significant trends, including a movement away from the use of whole plants and toward a greater reliance on purified and concentrated substances. A notable increase in uncontrolled or abusive use has been associated with the more purified drugs.

"Men and women feel such an urgent need to take occasional holidays from reality," Aldous Huxley noted in 1931, "that they will do almost anything to procure the means of escape. The only justification for prohibition would be success; but it is not and, in the nature of things, cannot be successful. The way to prevent people from drinking too much alcohol, or becoming addicts to morphine or cocaine, is to give them an efficient but wholesome substitute for these delicious and (in the present imperfect world) necessary poisons. The man who invents such a substance will be counted among the greatest benefactors of suffering humanity."

In one sense, humanity has already identified better substitutes for alcohol, morphine, and cocaine—the original natural sources from which these purified substances were derived: beer and wine, opium, and coca leaves. Even these drugs, of course, are potent and potentially troublesome. By comparison, the bulk of the "natural mind-alterants" included here are milder in their actions and less risky in their potential toxicity. In a number of cases, such as green tea, melatonin, ginkgo, and perhaps the smart drugs, their mind-altering properties are accompanied not by adverse health effects but potential health benefits, such as increases in immunity and reduced risk of heart disease and cancer.

Some of the substances considered here have just as long historical records as do alcohol, opium, and coca. Ephedra has been used in China for perhaps five millennia, both medicinally and as a stimulating, tealike beverage. The indigenous tribes of the South Pacific for three millennia have been using kava for many of the same purposes alcohol is used for elsewhere. A number of ancient herbalists remarked upon the use of valerian as a sedative, but only within the past few centuries has this been recognized as the herb's most important function. Other natural mind-alterants are more recent: melatonin was first isolated in the 1950s and has been on the market as a supplement for only about a decade. The smart drugs and nutritional supplements such as the isolated amino acids and choline are also recent developments.

As a whole, do these and the other substances described here qualify as Huxley's "efficient and wholesome substitutes"? Perhaps not, but they're a step in the right direction. The sociocultural factors relating to how conventional mind-alterants such as alcohol and coffee are promoted and used argue against any major shifts in consumption patterns. Nevertheless, many of the people who use these popular psychoactive drugs are open to information on alternatives, particularly if these new mood boosters and mind-alterants can be shown to offer similar psychoactive experiences and benefits but fewer drawbacks in terms of adverse health effects, hangover, and addiction potential.

ACTIONS AT A GLANCE

The following chart summarizes the principal actions for the herbs, amino acids, essential oils, smart drugs, and other natural mind-alterants that are covered in detail in subsequent chapters. Admittedly, the groupings into stimulants, mood brighteners, brain boosters, and so forth is somewhat arbitrary. Is ginkgo primarily used as a mood brightener rather than as a brain booster? Isn't kava more often taken as a relaxant than an inebriant? Perhaps. Natural substances tend to be complex both in their chemical makeup and their actions on the body and mind. The classifications in the chart are, however, useful tools for distinguishing among similar substances.

Although it is important to be as precise as possible in discussing various mind-alterants and their usual actions, it must be emphasized that the issue by its very nature is subjective, imprecise, and impressionistic. More so than the nutrients and smart drugs, plants are individual and may vary considerably in their active compounds from one specimen to the next. The properties of a mind-altering substance are not necessarily consistent from one

	STIMULANT	MOOD BRIGHTENER	BRAIN BOOSTER	RELAXANT	INEBRIANT	APHRODISIAC
STIMULANTS						
Green Tea	■	■	■			
Ginseng	■	■	■			■
Ephedra/Ma Huang	■	■				
Guarana	■	■				
Maté	■	■				
Kola Nut	■	■				■
Phenylalanine	■	■				
Tyrosine	■	■				
MOOD BRIGHTENERS						
St. John's Wort		■				
Rose Oil		■				■
Jasmine Oil		■				■
Neroli Oil		■				■
BRAIN BOOSTERS						
Vasopressin	■	■	■			
Deprenyl	■	■	■			■
Piracetam	■	■	■			
Hydergine	■	■	■			
Choline	■		■			
DMAE	■		■			
Pyroglutamate	■		■			
Ginkgo	■	■	■			■
Peppermint Oil	■		■			
Basil Oil	■		■			
Rosemary Oil	■	■	■			
RELAXANTS						
Valerian				■		
California Poppy				■		
Melatonin		■		■		
Tryptophan		■		■		
5-hydroxytryptophan		■		■		
GABA		■		■		
INEBRIANTS						
Kava		■		■	■	■
APHRODISIACS						
Yohimbé	■	■				■

batch, dosage, or individual to the next. Some substances that commonly cause a depressant action may be curiously stimulating to a few people. Ultimately, the experience of the user is primary. Despite what you think constitutes a substance's usual and customary properties, if your experience differs from others', accept it and adjust your usage as necessary.

THE NEED TO KNOW

What are the most important things to know before deciding whether to try an herb or supplement with potentially mind-altering properties? For each of the just-named natural substances, any number of questions crop up, chief among them:

- What exactly is this substance I'm thinking about taking?
- How has it been used in the past? And for how long?
- What have scientific studies discovered about its active ingredients and its effects on the body?
- What are its likely mind-altering or mood-boosting effects?
- Does it have any other potentially beneficial health effects beyond its ability to alter my mind or brighten my mood?
- What is its relative safety, toxicity, and addiction compared to other substances, natural or synthetic, used for similar purposes?
- What, if any, adverse side effects might I experience from using it?

- Are some forms of the substance preferable to others, or certain compounds more likely to be active than others? And if so, why?
- Where can I get it? How expensive is it?
- How do I take it? That is, what is the usual and customary dosage?

For some of the natural mind-alterants there is more information than for others. In some cases (such as the caffeinated herbs guarana, maté, and kola nut), this is because these substances' reputations have not yet spread much beyond their traditional populations. For a few substances (kava, green tea) there is a wealth of information on traditional uses but less scientific data pertaining particularly to mind-altering effects. For many of the natural mind-alterants there are a plethora of scientific studies, but definitive findings are lacking because the studies are suggestive, or conflicting, or only preliminary. In a few cases (particularly tryptophan), substances that were at one time the subject of promising research have become scientific pariahs, at least in the United States, as once-active fields of study have more or less come to a halt in recent years because of questionable regulatory actions. In some cases the information presented here is somewhat technical, such as that relating to chemical compounds found in natural mind-alterants. This is necessary to fully understand these substances' possible mechanisms of action in the mind and body and their range of safety concerns.

Safety is, of course, a major consideration. It is also one of the most difficult areas to address fully. The relative safety of any natural substance may vary from one individual to another. As with any drug, for example, it is possible for natural substances to cause an allergic reaction in a small minority of people. If your experience with a substance indicates you are one of those people, forget about the statistics and the averages. Avoid the drug and, if you want, try another with similar properties. Even if a mind-alterant causes seemingly minor side effects, don't settle for discomfort. Seek out other options, whether from the range of natural substances or from lifestyle changes (such as exercise and meditation) that can yield similar results over the long term.

Relative safety would be less problematic if the U.S. government more honestly evaluated the risks and benefits of herbs and supplements. Unfortunately the agencies entrusted with the mission of safeguarding public health and evaluating natural products, in particular the FDA, have little expertise when it comes to herbs and nutritional supplements. The situation in the United States contrasts unfavorably with that in Europe. For example, in Germany the government has created what's known as Commission E, a branch of the Ministry of Health. Commission E is made up of pharmacists, experts on toxicology, and doctors with training or clinical experience in herbal medicine. As a group, they evaluate botanical medicines and write official monographs on their findings. Commission E has issued more than three hundred monographs on almost two hundred herbs and herbal formulas. These detailed summaries are based on extensive literature searches, the results of scientific studies, and reports on traditional uses. Com-

missioners evaluate information based on the source and its reliability—the evidence from centuries of folk use is important but may not necessarily override experimental results, and vice versa. Final reports, which serve as the basis for regulatory status, include a detailed discussion of approved uses, contraindications, side effects, safety, and efficacy. An attempt is made to weigh benefits against risks, and those herbs or natural substances that are judged to have more risks than benefits can't be sold. (This is the case for approximately one in five of the substances investigated.) Regulations also address issues relating to which approved uses and safety concerns need to be included in the product label.

Despite attempts by botanical researchers and natural products groups to set up a similar system in the United States, no such formal regulations currently cover herbs or nutritional supplements in this country. The FDA regulates herbs and nutrients as "dietary supplements." Health claims are sharply limited and labeling requirements are chaotic. Herbs and supplements are subject to both less regulation and more control compared to over-the-counter medicines. Ultimately, it is American consumers who are the big losers. They are forced to rely on the claims of producers, articles in the popular press, hearsay from friends, and similarly incomplete types of information to find out whether a natural mind-alterant is safe and effective.

Consumers would definitely benefit if the German model ever became the standard for regulating herbs and supplements in the United States. In the meantime, the information that is proffered by regulatory agencies such as the FDA on herbs and supplements is often biased, out of date, or incomplete. Individuals can and should consider other sources of information, such as the specific comments on safety offered for each natural mind-alterant as well as the safe-use guidelines provided in chapter 19, and make their own determinations about whether to use any particular natural mind-alterant.

PART TWO

Stimulants

Green Tea

@

MELLOW YELLOW

Tea is the most widely consumed human-made beverage. Its use spans thousands of years and may even extend to prehistoric times. Tea is currently drunk by an estimated half the population of the world—by people in Asia, the Middle East, Europe, North and South America, Australia, and much of Africa. Its principal active ingredient, caffeine, rivals alcohol for the title of the most commonly used and socially accepted mind-altering drug in much of the world, and particularly in North America, Great Britain, and the Far East. Tea is valued for its ability to elevate mood, increase energy levels, prevent fatigue, and improve work capacity. Like alcohol, tea may also be beneficial to health when used in moderation. Alcohol's relaxing effects on the body may reduce some people's risk of heart attack, but it is not tea's prominent stimulant effects that are cited as particularly healthful. Rather, it is certain compounds found in especially high percentages in one form of tea, green tea, that may someday make doctors recommend

not "an apple a day" but "a few cups of green tea a day" for health and longevity.

BLACK, GREEN, AND OOLONG TEA

Tea is derived from the leaves and delicate young leaf buds of an evergreen bush (*Camellia sinensis*) with fragrant white flowers. Tea plants are hardy and reliable herbal partners with humanity, capable of growing in tropical and subtropical climes. Bushes can thrive at altitudes up to about 7,000 feet, live an average of twenty-five years, and offer a harvest of leaves several times each year. Tea plants can grow to twenty-five to thirty feet tall or be kept pruned to three feet to allow for easy hand-picking of the leaves. Tea production is a mostly low-tech process with basic steps that haven't changed much in thousands of years.

Slight variations in the method of tea production result in three distinct types of tea:

Black tea is the familiar dark brew that most English-speaking peoples drink. The first step in its production is to wither the freshly picked leaves by spreading them in a thin layer on racks or trays and exposing them to the sun or some other heat source, usually for ten to twenty hours. The limp leaves are then rolled, which releases juices and enzymes from leaf cells and exposes them to the air, and put under damp cloths or spread onto tables or on the floor in a large room that is kept cool and damp. This allows the tea to start to ferment, a process that oxidizes approximately 60 to 70 percent of certain bitter-tasting compounds in the leaves and allows new, unique by-products to form by condensation. The leaves darken in color and then turn almost black when a final firing or rapid-drying is done to stop the fermentation process.

Green tea is made from the same plants and leaves as black tea but is processed in a way that prevents fermentation. The freshly picked leaves are typically quickly exposed to steam or low heat to soften them and deactivate enzymes. The leaves are then rolled and gently heated or dried before any oxidation can occur, allowing them to remain fresh and green.

Oolong tea, from a Chinese word for black dragon, is treated in a way that puts it halfway between black and green—partly fermented but for not as long as black tea is. Somewhat lighter in color than black tea, oolong is also known as red or yellow tea.

An estimated 70 to 80 percent of the world's tea crop is fermented into black tea, with green tea accounting for 15 to 25 percent and oolong about 5 percent. Black tea represents some 98 percent of tea exports, however, since many of the tea-importing countries acquired their tea habit in emulation of the British, who have always drunk black tea. India, which now produces about a billion pounds of tea per year, and Sri Lanka are major exporters of black tea. Much of the tea that is grown in China and Japan is processed into green tea for domestic consumption. (China exports some 90 percent of its black tea but only 20 percent of its green tea.) Tea is also being grown in Africa, the Middle East, and South America. The United States boasts a single plantation, on an island off the coast of South Carolina.

Only within the past few years has a market for green tea begun to develop in North America and Europe, primarily through sales in natural foods stores. Health-conscious consumers of green tea prefer it to black tea for the former's higher content of certain biologically active compounds that have recently been demonstrated to quite possibly lower the risk of cancer, heart disease, and other illnesses. Black, green, and oolong teas all have the same amount of caffeine in the final product, though as we'll see, differences in how black and green tea are brewed can affect average caffeine levels.

THE ASIAN BEVERAGE

Tea is thought to be native to China, India, or the area around present-day Thailand and Burma. Its cultivation in China goes back to ancient times, though exactly how ancient is not known. Prehistoric humans may have chewed tea leaves, or possibly even added them to boiling water. A Chinese legend says that the first cup of tea was drunk by Emperor Shen Nong around the year 2737 B.C.E. He was said to have recommended that his people boil their water before drinking it, and while his servants were boiling his drinking water one day some tea leaves blew into the pot. The Emperor "tasted it and pronounced it good," as the legend goes, and the brewing of tea took off from there.

A later Japanese myth also traces tea drinking to China, but says that Bodhidharma, the Indian prince who became a founder of Zen Buddhism around A.D. 500, is almost literally the father of the tea plant. Legend has it that Bodhidharma traveled to China, established himself in a cave temple, and began a nine-year period of meditation during which he vowed not to sleep. Before completing the marathon meditation, however, Bodhidharma did fall asleep. Upon awakening he was so angry and disappointed in himself that he cut off his eyelids so as never to fall asleep during meditation again. He threw his eyelids on the ground, where they took root and grew into the first tea bush, a plant that could banish sleep. Though picturesque, this legend has the drawback of placing the advent of tea drinking more than a century after the date widely accepted by modern scholars as the earliest confirmed reference to tea: in A.D. 350, when a new edition of an ancient Chinese encyclopedia/dictionary was published with an entry on tea.

China introduced Japan to tea drinking, though the Japanese didn't begin to cultivate tea until some time in the seventh or eighth century. It took centuries more before tea drinking became popular. Tea was at first appreciated more as a medicinal herb, useful for treating coughs, colds, and breathing ailments. Following Bodhidharma's example, Buddhist monks also recognized tea as a useful beverage for staying awake during long periods of meditation. Tea allowed meditators to attain an apparently contradictory state: tranquil yet alert, relaxed yet focused. The herb's practical use for meditation gradually transformed into the ritual tea ceremony, which began to be formalized in China around the twelfth century. It didn't attain its height as a social function and cultural institution until the sixteenth century, when the Japanese tea master Senno Rikyu enumerated formal rules that emphasized the importance of mindfulness, cleanliness, attention to the tea and the utensils, and respect between guest and host. The tea ceremony was an embodiment of Zen Buddhism, a practical demonstration of how harmony and beauty are to be found in everyday life.

By the time the tea ceremony and drinking green tea had become well established in Japan, tea also began to make inroads into European culture.

TEA COMES TO EUROPE

The earliest reference to tea by a European appeared in the travel tales of a Venetian writer in 1559. It took another century, however, before tea started to be imported into most European countries in large enough quantities for it to become a popular beverage. The Portuguese and Dutch were familiar with tea by the end of the sixteenth century, while the first reference to tea drinking by an Englishman is in 1615. During the 1640s it began to become a fashionable drink among the royalty and the upper classes in England. Sometime in the 1650s tea began to appear in the earliest London coffeehouses, new establishments that had opened to offer two other stimulating, tropical beverages (coffee and cocoa) new at the time to the English public. One coffeehouse ad extolled tea for its ability to "removeth lassitude, vanquisheth heavy dreams, easeth the frame, and strengtheneth the memory."

Poised on the edge of the Industrial Revolution, England was quick to embrace tea, coffee, and cocoa for a variety of reasons that involved political, economic, and technological factors. These bitter herbs all needed sweetening to be palatable as drinks, and the new trade in sugar reinforced the use of these stimulants. Hot tea also began to replace malt liquor and home-brewed beer as the beverage that the working class took with their meals and even throughout the day, a switch in cultural drug preferences that was in some ways a nutritional loss (tea and white bread represented an almost starvation diet for many) but was in tune with the economic zeitgeist.

The need for large amounts of imported tea, sugar and spices, and coffee stimulated foreign trade, shipbuilding, and navigation, and promoted the development of government-protected trading companies, such as the British East India Company (chartered by Elizabeth I in 1600). These monopolistic merchant groups with their fleets of heavily armed ships were to play prominent roles in the political economy and the colonial expansion of Britain for more than two centuries. Though the British favored coffee to tea in the seventeenth century, empire building took precedence over culinary preferences in England, and tea swept past coffee as the beverage of choice. The British East India Company's control of the tea trade ensured that by the early 1700s British subjects would come to drink tea to the point of addiction, and indeed to this day tea remains the most popular beverage not only of England but of much of its former empire, including Scotland, Ireland, India, and Australia. The British East India Company's government-protected monopoly on Chinese tea ended in 1833, after which the British began to establish large tea plantations in India, soon thoroughly dominating the area's economy and political system and turning India and Ceylon (now Sri Lanka) into subservient colonies.

Britain's chief early competitor as tea consumer and shipper was Holland. The Dutch East India Company was importing tea to Holland by the mid-seventeenth century, and in 1679 a publication by a Dutch author "on the most excellent tea herb" recommended it as well as the three other stimulants (coffee, chocolate, and tobacco) new at the time to Europeans. By the mid-nineteenth century the Dutch had also shifted from mere shipping to controlling tea growing and production, having established plantations in Java (now in Indonesia).

The Dutch were also major dealers in coffee, and tea never became quite the national obsession in Holland that it became in Great Britain and, through overland shipments, in Russia. The seventh duchess of Bedford is credited with originating the British custom of a midafternoon tea break around 1840. In the eighteenth and nineteenth centuries, tea insinuated itself into many aspects of British society, forming what has been termed a "tea complex" with economic and social implications. As Sidney W. Mintz has noted in *Sweetness and Power: The Place of Sugar in Modern History,* drinking tea, eating bread smeared with treacle, and baking sweet cakes "were all acts that would gradually be assimilated into the calendar of work, recreation, rest, and prayer—into the whole of daily life, in sum—as well as into the cycle of special events such as births, baptisms, marriages, and funerals."

Tea's influence was less pervasive in the United States, in part because of a role it played in the American Revolution. Wishing to remind cheeky colonials of their place, as well as to preserve the monopoly of their trading company, in 1773 the British Parliament passed the Tea Act. The effect of this law was to enforce a seemingly minor and heretofore mostly ignored tax (actually passed in 1767) on tea imported into the American colonies. In December of 1773 angry patriots stormed three British ships in Boston Harbor and dumped chests of tea into the water. Over the next twelve months similar acts of rebellion against British tea took place in other colonial ports. The British reaction, including closing Boston Harbor as a port, inflamed public opinion and compounded the Brits' mistake. Within three years the colonies would be banding together in revolution against "taxation without representation" and declaring their independence from England—and from tea.

Tea subsequently became associated in the minds of many Americans with British oppression, and the tea market in America never really recovered from this early public relations disaster. Coffee rushed into the stimulant vacuum and remains much the preferred drink in the United States to this day. Americans drink about four times as much coffee as tea, while in Great Britain the figure is reversed: tea remains about four times as popular as coffee.

Americans have looked more favorably upon tea in the twentieth century as it has adapted to the national preference for cold drinks and instant gratification. Iced tea was known well before the oft-given date of its "invention" in 1904 at the Louisiana Purchase Exposition in St. Louis, but it was there that its popularity took off and word began to spread about it. Around the same time, the invention of the tea bag made brewing tea quicker and easier. Much of America's current consumption of tea (approximately eight gallons per person per year) is accounted for by iced tea, ready-to-drink bottled teas, and instant powders. Overall, tea shows signs of gaining rapidly in popularity in the United States, in part because of the growing evidence that it is a much more healthful beverage when compared with coffee.

THE MIND-ALTERING ALKALOIDS

Tea contains a few vitamins, minerals such as fluoride and manganese, small amounts of an aromatic essential oil, and biologically active substances known as flavonoids or polyphenols. Tea's mind-altering properties, however, are due to a group of related alkaloids known as methylxanthines. These are the same compounds—caffeine, theophylline, and theobromine—that also account for the stimulant properties of coffee, chocolate, cola, and the exotic herbs guarana, maté, and kola nut (see chapter 5).

Tea leaves actually have a higher caffeine content (1 to 4 percent) than coffee beans (1 to 2 percent) on a dry weight basis, making the leaf dust left over from tea production useful as a source of extracted caffeine for adding to soft drinks. Caffeine, however, is leached into brewed coffee more efficiently than it is into brewed tea, and tea is made with much more water per weight than is coffee. Thus, an average cup of black tea brewed five to ten minutes contains 50 to 75 mg of caffeine, while a cup of coffee ranges from 75 to 150 mg, depending on a variety of factors such as length and method of brewing. A cup of green tea, if it is brewed in the traditional two-to-three-minute fashion, contains only 20 to 30 mg of caffeine.

Tea has higher concentrations of theophylline than any other plant. While theophylline can boost the heart rate and stimulate the central nervous system, possibly to an even greater degree than does caffeine, theophylline is present in tea in much lower amounts than is caffeine. The amount of theophylline in a cup of tea—less than 1 mg—has no physiological effect. Tea also contains similarly inconsequential amounts of theobromine.

A CLEAR AND LIVELY SPIRIT

A well-brewed cup of green tea is a pleasure to imbibe. Its pale, yellowish green color and clean, fresh fragrance nudge the senses rather than clobber them. Its taste, preferably unsweetened or only lightly sweetened, is delicate yet complex—an expert taster can distinguish subtle taste notes in a thousand varieties, much like a master wine taster.

Green tea's effects on the mind are also subtle. Tea does not announce itself with the rush and bustle that coffee does, but rather quietly tiptoes onto the stage and mostly stays in the background. Tea awakens the mind and refreshes the spirit. Successive cups have cumulative gradations of effect, not just greater and greater stimulation.

As the Japanese discovered, green tea is the perfect complement for meditation or quiet contemplation. It keeps the mind alert without pumping the body too full of energy. Tea is widely appreciated by students because it improves concentration and alertness and seems to stimulate mental activity. Drinking green tea in a group increases sociability and prompts friendly conversation. Author C. R. Fay, referring to the British, noted that "Tea, which refreshes and quietens, is the natural beverage of a taciturn people." (He went on to note that "being easy to prepare, it came as a godsend to the world's worst cooks.")

Green tea also provides a gentle boost in mood, providing the drinker with a positive and optimistic outlook. "The spirit of the man who drinks tea will become clear and lively," as an ancient Chinese author put it.

TEA VERSUS COFFEE

Tea and coffee are often consumed for similar purposes, and they share the active compound, caffeine, responsible for most if not all of their mind-altering properties. The different effects on mind and body from drinking tea and coffee are not stark but are nevertheless worth noting. Many drinkers note that tea seems to cause less of a physical rush than coffee. Some even describe green tea's effects as calming rather than stimulating, while few people seem to find coffee relaxing, despite coffee industry ads to the contrary. Tea seems to have more of a cerebral effect, while coffee promotes physical activity.

In part, differences between the beverages may be attributed to average variations in the caffeine content. A cup of brewed tea contains not only less caffeine than coffee, however, but fewer other potentially harmful compounds. While coffee pharmacology is undeveloped, researchers say that roasted coffee beans contain the oil caffeol, creosote, phenol, tars, and other potentially toxic or carcinogenic compounds that aren't found in tea. (Indeed, green tea not only contains no aromatic hydrocar-

bons, such as tars, but the polyphenols in green tea may actually protect against these substances' cancer-causing effects.) The aromatic hydrocarbons in a cup of coffee may also be more harmful to long-term health than is the caffeine, according to a 1985 study. Though not all studies, for example, have confirmed a possible link between coffee and pancreatic cancer, regular and decaf coffee have been tied to the condition but not tea. Researchers suspect that chemicals in coffee other than caffeine may be responsible for raising some coffee drinkers' (including decaf coffee drinkers') blood cholesterol levels and heart attack risk. Corresponding increases have not been found among tea drinkers. Coffee also seems more likely than tea to cause stomach irritations, digestive ailments, and fibrocystic breast condition. According to Andrew Weil, M.D., a renowned authority on plant drugs, "Tea is not nearly so irritating to the body as coffee, and cases of dependence on tea are less common in our society."

THE HEALTH-BENEFITING POLYPHENOLS

In ancient China tea was considered a potent medicine. Traditional healers recommended it to relieve headaches, soothe colds and coughs, and treat diarrhea, asthma, and other conditions. A number of these applications have survived to modern times, though with isolated tea constituents recognized as the active agents (such as caffeine to help relieve headache and theophylline for asthma). While therapeutic uses of whole tea have faded from the current scene, green tea in particular is now gaining increased recognition for its potential to counter bacteria and viruses, boost overall immunity, and prevent major debilitating diseases, including cancer and heart disease.

Chemical analysis of the beneficial active compounds in green tea has identified the major ones as polyphenols, particularly the catechins. (Though catechins are technically a subset of polyphenols, herbal companies often use the terms *polyphenols* and *catechins* interchangeably.) The principal green tea catechins are epicatechin, epicatechin gallate, and epigallocatechin gallate (EGCG). EGCG is currently considered the most physiologically active of the catechins. These green tea compounds are potent antioxidants, capable of neutralizing free radicals and thus protecting the body from harmful effects ranging from cancer to aging. Studies have determined that catechins may be twenty to thirty times more powerful in their antioxidant action than are vitamins C and E, well-known radical quenchers.

While black tea has some of the same beneficial compounds as green tea, as well as some unique ones, green tea is generally thought to have higher levels of the most beneficial compounds. A 1996 study conducted by Italian researchers determined that green tea was six times more powerful as an antioxidant when compared to black tea. Also, the black tea–drinking British do not have especially low rates of cancer or heart disease. On the other hand, a number of studies that have linked health benefits with tea drinking have focused on populations that drink black tea.

For example, a 1993 Dutch study found that men with the highest overall intake of flavonoids, which in the Netherlands is mainly from tea drinking, have dramatically reduced rates of heart disease.

Green tea's anticancer effects have been confirmed in a number of studies, both of the population and the clinical trial variety. Researchers have found that green tea protects animals from lung tumors, from leukemia after being exposed to radiation, and from skin tumors. The results of population studies vary, but most indicate that green tea may help protect against cancers of the lungs, skin, liver, pancreas, and stomach. Surveys indicate that green tea consumption may be an important factor in why Japanese smokers have a much lower death rate from lung cancer compared to American smokers. Recent findings suggest that EGCG may help shrink tumors by blocking the action of an enzyme that promotes the spread of cancer.

Drinking green tea may also help prevent heart attacks, strokes, and other forms of cardiovascular disease. Green tea inhibits the aggregation of platelets, the small, sticky blood particles that play a major role in inducing blood clots to form. When platelets encounter a rough area on the inside wall of an otherwise intact blood vessel, it can encourage fatty buildup and increase the risk of heart attack. The catechins' anti-clumping effects may rival that of aspirin, and another compound in green tea has also been shown to indirectly inhibit platelet stickiness. The antioxidant activity of green tea compounds is also thought to protect certain blood lipids from being oxidized; it is this oxidation process that promotes atherosclerosis. Green tea also helps to lower blood cholesterol levels and possibly reduce high blood pressure.

Among the studies that have linked cardiovascular benefits with green tea consumption are two Japanese epidemiological studies. The first, done on 6,000 Japanese women over the age of forty, tied fewer strokes to increased consumption of green tea. The second, published in the *British Medical Journal* in 1995, found that among 1,371 Japanese males, those who drank green tea had statistically significant reductions in total cholesterol and triglycerides (blood fats) and higher HDL (good) cholesterol. Both studies found that the heart health benefits were greatest for subjects who drank at least five to ten cups of green tea per day.

The results of international symposia on green tea's health benefits indicate that, in addition to protecting against cancer and heart disease, green tea may help:

■ Regulate blood sugar imbalances. Drinking relatively large amounts of green tea (five to ten cups per day) seems to normalize the release of insulin from the pancreas and help prevent large swings in blood sugar levels.

■ Prevent tooth decay and gum disease. Green tea extract has become a popular ingredient in toothpastes, and drinking green tea seems to inhibit the spread of the bacteria that can cause plaque to build up and cavities to form. The reason may be related to the catechins' ability to bind to tooth surfaces and to the fact that green tea contains fluoride, a proven tooth-decay preventive. Relying upon green tea consumption to replace proper dental hygiene, however, is hardly recommended. Chairman Mao bragged about never having to brush his teeth because he rinsed his mouth out with tea, but according to the memoirs of Mao's personal physician, Mao suffered from severe dental problems as a result.

■ Aid in weight loss. Caffeine's noted ability to increase metabolism, raise body temperature, and increase the rate at which calories are burned has prompted researchers to test it for weight loss. Some studies have shown positive results from taking caffeine supplements or from drinking caffeinated coffee. Another placebo-controlled study found that overweight women who complemented their low-calorie diet by taking tea supplements lost three times more weight after a month than those who didn't take the supplement.

While the mildly stimulating effects of the caffeine in green tea account for some of its potential as a weight-loss agent, researchers have also found that the polyphenols in green tea can promote the burning of fat and help to regulate blood sugar and insulin levels. A 1996 study determined that green tea polyphenols significantly increased the fat-burning properties of both caffeine and ephedrine, the stimulating alkaloid from the herb ephedra (see chapter 4). Thus, green tea may be a better source of caffeine than coffee for those looking to lose a few pounds, as it has relatively low levels of caffeine and it contains other compounds with potential weight-loss effects not found in coffee.

Weight-loss products containing green tea go by names like Thermo-Lift Powder and

ThermoLoss. Read labels carefully for caffeine content to avoid consuming excessive amounts of caffeine. Only 100 to 150 mg of caffeine per day is sufficient to boost the effects of ephedrine and other weight-loss factors.

SAFETY AND SIDE EFFECTS

As common food constituents, polyphenols and catechins are considered to be safe and nontoxic. It's estimated that Americans consume approximately one gram of various polyphenols every day in fruits and other foods. The tea compounds that do have potentially adverse health effects are methylxanthines, such as caffeine.

Most of the potential adverse health effects associated with tea drinking can be traced to the stimulant powers of the methylxanthines, particularly caffeine, because brewed tea has such low concentrations of theophylline and theobromine. Excessive caffeine consumption may cause overstimulation in the form of restlessness, anxiety, tremors, and insomnia, as well as a variety of other symptoms, including abdominal pain, high blood pressure, and heart palpitations. Caffeine is potentially addictive, both psychologically and physically (leading to withdrawal symptoms such as headache, fatigue, and irritability when it is withheld). See chapter 5 for a more complete discussion of caffeine and other xanthines.

Because tea typically contains lower levels of caffeine than coffee, addiction to tea is less prevalent in North America than is addiction to coffee. Still, a particularly strong cup of black tea may exceed 80 mg of caffeine, and consuming a half-dozen or more such cups per day may well lead to dependence. Famous tea addicts include Dr. Samuel Johnson, who would drink as many as thirty cups in a sitting, and tea addiction is not unheard of in England, Ireland, and other countries where black tea is consumed in large amounts. Green tea usually has lower levels of caffeine than black tea (see "Taking Green Tea," below), and the adverse effects of caffeine seem to be less common in countries where the tea of choice is green. Even in ancient China, however, drinking too much tea was recognized as causing problems. As one traditional healer said, "Tea has a cooling effect, and if too much is taken fatigue and exhaustion result."

A number of studies, including one done on women in China, indicate that tea drinking may worsen the symptoms of premenstrual syndrome, particularly irritability, tension, fatigue, and tenderness of the breasts. Compared to abstainers, women who drank in excess of four and a half cups of tea per day were almost ten times as likely to suffer from PMS symptoms. Because coffee and cola have also been implicated in aggravating PMS, it is likely that caffeine is responsible.

At least two studies have indicated that Asian populations that drink large amounts of hot, salty tea have an increased risk of cancer of the esophagus, the muscular tube that connects the throat to the top of the stomach. The evidence is mixed, however—another study involving almost 2,500 Chinese found that women who were regular drinkers of green tea had a 60 percent lower risk of esophageal cancer than women who didn't drink green tea, once smoking, alcohol, and dietary factors were taken into consideration. It is possible that the custom of drinking tea scalding hot increases the risk of cancer of the esophagus, not some compound in the tea itself.

Health authorities have also pointed the finger at tannins, astringent compounds found in tea and other plants, although the association between tannins and esophageal cancer is not firmly established. Some findings indicate that tea-drinking societies that add milk to their tea, like the British, have lower rates of esophageal cancer than those societies that drink tea black. This has led scientists to speculate that milk binds or chelates with the tannin in tea, allowing it to be excreted from the body without adverse effects. (Adding milk to green tea, on the other hand, may reduce the absorption of beneficial polyphenols, according to the 1996 study that compared the antioxidant effects of green and black tea.) According to plant researcher Memory Elvin-Lewis, Ph.D., however, writing in the trade journal *HerbalGram,* "There is no evidence to suggest that black tea–drinking areas of the world have a disproportionately higher incidence of esophageal cancer any more than green– or herbal tea–drinking (if there is a region) have less." He notes that plant tannins have many beneficial medical effects and concludes, "I believe that concerns regarding tannin in teas are highly exaggerated."

TAKING GREEN TEA

Green tea is now widely available in numerous forms. You can buy it either loose or in tea bags for brewing into a hot or cold beverage. Green tea extract supplements, mostly in capsule form, have also become extremely popular in recent years.

Green tea's caffeine levels are a major consideration for some people. Green tea capsules are typically promoted for their antioxidant rather than stimulant properties. Caffeine may be present, however, in varying levels. Some capsule producers add extra caffeine to promote the "energizing" effects of the product. Others remove some of the caffeine to promote the extract as more healthful. Most extract products have relatively low levels of caffeine, such as 10 to 20 mg per capsule. Checking labels is useful, though the caffeine level is not always stated. A phone call to the product manufacturer may be necessary.

Polyphenol content of dried tea leaves ranges from 15 to 30 percent. Polyphenols may be concentrated, however, to more than 50 percent in green tea extract products. For comparison, keep in mind that a cup of brewed green tea probably contains about 20 to 30 mg of polyphenols. Thus, a 200 mg green tea extract capsule that has 25 percent polyphenols is equivalent to drinking about two cups of green tea. An average daily dose of green tea polyphenols for their health-promoting properties is 50 to 100 mg.

Though green tea leaves have the same amount of caffeine as black tea leaves, two factors can noticeably affect caffeine levels:

Length of Brewing

Ancient peoples probably added the fermentation step to their traditional tea production (perhaps after accidentally allowing some leaves to ferment) when they noticed that black tea was less bitter and astringent than green tea. To avoid this bitterness in green tea, the traditional method is to brew it for only two to three minutes. This yields a tea with about half the caffeine levels (20 to 30 mg) of a tea that is brewed for the standard five minutes or longer.

Grade of Tea

Tea of all colors comes in various grades, depending upon such factors as when the leaf was picked (early leaves and the growing buds are considered prime), the size of the leaves, whether the leaves are whole or broken, and the presence or absence of twigs, stems, and other less desirable parts of the plant. High-quality green teas, such as gunpowder (considered the highest grade of Chinese green tea, in which choice leaves are rolled up into little balls) and Japanese matcha and sencha, are made from young leaves that brew into a light, delicately flavored tea. Chinese Imperial and Japanese Yamashire are good-quality green teas made from older whole leaves. High-grade Asian green teas can be difficult to find in North America, where most green tea is sold in tea bags. (Tea bag tea has a reputation for using primarily lower grades of tea, including those that contain broken leaves and "fannings and dust," small tea particles. While many commercial black-tea bags are made from fannings and dust, specialty producers now offer higher-quality black-tea bags. A few natural foods companies also offer green-tea bags made from higher grades of tea; check labels.)

Lower grades of tea brew more quickly into darker, stronger-tasting teas. One advantage to these lower grades of green and black tea, however, is that they result in beverages with reduced caffeine levels, because caffeine is naturally present in higher amounts in leaves than in the more woody parts of the tea plant. For example, *bancha* (literally "three tea," for three years old at harvest) and *kukicha* (twig tea), the low-grade Japanese green teas that have become popular in the United States in part due to early macrobiotic advocates, are naturally low in caffeine—a two- or three-minute brew provides only 5 to 15 mg of caffeine.

Decaffeinated green teas are coming on the market, though it is possible that the decaffeinating process also removes some of the healthful polyphenols.

If you brew green tea, don't drink it scalding hot, which may reduce its benefits or even be harmful (possibly increasing the risk of cancer of the esophagus). In North America, many people add sweeteners to green tea, but if you brew it briefly to limit the bitterness, you can emulate traditional Asians and appreciate its subtle flavor unsweetened.

You don't have to turn tea drinking into a ceremony to enjoy it. Even tea master Rikyu noted, "Tea is nothing other than this: Heat the water, prepare the tea, and drink it with propriety. That is all you need to know."

The Ginsengs

◉

HERBAL ENERGY TONICS

Ginseng has long been one of the most widely recognized and best-selling medicinal herbs on the market. Siberian ginseng/eleuthero is a Russian import gaining increased favor in the North American market. What these herbs have in common is enduring respect among traditional users as strengthening and balancing, or tonic, substances. Their reputations for being safe and reliable herbs for increasing physical energy and mental stamina have carried over into modern times. In some cases, ginseng and Siberian ginseng/eleuthero may also help to brighten mood, promote sexual vigor, or even relax mind and body.

This concept of a system-strengthening or tonic substance is somewhat foreign to Western medicine and can create confusion—how can an herb be a "vitalizer" and "rejuvenator" that increases energy levels in one person and a sedative that is calming or anxiety-reducing to another? Actually, tonic herbs such as ginseng

and Siberian ginseng/eleuthero are thought to have slightly different effects depending upon the person's circumstances and condition. Tonics nourish the body and bring the system back into balance, so that, for example, high blood pressure is lowered yet low blood pressure is raised.

Tonics are everyday herbs taken to help the body function under stress and to resist disease. From the Asian perspective, the best tonics are rare "superior" substances. Superior herbs like ginseng that can help someone maintain optimal health on a day-to-day level are of greater value than single-bullet medicines that merely remedy a specific ailment or relieve a certain symptom. Practitioners of traditional Chinese medicine categorize tonic herbs according to bodily energy systems or groups of organs they affect, as well as other subtle characteristics. Some herbs, including certain types of ginseng, are considered energy tonics with whole-body benefits: they normalize the body's systems and thus enhance health and vitality. In the West, tonic herbs are appreciated not only as well-person nourishers but as remedies for conditions such as nervous exhaustion, debility following an illness, reduced resistance to disease, restlessness and anxiety, and lack of sleep.

In the late 1940s Russian plant scientists developed a new term, *adaptogens,* for natural tonic substances such as ginseng and Siberian ginseng/eleuthero. According to the current definition, to be considered an adaptogen a substance has to be:

- Safe and nontoxic, causing no more than minimal side effects.
- Nonspecific in its action. An adaptogen increases resistance to a wide range of biological, environmental, and other physical factors. It should boost the body's overall immune function by various criteria rather than one specific action, such as an increase in the number of certain immune cells.
- Normalizing in the body. No matter what the disease state, an adaptogen should restore to balance all bodily systems while aggravating none.

By promoting the body's ability to adapt to new conditions, adaptogens aid the body in its struggle against stress. Whether due to pressures at work or an unstable relationship, stress can lead to some of the most common ailments in modern society: insomnia, headaches, fatigue, depression, and lack of energy. The long-term effects of unrelieved stress may contribute to such debilitating conditions as heart disease and immune system malfunc-

tions. Stressful conditions especially challenge mind and body, putting an extra burden on the nervous and cardiovascular systems and on endocrine organs such as the adrenals, the small glands on top of the kidneys that play a prominent role in setting the body's metabolic rate and allowing the body to respond to challenging situations.

Though scientists have conducted thousands of studies on tonics such as ginseng, exactly how these substances work is still unclear. In most cases researchers have yet to fully determine which of the numerous chemical constituents found in these plants are responsible for the tonic effects. Many of the plants contain unique compounds with complex and varied actions. Some herbs also share potentially therapeutic nutrients such as vitamins, minerals, and trace elements. In general tonics increase cells' ability to create, store, and use energy and to process wastes; promote efficient oxygen use; provide nutrients crucial to bodily processes; and detoxify blood and tissues. Tonics smooth out swings in blood sugar levels, hormone synthesis, and biorhythms. They may also have beneficial effects on the levels of neurotransmitters such as serotonin and noradrenaline.

Many people find that tonifying, adaptogenic herbs taken over the long term are a better choice than immediate-acting nervous system stimulants such as caffeine or ephedrine to increase daily energy levels and overcome ongoing fatigue. Fatigue that is not directly tied to physical exertion may be caused by an underlying health problem or condition, dietary deficiencies, hormonal changes, or even abuse of caffeine or other stimulant drugs. Identifying and addressing the underlying cause is crucial, and adaptogens can often be used as part of a long-term strategy and in conjunction with other natural substances to reenergize the body.

"Ginseng is the only plant used routinely by so great a number of more or less healthy individuals for stimulation, added energy, and a sense of well-being—a panacea for the healthy who want to remain well for a long time and if possible become healthier," say Walter H. Lewis and Memory P. F. Elvin-Lewis in *Medical Botany*. Though the herb is definitely not a panacea in the mythical (and essentially Western) sense of being able to cure all ailments, it has diverse effects on the body that can provide numerous benefits. Ginseng is a favorite remedy in Asia, where older people in particular take it regularly to increase vitality as well as to enhance longevity. Its popularity in North America continues to climb as well, with higher-quality products reaching the market and a growing interest in a native species of ginseng.

Some of the confusion that surrounds this herb can be traced to the loose usage of the term *ginseng* itself. In reality ginseng is not a single herb. The "true ginsengs" are those half-dozen or so in the small *Panax* genus with notable medicinal uses in Asia. The two most prominent of these species are from Asia (*Panax ginseng,* usually referred to as either Chinese or Korean ginseng, depending upon its origin) and North America (*Panax quinquefolius,* called American ginseng though much of it is grown in Canada). A lesser-known true ginseng is *P. pseudoginseng,* known as *sanqi* or *tienchi* by the Chinese. The Chinese use pseudoginseng in various remedies, mainly to reduce internal and topical bleeding, but this ginseng hasn't caught on in the West.

Ginseng is a perennial ground plant. After two to three years it bears small flowers, white to yellow green in color, and red berries; the sometimes human-shaped root is pulled from the ground to make herbal medicines.

The Chinese have long revered ginseng as the king or prince of herbs. Use of Asian ginseng in China is thought to go back at least three thousand to four thousand years, principally as a system-strengthening herb. The word itself connotes a tonic—*gin* (*jen*) basically referring to "form of man" and *seng* (*shen*) to "essence of the earth" or "a strengthening root." Emperors sought and hoarded ginseng much as monarchs elsewhere yearned for gold. Ginseng is mentioned as the most desirable tonic herb in Chinese medicinal texts that date back to before the birth of Christ. Much ritual and folklore came to surround ginseng. Men embraced it to preserve their virility, the healthy to maintain overall vitality, the ill to help promote recovery. Ginseng was also appreciated in India, where an ancient text notes, "This herb will make thee so full of lusty strength that thou shalt, when thou art excited, exhale heat as a thing on fire."

Today, cultivated Asian and American ginseng is one of the world's most lucrative legal crops, with the final product often bringing in more than $50 per pound. In parts of

Asia locals have so completely foraged the wild plant that some wildcrafted Asian ginseng with desirable qualities is now rare enough to command hundreds of dollars *per ounce*. Much of the world's supply of *Panax ginseng* is cultivated in South Korea and China.

AMERICAN GINSENG: A VALUABLE EXPORT

The American species of ginseng was known by the Cherokees, Mohawks, Iroquois, and numerous other tribes, who used it to treat various conditions and to boost alertness, promote longevity, increase appetite, or enhance fertility. The first European to find American ginseng in North America was a Jesuit priest who located a plant in 1716 in Canada, near Montreal. American ginseng was soon discovered to grow widely in the forests of eastern and midwestern United States. Almost immediately a vigorous export trade in American ginseng developed, primarily to Asia, with Americans as diverse as Daniel Boone and John Jacob Astor eventually becoming involved in the enterprise.

Shipping of American ginseng to Asia continues to this day. All American ginseng was wildcrafted until the 1870s, when overharvesting had so reduced wild supplies that growers began to cultivate ginseng. Today more than 90 percent of the American ginseng that is cultivated in the United States is grown on farms (some is also "woodsgrown"—cultivated in forests) in Wisconsin, almost exclusively for export to China. American ginseng

is so highly valued there that the Chinese have even begun to grow it themselves.

In 1989 Chinese researchers compared the composition and content of the essential oil from *P. quinquefolius* grown in China to that of *P. quinquefolius* imported from the United States. They determined that the oils were similar.

WORKING THROUGH MYSTERIOUS CHANNELS

Ginseng's actions on the body are diverse. Researchers have determined that it can regulate blood pressure, increase hormone and enzyme secretion, maintain blood sugar levels, enhance the body's use of oxygen, and boost heartbeat and metabolic rate. Ginseng may also affect neurotransmitter levels and blood flow to the brain, protect the body's cells from damage due to radiation and exposure to toxic substances, and nourish the thymus and spleen. Animal studies have found that ginseng can help protect against infection by stimulating certain parts of the immune system, enhancing particularly the natural killer white blood cells. One of the herb's most valuable properties relates to how it promotes better functioning of the adrenals by maintaining their ability to produce certain hormones.

Studies done on rats and mice have found that animals given ginseng can swim for a longer duration and more readily adapt to adverse conditions. Many people who take ginseng notice that it significantly reduces fatigue and enhances endurance. Ginseng is generally not regarded, however, as strictly a central nervous system stimulant. Most people don't feel notably aroused after taking ginseng, in contrast to, for example, their experience after taking herbs with caffeine or ephedrine. Ginseng rarely causes nervousness or insomnia, either. Indeed, some people may not find it stimulating at all, or will actually find it to have a calming effect.

Experiences with ginseng tend to confirm its famous tonic property. People report that ginseng improves athletic performance under stress and increases their ability to run or swim faster and longer. Ginseng is not so much an immediate libido booster but rather a restorative for the sexual system. The elderly and those who are weak or recovering from illness are more likely than the young and healthy to notice a boost in mood and overall vitality. Indeed, in China ginseng is taken more frequently by the elderly than by young people.

Ginseng has attracted quite a bit of scientific interest. Hundreds, even thousands, of studies have been done, with the vast majority focusing on Asian ginseng. Yet much of the scientific community continues to regard the herb with skepticism. Partly this is because most of the research has been done on animals rather than on humans, and the studies have been published in obscure foreign medical journals. In many instances when the studies have been examined closely they've been found to be lacking in some regard—poor controls, questions about the composition of the herb, funding from ginseng trade associations,

and so on. Another part of the problem, however, is that ginseng doesn't fit well into the Western model of drugs. It has an exceedingly complex chemical structure, with the effects being due to a synergy of the parts rather than one or two simple-acting compounds.

Scientific research has confirmed that the conception of ginseng as a one-dimensional nervous system stimulant does not do justice to the herb. For example, Japanese researchers in 1991 found that an extract of Asian ginseng caused an increase in spontaneous motor activity and low dopamine utilization in old rats, but a decrease in the spontaneous motor activity and high dopamine utilization in young rats. A number of studies have found that ginseng does not cause increases in insomnia, anxiety, and aggressive behavior, a property more usually associated with relaxant rather than stimulant substances. Ginseng has been shown to help to stabilize sleep and wakefulness in more than one study. For example, the authors of a 1990 study found that ginseng decreased wakefulness and increased slow-wave (deep) sleep. They concluded, "It is speculated that the well-known health-improving effect of the ginseng may be, at least in part, related to an enhancement of sleep." Another study, done on rats and mice in 1991, found that daily doses of *Panax ginseng* for five days had anxiety-relieving effects that were comparable to those induced by diazepam (Valium). A 1988 study, also on mice, found that ginseng compounds suppressed "aggressive episodes (offensive sideways posture and attack bite)" in a dose-dependent manner. Researchers have found that low doses of ginseng can increase blood pressure while high doses can lower it.

Some studies have had positive results using ginseng to increase aspects of mental performance. For example, in a 1987 study done on rats, scientists found that low doses of ginseng (10 to 30 mg per kg of body weight) had positive effects on mental performance while much higher doses greatly increased locomotor activity. "The results show that ginseng at appropriate doses improves learning, memory, and physical capabilities," the researchers concluded. Other studies on animals and humans (radio operators, nurses, students, and others) have found that ginseng tends to improve reaction time, problem solving, attention and alertness, and logical deduction.

For many people ginseng's effects fall somewhere between those of green tea and ginkgo. You may notice a strong and immediate stimulant effect from taking it (especially if the ginseng is high quality and potent), or you may experience more of a subtle long-term boost in energy levels by taking it on a daily basis for two or three weeks. Like other adaptogenic herbs, ginseng is often taken regularly or in cycles for its long-term effects on health and longevity. People generally stop taking ginseng and other tonic herbs during periods of acute illness.

GINSENG'S COMPLEX CHEMISTRY

The root of the ginseng plant seems to have representatives of every major type of poten-tially bioactive compound known to humanity: vitamins, minerals, and trace elements; amino acids, peptides, and proteins; monosaccharides, polysaccharides, and other sugar compounds; lipids and fatty acids; essential oils; alkaloids; flavonoids; and more. Among the key ingredients are certain saponins or glycosides, particularly the ginsenosides, first discovered in the early 1960s. About two dozen ginsenosides have been identified in wild ginsengs, amounting to a total of approximately 3 to 6 percent of the dried root. Cultivated ginsengs have about a dozen various ginsenosides, though some of the others may be found in minute amounts.

The ginsenosides are identified by a capital R followed by letters and sometimes numbers, such as Ra, Rb_1, Rg, and so forth. Asian and American ginsengs have been found to have different ginsenoside profiles. Asian ginseng has higher quantities of certain ginsenosides (such as Rg_1 and Rg_2) that have been found to be stimulating. American ginseng has higher concentrations of ginsenosides (such as Rb and Rc) that have been found to be calming. Interestingly, this scientific analysis matches two of the prevailing views of practitioners of traditional Chinese medicine. One, they have long contended that Asian ginseng is, in the words of the Chinese, *yang* (warming, energizing) and American ginseng more *yin* (cooling, calming). The contrasting properties of the two ginsengs explain in part Chinese interest in importing American ginseng: it is better suited for certain individuals (some women and elderly; anyone who is especially energetic or hyperactive), conditions (it affects the respiratory and digestive systems more so than the circulatory), and circumstances (tropical climates, hot weather). And two, from the Chinese perspective the whole ginseng plant is more effective than any of its individual components. Because of the variations in ginsenosides, and because some of the ginsenosides can even have opposite effects depending on dosage—stimulating in small amounts and relaxing in larger—it is impossible to narrow ginseng's effects down to a few of its many parts.

It should be noted that analyses of commercial ginseng products done over the past thirty years have repeatedly found tremendous variations in quality and potency. Ginseng products can vary considerably, both in their total ginsenoside content and in the ratio of the ginsenosides present. Although products have improved in recent years with the advent of standardization, better manufacturing controls, and the development of more reputable companies, as recently as 1994 an analysis of fifty commercial products determined that ginsenoside content varied from 0 percent (in six of the samples) to 9 percent. The respected American Botanical Council of Austin, Texas, recently analyzed over four hundred commercial ginseng products. Early reports indicate that more than half of the products are accurately labeled.

While the ginsenosides account for much of ginseng's action, and these variations can help to explain why products have different effects, other compounds found in ginseng, such as panax acid, have been found to affect metabolic rate or influence the function of the heart, brain, or other organs. Some herbalists believe that tonic herbs such as ginseng, with

their diverse and complex effects, suffer in their overall function when compounds are removed in the making of certain extracts.

A BUYER'S GUIDE TO GINSENG

It is possible to wildcraft American ginseng, though learning its habitat and locating specimens can be a real art that takes years to develop. Also, wild ginseng is vulnerable to overforaging, as the whole plant is uprooted to harvest it. Wild American ginseng has been harvested almost to extinction in much of its native habitat in the northeastern United States. Wildcrafters should thus adopt a conservationist approach to wild ginseng: plant seeds from the harvested plant, leave young plants alone, and so forth. Finally, some states require anyone who wants to wildcraft ginseng to obtain a permit and adhere to certain restrictions. Find out about the appropriate regulations and environmental considerations before attempting to wildcraft ginseng.

Asian and American ginseng products come in a wide variety of forms, including the root (whole, sliced, or powdered) and in capsules, tablets, tea bags, tinctures, standardized extracts, and even soft drinks. Roots should be at least five to six years old to have sufficient levels of ginsenosides. Potency varies considerably, depending on the type, how it was cultivated, its place of origin, and storage factors.

Preparation can be crucial in determining the herb's effects. Different methods of processing can cause color variations in ginseng, from white to red. The whitest product is derived by peeling the yellowish root and allowing it to dry. Ginseng turns its most reddish color when the peel is left on and the root is slowly steam cured and then dried. Red ginseng is hard and resistant to pests. Studies have found that steaming acts as a preservative for some ginsenosides and even creates a few new ones, giving red ginseng (especially red Korean ginseng) a higher total content of saponins compared to white. The different colored ginseng preparations have varying properties:

White ginseng is considered relatively mild and neutral, less warming and stimulating to the body than red, but less cooling than American ginseng.

Red ginseng is widely considered to be more yang, warming, and stimulating than white, with red Korean ginseng being especially potent. Red ginseng is most appropriate for persons who need invigoration, such as some elderly, and least appropriate for charged-up younger people.

Whether red or white, judging root quality is difficult for novices. Considerations include overall appearance as well as shape (slim, human-shaped roots are favored over fat ones, though this may be more of a traditional belief than a factor with a basis in scientific analysis) and age (since the plant dies back to the ground each year, a series of stem scars in the form of rings at the top or "neck" of the root can indicate age, with the best roots being at least five to six years old). Most people prefer to rely on capsules of the whole, dried herb; whole-plant extracts that are standard-

ized for 5 to 9 percent of ginsenosides; or on popular concentrated extract products such as Ginsana and Ginsun.

The various types of ginseng are often combined with other adaptogenic herbs (look for products with names like Chisandra Adaptogen, Metamorphosis, and Ginseng/Schizandra Supreme), with energizing herbs (Energia, ReZoom, Natrol High, Pure Energy), or with stress-reducing nutrients such as vitamin C and B complex (B-Stress). The different types of ginsengs are also combined; ginseng-only combination products go by names like Ginseng Extracts, Eight Ginsengs, Nine Ginsengs, and Wild Ginseng Supreme.

SAFETY CONCERNS

Ginseng is generally considered to be safe even for long-term use. Especially compared to alkaloids, glycosides tend to be fairly nontoxic. Lethal-dose tests have found that tonic herbs such as ginseng are many times less toxic than prescription or even over-the-counter drugs.

A 1979 report in the *Journal of the American Medical Association* on so-called ginseng abuse syndrome, characterized by irritability, nervousness, and other adverse effects, is frequently cited in media reports on ginseng. The original data in this study, however, has been seriously questioned—exactly what subjects were taking and in what doses and potencies was not validly determined. Admittedly, people who take as much as 15 g of ginseng a day may suffer from ginseng abuse, but this dosage is much higher than suggested doses and warnings about ginseng abuse syndrome now seem wildly exaggerated.

Taking some types of ginseng every day for long periods of time may also cause adverse effects. Red Korean ginseng in particular may cause overstimulation in some people. Practitioners of traditional Chinese medicine often recommend that ginseng users cycle off the herb every three to four weeks, or not take the herb for longer than two to three months. The Chinese also usually take ginseng in formulations with other, balancing herbs.

Though ginseng may occasionally cause insomnia, no long-term adverse effects from taking average doses have been identified, and few contraindications exist for ginseng. The primary ones are that ginseng is best used with caution by anyone with high blood pressure or cardiovascular disease. Because the structure of some of the ginsenosides is chemically similar to certain steroidal hormones, the exact range of their effects on growth and development among children is not known and ginseng is therefore generally not given to them, nor taken by pregnant or lactating women. Some herbalists even caution that women during their childbearing years should not take large doses of ginseng on an ongoing basis, though no studies have established related problems.

In mid-1997 health officials in a number of states took steps to discourage the sale of alcohol-based ginseng products to children. In Massachusetts, for example, the state Alcoholic Beverage Control Commission sought a voluntary recall of a chocolate-flavored gin-

seng extract that some convenience stores were apparently selling as point-of-purchase snack items. An official noted that some of the vials contained more alcohol than a beer or a wine cooler.

TAKING ASIAN AND AMERICAN GINSENG

Many herbalists recommend experimenting with ginseng and other tonic herbs, starting with low doses and taking note of how your body reacts. Herbalists may also be able to help tailor an herbal regime for your body and your activity level. For example, if you often feel cold and tired, an herbalist might recommend red Asian ginseng preparations. If you're relatively strong, young, and healthy, red might be overstimulating. White Chinese ginseng or American ginseng might be better for those athletes and people under age forty-five who want to take ginseng every day.

Doses of ginseng vary widely, and it is a good idea to check the label for the manufacturer's recommendation. An average one-time stimulant dose of Asian or American ginseng capsules standardized for 8 percent ginsenosides is 150 to 300 mg. If you intend to take ginseng on a daily basis for its cumulative effects, the dosage is perhaps half of the stimulant dose and divided so that it is taken one to three times daily. An increase in energy and mental sharpness may not be noticed for two weeks or so.

SIBERIAN GINSENG/ ELEUTHERO: GINSENG'S RUSSIAN COUSIN

Siberian ginseng (*Eleutherococcus senticosus,* or *Acanthopanax senticosus* to the Chinese) is not in the *Panax* genus though it is in the same plant family (Araliaceae) as the Asian and American ginsengs and has effects and uses somewhat similar to them. Most herbalists and researchers prefer to call Siberian ginseng by the name eleuthero, believing that the only true ginsengs are those in the *Panax* genus and that "Siberian ginseng," a name apparently created by American marketers in the 1970s, is more of an advertising ploy than an accurate description of the plant. At least one herbal company has begun to use the Chinese term for Siberian ginseng root, *ciwujia*. However, because the vast majority of North American companies that market *Eleutherococcus senticosus* products refer to the herb as Siberian ginseng, for better or worse that's the name we'll prefer here.

Siberian ginseng rivals the *Panax* genus ginsengs as one of the most popular tonic herbs. Many athletes, students, workers with stressful jobs, and others are now taking Siberian ginseng on a daily basis to strengthen bodily systems and improve overall health. Those who use Siberian ginseng note that it often has a positive effect on mental alertness, work quality, and physical performance. Natural health practitioners say that Siberian ginseng supports the adrenal glands' ability to balance hormones in response to stress. Like other tonics, Siberian ginseng has a normalizing effect on bodily functions such as blood pressure and blood glucose levels, tending to raise them when too low and lower them when too high. It improves adaptation to extremes in elevation and climate. It is said to be especially helpful for people who suffer from frequent bouts of illness, lack of energy or appetite, or depressed mood.

Siberian ginseng is derived primarily from the roots but also from the bark, stems, and sometimes the leaves of a relatively common thorny shrub native to the taiga forests of northeastern Asia, including parts of Russia, Korea, and China. Plant historians are still debating Siberian ginseng's role in traditional Asian folk medicine, with some contending that its use as a tonic herb is relatively recent and others believing its historical popularity rivals that of Asian ginseng. (The disagreement hinges on whether certain remedies in ancient medical texts refer to Siberian ginseng or to some other plant.) A Russian who, in the mid-1850s, was the first modern botanist to collect and study Siberian ginseng eventually recognized it as a member of a new genus, *Eleutherococcus* or "free-berried shrub." *Eleutherococcus* is now known to contain more than two dozen species of trees and shrubs in addition to *E. senticosus*.

Siberian ginseng's modern history really began only when it came to the attention of the plant researcher Izrail I. Brekhman in the 1950s. Brekhman and other Soviet Union scientists at the Institute of Biologically Active Substances in Vladivostok had devised ways to test mice for the tonic effects of Asian ginseng. (Essentially the researchers measured how long mice could swim or climb a rope until they were too exhausted to continue.) These studies confirmed an increase in endurance among animals administered ginseng.

The Soviet scientists then began to test other herbs for tonic effects. In particular they were looking for strengthening herbs that might be cheaper and more widely available than Asian ginseng. After many years of studying the chemical composition of Siberian ginseng and testing it on animals and humans, Brekhman concluded that Siberian ginseng was even more effective than Asian ginseng as a tonic. (Admittedly, the social and political environment in which Brekhman and his colleagues worked must be considered in evaluating this conclusion, as Soviet officials no doubt preferred the idea of a home-grown tonic herb to continued reliance on an expensive Chinese import.)

Like Asian ginseng, Siberian ginseng has been shown in some studies to cause animals to swim greater distances under stress, live longer after being exposed to radiation, and improve in immune response. Animal studies have also established disease-preventative properties in Siberian ginseng. For example, a 1992 Russian study that induced nervous system tumors in rats found that Siberian ginseng reduced the cancer occurrence rate and increased survival time, though the effect was less pronounced compared to a ginseng preparation. A 1996 study by Japanese researchers determined that Siberian ginseng can help protect against gastric ulcer.

Chemical analysis has isolated various types of compounds in Siberian ginseng, including polysaccharides, essential oils, glycosides, and flavones. Foremost among the many Siberian ginseng constituents that may affect the mind and body is a series of more than a dozen compounds known as eleutherosides. The eleutherosides occur in tiny amounts (generally less than 1 percent) in the plant's roots and stems; some are also found in low concentrations in the leaves. Much like the ginsenosides isolated from the *Panax* ginsengs, the eleutherosides have been designated with letters such as eleutheroside A, eleutheroside B, and so forth. Studies have determined that the eleutherosides and the ginsenosides cause some similar effects on the body, such as reducing the adverse effects of stress. As a group, however, the eleutherosides vary quite a bit in their chemical makeup, and all are quite distinct from the ginsenosides. Also unlike the ginsenosides, the eleutherosides are not unique to Siberian ginseng and can be found in various other plants.

Exactly how these compounds (or the whole herb—Siberian ginseng appears to be like other ginsengs in that the isolated components do not have the same tonic action as the whole plant) affect the body is still being determined. Siberian ginseng may be especially effective at balancing neurotransmitter levels, an action that can explain its reputation for alleviating emotional complaints and enhancing overall feelings of well-being.

Though the vast majority of the more than 1,500 studies done on Siberian ginseng has been published in Russian scientific journals, researchers in China, Japan, and Europe have also performed clinical trials over the past few decades, generally reporting positive results. For example, a 1987 double-blind, placebo-controlled German study on thirty-six human subjects found Siberian ginseng enhances the body's overall resistance to infections and immune-related ailments. Various other studies that have tested for factors such as work capacity and quality, fatigue, and sleep requirements have determined that Siberian ginseng has potentially positive effects on energy levels and resistance to stress and disease.

Sports- and exercise-related benefits remain controversial. A recent study done on twenty experienced distance runners failed to confirm any potential effects on exercise performance, as measured by heart rate, oxygen consumption, and other physical factors, from taking a liquid Siberian ginseng extract every day for eight weeks. This study can be criticized on the grounds that the subjects already were especially fit, making it difficult to measure any effects from taking a tonic herb such as Siberian ginseng. Some studies done on average people have found increases in physical endurance from taking Siberian ginseng.

Siberian ginseng is generally thought to be less overtly stimulating to the nervous system than is Asian ginseng. Some practitioners of traditional Chinese medicine contend that Siberian ginseng's energy is more compatible with women than is Asian ginseng's, and that Siberian ginseng is preferable as an immune-enhancing herb for those who wish to take a tonic herb on a daily basis.

Adverse side effects from using Siberian ginseng are rare. It is considered to be safe for daily consumption even in doses many times larger than average, though some people have been known to experience insomnia, headache, and other mild side effects from taking high amounts. Animal studies have not shown any danger of Siberian ginseng causing cancer or birth defects. Extrapolating from lethal-dose research done on mice, authorities have estimated that a 150-pound human would have to swallow almost five pounds of powdered Siberian ginseng before the effects of the herb were likely to be fatal.

Herbal producers often combine Siberian ginseng with other adaptogenic herbs, such as Asian or American ginseng, astragalus (*Astragalus membranaceus*), and schisandra (*Schisandra chinensis*). Companies have also begun to offer Siberian ginseng products that are standardized for one or more of the eleutherosides, particularly eleutheroside B (also known as syringin) and eleutheroside E.

Because Siberian ginseng has a more extensive root structure than does Asian and American ginseng, growers can partially harvest Siberian ginseng's roots without killing the plant. Siberian ginseng grows faster than *Panax* ginsengs; herbal companies have also begun to cultivate Siberian ginseng in North America. Thus, Siberian ginseng is usually less expensive than these ginsengs. As is true of other ginsengs, wild plants are considered superior to cultivated ones. High-quality, wild-crafted Siberian ginseng, however, is becoming rarer, and adulterated and/or mislabeled products have been identified in recent years, so purchase only from reputable, quality producers.

Taking Siberian Ginseng/Eleuthero

An average dose of Siberian ginseng in capsules is 500 to 750 mg one to three times per day. The dosage is lower for products standardized for one or more of the eleutherosides—often 100 to 200 mg up to three times daily, but check dosage instructions on the package label. In liquid extract form an average dose is one to two dropperfuls up to three times per day.

Siberian ginseng leaves make a somewhat more palatable tea than does Asian or American ginseng. You can find Siberian ginseng in tea bags, instant tea granules, and the like.

CHAPTER 4

Ephedra/ Ma Huang

◎

TRADITIONAL MEDICINE AND MODERN STIMULANT

Ephedra is currently one of most controversial herbs in North America, with
many medical authorities and regulators calling for states or the federal government to ban
its sale. Even within the supplement industry,
ephedra's inclusion in "natural high" products, first formulated in the early 1990s and
now widely promoted to teens and young
adults, has caused a rift between established
herbal companies and upstart marketers.
Meanwhile, tens of millions of people regularly take conventional, over-the-counter products that contain ephedra-based compounds.
A closer look at this widely misunderstood
herb shows it to be neither the killer its critics
claim nor the safest stimulant around.

A BOTANICAL RELIC

You won't find ephedra in many gardens. Like
horsetail, which it resembles, ephedra is a
botanical relic. It even looks primitive, with its
lack of showy features—such as flowers or
even leaves—that today's gardeners value in
an evergreen shrub. Actually, if you look
closely, ephedra does have tiny leaves and it
also bears cones from the joints in its woody,
green stems. The forty-odd species of the
genus *Ephedra* are native to arid regions of
Asia, the Mediterranean, North America, and
elsewhere.

The most well-known of the ten North
American species is Mormon tea (*E. nevadensis*), found throughout much of the Southwest
and as far north as southern Oregon. Native
Americans in the Four Corners area used *E.
nevadensis* medicinally and introduced it to the
Mormons when Brigham Young led them into
Utah in the late 1840s. Mormon tea is much
less stimulating than coffee and tea, which the
Mormons regard as unhealthy. Mormon tea is
also known as cowboy tea and teamster's tea,
names that refer to other groups that favored
it in the mid-nineteenth century. In other parts

of the West it was often called whorehouse tea, as it was commonly served in those institutions, apparently in the mistaken belief that it could help to prevent syphilis and gonorrhea.

It is a Chinese species of ephedra, *E. sinica,* that has become known worldwide for its many medicinal and mind-altering properties. The Chinese refer to *E. sinica* as ma huang. *Ma* refers either to the astringent taste or to its hemplike stems; *huang* means yellow. (Technically, ma huang is the dried young stems of the plant, while *ma huanggen* is the root and rhizome. The latter has only a minor traditional use, as a remedy for profuse night sweating. In the natural product industry, *ephedra* and *ma huang* are used more or less interchangeably to refer to *E. sinica.*)

Ma huang ranks as one of the world's oldest medicines, having been used for its therapeutic properties for as many as five thousand years. The Chinese prescribed ma huang tea as a traditional remedy for colds, hay fever, nasal congestion, bronchial spasms, and asthma. The traditional healers of India also valued ephedra for similar purposes, and India remains today a major exporter of the herb to the West. Over the past century, scientific investigation of ephedra has confirmed the wisdom of using the plant as a decongestant and asthma reliever.

IN SEARCH OF HERBAL ADRENALINE

The modern history of ephedra begins in 1887, when a Japanese chemist first isolated one of the herb's most active compounds, the alkaloid ephedrine. The discovery didn't garner much scientific interest, however, until 1924, when a Chinese researcher, K. K. Chen of the Peking Union Medical College, became interested in the pharmacological properties of ephedrine. Familiar with ma huang's reputation as one of humanity's oldest medicines and as an herb for relieving respiratory complaints, he began to investigate whether ephedrine would be able to substitute for the hormone adrenaline as an anti-asthma drug. Adrenaline had been isolated in 1897 by an American physician from the adrenal glands of sheep. (The pharmaceutical firm Parke-Davis subsequently obtained a trademark on the name Adrenalin. Because of the confusion between adrenaline and Adrenalin, most scientists refer to the hormone by its scientific name, epinephrine; the more familiar adrenaline will be used here.) Physicians soon realized that adrenaline was one of the most effective treatments for asthma. In addition to increasing heart rate and muscular strength, adrenaline also dilates bronchial tubes, allowing the lungs to take in more oxygen and the person to breathe more deeply. This effect is important to asthma sufferers, whose bronchial tubes constrict and thus interfere with free breathing. The drawback to using adrenaline as an asthma treatment, however, is that it is ineffective when taken orally and even when injected its effects are short-lived. Chemists working on this problem hoped to produce a synthetic adrenaline derivative that would be orally active and longer lasting.

Chen's research was groundbreaking. He

determined that ephedrine was chemically and functionally similar to adrenaline. Like adrenaline, ephedrine dilates bronchial passages; ephedrine differs in being active orally and for an increased duration. After 1927, when synthetic ephedrine was first developed, clinical use of ephedrine as a bronchodilator took off. Ephedrine became the first compound derived from a traditional Chinese herb to gain scientific respect and widespread clinical use in the West.

In addition to clearing the airways and relieving nasal congestion, ephedrine was quickly recognized as a major central nervous system stimulant. Tests showed that it boosted metabolism, raised blood pressure, and increased the flow of blood through the heart (and sometimes the heart rate itself). Asthma sufferers who took ephedrine noticed that it frequently caused them to become nervous and restless and to suffer from insomnia. By 1930 researchers had developed an ephedrine-like synthetic compound that also enlarged bronchial and nasal passages and was claimed to have fewer side effects. The substance was amphetamine, and by the early 1940s proprietary products such as Benzedrine had replaced ephedrine as the asthma treatment of choice. The medical community embraced amphetamine enthusiastically and it was widely used by soldiers, housewives, businesspeople, and others as an endurance enhancer, weight-loss agent, and mood brightener. Amphetamine's stimulating effects on the central nervous system (in reality much more marked than ephedrine's) and abuse potential were to be responsible for its own downfall as a ther-

apeutic drug by the 1970s. Meanwhile, a few ephedrine-containing medications, such as Primatene tablets, are still marketed for certain types of asthma. Pharmacological researchers have developed a number of other prominent asthma drugs, such as albuterol (Ventolin), by using the chemical structure of ephedrine as a model.

Ephedrine's other main uses, as a cold remedy and a nasal decongestant, have been taken over by the related alkaloid compound pseudoephedrine. Like ephedrine, pseudoephedrine occurs naturally in some ephedra species and can also be produced synthetically. Pseudoephedrine's slight difference in structure from ephedrine causes the two alkaloids to have minor differences in bodily effects. Compared to ephedrine, pseudoephedrine is less effective against asthma but has the same ability to constrict blood vessels of the mucous membranes in the nose, leading to decongestion and relief of cold symptoms. Pseudoephedrine is somewhat less likely to stimulate the central nervous system and to increase blood pressure than ephedrine. Pseudoephedrine is now found in dozens of popular over-the-counter medications, such as Contac, Sudafed, Actifed, Vicks Vatronol, Dristan Cold and Flu, and Benadryl Cold Tablets. The FDA has approved the use of ephedrine and pseudoephedrine in over-the-counter drugs as bronchodilators and nasal decongestants. Infrequently, doctors use ephedrine-based drugs to treat certain allergic disorders, narcolepsy (the sleep disorder characterized by excessive daytime sleepiness), minor irritations of the eye, motion sickness, and incontinence.

One popular current use for ephedra products that the FDA has assuredly not approved is for weight loss. Studies on both animals and humans have demonstrated that ephedrine can lead to weight loss, partly because of its ability to suppress appetite and partly because it boosts metabolic rate and the burning of calories. Researchers call this latter process that ephedrine promotes *thermogenesis*— the metabolizing of fat leading to energy loss through heat.

Most of the research on ephedrine and weight loss has been done on animals, but a few studies have used humans. For example, a double-blind 1992 Danish study found that dietary changes plus a combination of 20 mg of ephedrine and 200 mg of caffeine led to the same amount of weight loss as those who were on a diet-plus-placebo program. The ephedrine/caffeine group, however, was able to lose more body fat and less muscle mass compared to the placebo group. A double-blind trial published in 1994 determined that ephedra/caffeine compared favorably to dexfenfluramine (Redux), the controversial serotonin-enhancing weight-loss drug that in September 1997 was voluntarily withdrawn from the market, in promoting weight loss in obese patients. Among all the subjects in this trial, ephedrine/caffeine led to 20 percent more weight loss than Redux, while among subjects who were more than 40 percent overweight, ephedrine/caffeine led to 29 percent more weight loss than Redux. A 1996 study found that the combination of 30 mg ephedrine, 100 mg caffeine, and 300 mg aspirin increased postmeal thermogenesis.

Studies have generally found that the combination of ephedrine and caffeine is more effective at promoting thermogenesis than either alkaloid on its own. Using ephedrine and caffeine to promote weight loss, however, has a number of notable limitations. It doesn't work at all for some people. The dosages required are frequently high enough to cause overstimulation, at least initially (side effects such as nervousness tend to diminish with continued use, and it is best to start with low doses and gradually increase levels as needed). Also, many of the best potential candidates for the treatment, severely obese people, suffer from medical conditions such as high blood pressure that can be worsened by taking an ephedrine/caffeine combination. Finally, pill-based weight-loss programs, whether the substance is a natural dietary supplement or a prescription drug, rarely lead to long-term weight loss unless they are accompanied by healthful lifestyle changes, particularly a low-fat diet and regular exercise or physical activity.

The FDA has approved as a weight-loss agent a synthetic compound, phenylpropanolamine (PPA), that is chemically similar to ephedrine. PPA is "approximately equal in potency to ephedrine but usually causes less central nervous system stimulation," according to the AMA's *Drug Evaluations* (sixth edition).

WHOLE PLANT OR ISOLATED ALKALOID?

The stimulating and mildly mind-altering effects of ephedra have been well established since the 1930s, when ephedrine served as a reference standard for the scientific testing of stimulant drugs. Ephedrine's effects are known to be much like adrenaline's because ephedrine stimulates various receptors of the sympathetic nervous system, promoting the activity in the body of adrenaline and the related neurotransmitter noradrenaline. These chemicals affect the activity of the heart, muscles, brain, and other parts of the body, especially when the body is exposed to a stressful or threatening situation. The predominant effect is to increase the readiness to act in some way—to fight or take flight, for example. Energy is diverted from the center of the body to the surface. The heart pumps more blood, but it goes not to the digestive system and the internal organs but to blood vessels in the skeletal muscles, temporarily increasing their strength. The body begins to sweat, the pupils dilate, and airways in the lungs expand. If somebody throws something at you, you're ready to duck.

All this nervous system stimulation also has a pronounced effect on the mind. For many people, ephedra will cause a mild to moderate increase in alertness, concentration, and mental clarity. It will alleviate perceptions of fatigue and enhance endurance, at least for a few hours. People may become more talkative and outgoing.

Of course, exactly what types of cerebral effects ephedra causes and how strong they are will depend on various factors, including the body's overall health, individual susceptibility to ephedra, other drugs consumed, and so forth. Which alkaloids predominate in the herb and total dosage are major considera-

tions, ones that are often difficult for the consumer to control because of limited label information. The alkaloid content of ephedra species varies from almost 0 percent (North American species of ephedra, including Mormon tea, are virtually alkaloid-free) to 3.3 percent (some batches of ma huang). Ephedrine is the principal alkaloid in ma huang, accounting for up to 90 percent of the alkaloid content, depending upon where it was grown and other factors. In addition to pseudoephedrine, other ephedra alkaloids include norephedrine, N-methylephedrine, and norpseudoephedrine. Low percentages of norpseudoephedrine and norephedrine are also found in another plant with ephedralike properties, khat (*Catha edulis*), a traditional stimulant of the Middle East and northern Africa. The action of the ephedra alkaloids are similar to one another though they can differ in degree.

Ephedrine doubtless accounts for much of the action of ma huang, though some herbalists contend that there are noticeable differences between taking ephedrine and taking the whole plant. According to Simon Mills, author of *Out of the Earth: The Essential Book of Herbal Medicine,* the hypertensive (blood pressure–raising) effect of ephedrine is, in the whole plant, largely eclipsed by the action of pseudoephedrine. He says, "With no doubt the contribution of other constituents, this means that the whole herb does not have the same hypertensive effects as the isolated ephedrine." Herbal authority Rudolph Weiss, M.D., also has written that the whole plant is safer and better tolerated than its isolated alkaloids. In addition to its alkaloids, constituents of ephedra species include saponins, essential oil, and other compounds that may have anti-inflammatory or other physiological effects.

Much of the current controversy over ephedra has been provoked by the recent explosion of interest in and sales of products that are promoted as "natural highs" and as nontoxic alternatives to "ecstasy," a synthetic amphetamine derivative, and to other controlled substances. Most of these natural highs are formulated products that combine ephedra with caffeine-containing herbs plus other potentially stimulating herbs, such as ginseng (see chapter 3). Some of these products, perhaps most, may have both ephedra and added (usually synthetic) ephedrine. Typically these products are sold not by established herbal or dietary supplement companies, nor are they available in most natural foods stores. Rather, they're formulated by marketing companies that rely on flashy ads, psychedelic packaging, and mail-order sales or multilevel marketing. Some are also sold at rock concerts, head shops and sex shops, over the Internet, and at all-night raves frequented by teens and young adults. Products go by names like "herbal ecstacy [sic]," Cloud 9, Tribal Trance, Ultimate Xphoria, and Planet X.

The hype surrounding these products has scaled new heights, even in an industry not known for its reserve. Ads promise that taking these products will create "natural euphoric pleasures" and "electrify your senses." One product is touted as a "party prolong" that "zooms your mood to mach 5, heightens sensitivity to light, music, and tactile stimulus—completely natural and safe!" Products are claimed to be nontoxic, and explicitly or by implication, safer than alcohol, ecstasy, and other drugs often abused.

Do these products deliver on the hype? Yes and no. It is true that some people, when they take high levels of potent nervous system stimulants such as ephedrine and caffeine in combination, may experience not only marked stimulation but quite possibly mild euphoria if not ecstasy. One user describes the experience of taking a large dose (more than recommended on the product label) as providing "a cocainelike rush." Much of the sales pitch for these products is made up of testimonials from satisfied users, along the lines of how the product causes "tingly and floaty mind-expanding euphoria."

But these nirvanalike experiences are not necessarily typical, and in many other respects the products are misleading and possibly even dangerous.

On the most basic level, these products bear little resemblance to the drug ecstasy, also known as XTC and MDMA (an abbreviation of its scientific name, methylene-dioxy-methamphetamine). Ecstasy has a reputation primarily as a euphoriant that gained considerable notoriety in the early 1980s when it became a popular party drug. For some people it is also an empathogen, a substance that increases the capacity to understand and be sensitive to another's feelings and thoughts. By helping to lower inhibitions, reduce defensiveness, and promote feelings of intimacy and closeness with other people, empathogens can play a role in relationship building. Mental health counselors sometimes suggest empathogens if a subject is particularly closed and withdrawn, and ecstasy was used for this purpose by a few psychotherapists and other mental health professionals during counseling sessions.

Unlike ecstasy, which is thought to work by affecting serotonin levels, the ephedra/caffeine natural highs are basically central nervous system stimulants. They may make you a better talker, but they're unlikely to promote contemplative listening. Despite the hype about the ephedrine/caffeine ecstasy alternatives, you're more likely to have positive empathogenic effects by taking kava (see chapter 17).

In terms of safety, government regulators obviously consider real ecstasy much more of a health threat. The Drug Enforcement Administration classified ecstasy as a controlled substance in 1985, claiming that its use could permanently damage nerve cells in the brain. Further scientific investigation was vastly curtailed. Therapists no longer use ecstasy, though it remains a popular street drug.

It is possible, however, that the ephedrine/caffeine drugs may pose health risks to some people that are at least as great as the risks of low doses of real ecstasy. This is due to the fact that the advertised effects from the natural "X-products" are predominantly available only at very high dosages. Until regulators began to crack down, typical dosage suggestions read

like this: "Suggested serving: 3–5 tablets or as directed by a medical professional. Caution: Do not exceed 10 tablets in 24 hours without first consulting a health practitioner." When the products are hand-sold at concerts and the like, buyers are typically told that they need to take a dose of five to ten tablets to get high. But most herbalists, health authorities, and government regulators agree that such high doses vastly increase the odds that users will experience adverse side effects. For most people these ill effects may be just nervousness or insomnia, but an unlucky few may experience potentially more serious effects such as a dangerous increase in blood pressure.

Recently, presumably in response to deaths attributed to the products, adverse publicity, and regulators' concerns, a number of major natural-high producers have changed their package labels to caution against taking high doses or exceeding the recommended dosage. One prominent product now warns against taking more than one tablet in seventy-two hours. Though this makes these products vastly safer (assuming users follow the recommendations), it also presents an obvious "truth in advertising" problem: taking such limited quantities usually offers the approximate "ecstatic high" of drinking a strong cup of coffee.

The question of dosage is especially worrisome because these products typically don't offer any idea of exactly how much ephedrine and caffeine can be found in each tablet. Yet this information is vital for consumers. These two alkaloids account for virtually all of the products' effects on the nervous system and the brain (with the possible exception of those products that contain yohimbine, another potent stimulant alkaloid; see chapter 18). Some products contain a half-dozen or more herbs that are promoted as working synergistically. But the levels of active compounds from these other herbs, such as kava, ginseng, and ginkgo (see chapter 11), are almost assuredly much too low to account for the products' dramatic psychoactivity. Multiple caffeine-containing herbs may be included. For example, "herbal ecstacy" contains, in addition to ephedra and other herbs, the common caffeinated herb tea (see chapter 2) and two exotic caffeinated herbs: guarana and kola nut (see chapter 5). Nary a mention of caffeine (much less milligrams of caffeine per dose) appears anywhere on the label.

Consumers who call, as I have, and ask marketers exactly how much ephedrine and caffeine are contained in their products are likely to be told that the information is "proprietary." One company said that they provided that information to government regulators but not to the general public. If labels offered this basic information, it would be possible to estimate how one tablet—or ten—would act on the body. Consumers would be able to judge, for example, whether most of the physiological effects were due to ephedrine, caffeine, or their combination.

When regulators have tested some of the natural-high products for ephedrine and caffeine content, not surprisingly the results have been all over the board. According to Gary Coody, a health official in the Texas Department of Health's division of drugs and med-

ical devices, in 1995 the department tested three batches of one ephedra-caffeine product for ephedrine content. Two batches averaged 10 to 11 mg of ephedrine per tablet, while the third averaged a whopping 45 mg of ephedrine. "Obviously, they don't have great manufacturing controls," Coody observed. Only one batch was tested for caffeine content, and it averaged 20 mg caffeine. The Department did not test for any other alkaloids.

In mid-1996 the respected herbal trade quarterly *HerbalGram,* a joint publication of the American Botanical Council (ABC) in Austin, Texas, and the Herb Research Foundation (HRF) in Boulder, Colorado, published the results of a test it commissioned on three natural-high products. Two of the products (Ultimate Xphoria and "herbal ecstacy") contain ephedra and caffeine-containing herbs; one (Cloud 9) contains only ephedra. Two leading independent labs were provided with blind samples of the three products, which were purchased at retail stores in Austin. The labs tested for ephedrine, pseudoephedrine, and four other ephedra alkaloids, plus caffeine. The chart on page 57 averages the two labs' test results.

The tests indicate that total ephedrine content among the natural-high products varies considerably, as does caffeine content. The two labs came up with figures within approximately 20 percent of each other for all but one of the measurements (19.8 versus 10.4 mg of caffeine in Ultimate Xphoria).

A final criticism is that, as herbal supplements, these faux-ecstasy products represent an incredible rip-off to consumers. Compared

	ULTIMATE XPHORIA MG/TABLET	HERBAL ECSTACY MG/TABLET	CLOUD 9 MG/TABLET
Ephedrine	17.4	7.0	39.2
Pseudoephedrine	11.2	8.5	0.5
Other Ephedra Alkaloids*	2.1	0.9	0.7
Total Ephedra Alkaloids	**30.7**	**16.4**	**40.4**
Caffeine	**15.1**	**20.5**	**0.2**

*The labs provided separate totals for norephedrine, norpseudoephedrine, N-methylephedrine, and N-methylpseudoephedrine. Because the figures for these four ephedra alkaloids were so low, here they are grouped together. SOURCE: American Botanical Council/Herb Research Foundation.

to other herbal products and dietary supplements, natural highs are inexplicably expensive. Typically they are sold in packets of only five to ten tablets, at a total cost of $15 to $30. Three dollars per tablet reflects a cost determined by hype and greed, not ingredients. Products from established companies can be found in natural foods stores with similar ingredients, though typically promoted as weight-loss agents. For example, in 1996 Thermogenic Enhancer from Vitamin Research Products provided 10 mg of ephedrine per capsule plus 40 mg caffeine (plus some other ingredients such as taurine). The cost for 180 capsules was approximately $20, or a little more than a dime per capsule. The VRP label offered explicit information about the total ephedrine and caffeine content.

- -
R E G U L A T O R S
C L O S I N G   I N
- -

Much of the controversy that has surrounded ephedra recently has resulted from the marketing of the ephedra/caffeine products. The natural-high combos really began to take off only in early 1995, while a few of the ephedrine/caffeine weight-loss products garnered critical attention in the early 1990s. The proliferation of these potent products has had repercussions throughout the established herbal industry. Some products' high dosage recommendations and lack of label information on ephedrine and caffeine content have put on the defensive even responsible members of the natural foods industry. By mid-1996, at least twenty states had taken steps to regulate select ephedra products, with officials in a few (notably Ohio, New York, and Texas) claiming that ephedrine-containing supplements were responsible for citizens' deaths—a seventeen-year-old high school football player in Ohio, a Texas woman in her early forties who died while playing tennis, and a Long Island college student who died on spring break in Florida. (Ohio's 1994 law that banned anyone but pharmacists from selling ephedra products was amended in late 1996 to exempt products that contain a maximum of 25 mg of ephedrine per serving or dosage unit. In early 1997, Texas officials also retreated from proposed regulations that would have classified as prescription drugs all ephedra-containing products.)

The FDA blames ephedra and ephedrine/caffeine combination products as the cause of at least twenty-two deaths since 1993 in the United States. Substantiation, however, in the form of the approximate dose ingested and definitive autopsy reports is lacking in a number of these cases. In others the deaths appear to be inconsistent with single overdoses of ephedrine. An analysis by a researcher for the Council for Responsible Nutrition (CRN), a Washington, D.C.–based dietary supplement trade group, found that six of the deaths might be attributed to ephedra and two were clearly tied to consumption of high levels of the herb. Producers of the ephedrine/caffeine natural-high products also note that when people at rock concerts, for example, take multiple illegal drugs and get sent to hospitals vomiting or babbling incoherently, it creates fewer problems for them to blame their condition on the legal ephedra product they took than on the ten lines of coke they also snorted.

The spate of adverse effects and deaths from ephedra led to a rash of herbal horror stories in the press in 1995 and 1996. *Consumer Reports* called for ephedra to be banned in an article on "Herbal Roulette." Major metropolitan papers including the *New York Times,* the *Boston Globe,* and the *Washington Post* weighed in with articles having titles like "The Unwholesome Tale of the Herb Market," which were uniformly critical of herbal safety and focused heavily on ephedra. "So far, at least 15 people have died in the United States after taking herbal products containing ephedrine," the *Times* intoned, not bothering to say whether these were overdoses, or even to offer any evidence or attribution. The television networks weighed in as well, with news features critical of natural-high products. Many of the media reports quoted state officials and "supplement critics" calling for an FDA ban on all ephedra-containing products. The FDA was typically portrayed as powerless because the 1994 Dietary Supplement Health and Education Act (DSHEA) deregulated the dietary supplement market, preventing the agency from controlling herbs and nutrients and allowing companies to make "unrestrained and unjustified claims."

In fact, the DSHEA hardly leaves the dietary supplement industry unregulated. Among other things it mandated an increased level of "good manufacturing standards" for the industry and explicitly referred to label cautions and warnings for dietary supplements. In addition, the FDA has full authority now—as it did before the law was passed—to determine that a product poses "an imminent hazard to public health or safety" and if so to remove it immediately from the market. What the DSHEA did do is shift the burden of proof that an ingredient in a dietary supplement is unsafe and poses a significant health risk from the manufacturer to the FDA. The DSHEA also mandated that the FDA hold public hearings whenever it decides that an existing dietary supplement (such as ephedra) should be banned or changed in its classification to a drug. This provision in the DSHEA was partly in response to what was viewed as arbitrary FDA actions against evening primrose oil and other dietary supplements prior to 1994.

In any case, the FDA has been avidly involved in questions regarding ephedra in recent years, though it has not called for the total ban ephedra's critics desire. A 1993 agency *Import Bulletin* stated, "There is no known food use for this herb. . . . Ephedrine is a strong reactive alkaloid and has been associated with elevation of blood pressure in humans. We have no information to support the GRAS [generally recognized as safe] status of ephedra or conditions of safe use." It also stated that "manufacturers should be aware of FDA's continuing interest in ephedra." More recently, in October 1995 and in February 1996, the FDA convened expert advisory groups to consider possible labeling requirements, dosage limits, and consumer warnings for ephedra supplements. Perhaps signaling a more open attitude toward herbal supplements, however, the FDA for the first time included representatives from the herbal and dietary supplement industries on one of its advisory committees.

The FDA has noted that a 1995 survey of ephedra products on the U.S. market found that only 15 percent of those reviewed did not contain a label warning relating to the potential adverse effects and contraindications for ephedra. The agency also said that its test found that products contained an average of 21 mg of ephedrine per dose (not necessarily per tablet). Alkaloid levels averaged from 6 to 8 percent (standardized extracts can concentrate alkaloids at higher levels than the 1 to 3 percent average of whole ma huang). Eight different supplements containing ephedra alkaloids accounted for 55 percent of the total 665 complaints related to all dietary supplements received by the agency since 1993, an FDA official said.

In April 1996, the FDA issued an alert

warning consumers not to purchase or consume ephedrine-containing dietary supplements with labels that often portray the products as apparent alternatives to illegal street drugs such as "ecstasy," because these products pose significant health risks to consumers. . . . Ephedrine is an amphetamine-like stimulant that can have potentially dangerous effects on the nervous system and heart. . . . Many of these ephedrine-containing products bear labels that appear to be targeted at adolescents and young adults and that imply the products can produce a "high." The agency considers this type of promotion and these claims to violate the Federal Food, Drug, and Cosmetic Act, even as amended by the . . . DSHEA, which governs the U.S. marketing of dietary supplement products.

FDA Commissioner David Kessler stated, "These are recreational street drugs masquerading as dietary supplements. . . . These are drugs, and should be regulated as such." (The recent Ohio law similarly targets herbal highs by prohibiting companies from claiming that any ephedra product "causes euphoria, ecstasy, a 'buzz' or 'high,' or an altered mental state; heightens sexual performance; or, because it contains ephedrine alkaloids, increases muscle mass.")

The FDA warning was clearly worded in a way that excluded ephedra-based supplements produced by the established herbal industry and marketed for purposes other than attaining euphoria. At the same time that it announced its consumer warning, the FDA also mailed threatening letters to a half-dozen manufacturers of ephedra-based "natural high" products.

The FDA advisory panels had difficulty reaching a consensus about how the agency should regulate ephedra. A "Special Ephedra Working Group" of the agency's ephedra advisory committee recommended reduced, industry-mandated dose limits and explicit labeling requirements. In fall 1996, however, the full Food Advisory Committee Meeting on Ephedra-Containing Dietary Supplements recommended more strict control of ephedra, including a government-mandated dose limit and label warnings against extended use of the herb. A minority of the panelists were in favor of declaring that no safe dose existed for ephedra, no health claims should be allowed on ephedra labels, and the herb should be reclassified as a drug.

In June 1997, the FDA finally acted upon these recommendations. The agency proposed that ephedra products could not be sold as dietary supplements if a serving or recommended dose exceeded 8 mg ephedrine in a six-hour period or 24 mg in a day. Supplement manufacturers would be prohibited from combining ephedra with other stimulants, including caffeine. Ephedra product labels would have to warn consumers not to take the supplement for more than seven days, a ruling that would effectively eliminate use of the herb in any weight-loss or muscle-building products. The label would also have to warn consumers that "taking more than the recommended serving may result in heart attack, stroke, seizure, or death." The FDA gave the public (and the herb industry) seventy-five days to comment on the proposed new rulings.

In recent years a number of the largest and most influential herbal and dietary supplement-industry trade groups have also been actively examining the issues surrounding ephedra and adopting more restrictive policies on the herb. These groups include the CRN, National Nutritional Foods Association (NNFA) of Newport Beach, California, and the American Herbal Products Association (AHPA). In mid-1996, these groups released a joint statement recommending that ephedra products provide no more than 12 to 15 mg of ephedra alkaloids per dose, a reduction from previous maximum levels of 20 to 30 mg recommended by some of the groups. Industry groups are also considering limits on the percentage of total alkaloids in ephedra extracts and a ban on added synthetic ephedrine. A 1994 advisory to the natural products industry stated, "The use of synthetic ephedrine as an additive to ephedra or ma huang products is inappropriate and adulterates these products." The advisory urged manufacturers to obtain certificates of analysis or to perform independent analyses to ensure that the raw material for their ephedra products did not contain added ephedrine. It is worth noting that a 1997 study of nine ephedra-based dietary supplements determined that none of them contained synthetic ephedrine.

The NNFA has also urged suppliers and

manufacturers to state on product labels the level of ephedrine and pseudoephedrine, and, if it is also present, caffeine. According to Anthony Young, NNFA general counsel, "NNFA also agrees with a suggestion FDA made earlier this year to all the associations that the ephedra alkaloid content in each unit dose be listed as ephedrine equivalents on the product label. We also suggest that the total xanthine alkaloids be listed as caffeine equivalents."

The NNFA disagreed with the ephedra proposal announced by the FDA in June 1997, noting that the association considered the seven-day duration of use and 8 mg potency limitations overly restrictive. In general, supplement industry opposition was not vociferous, perhaps because the ephedra controversy was perceived as clouding the reputation of the entire alternative health field. The safety questions have caused a number of companies to either phase out ephedra products or promote supplements as ephedra-free. A few herbal companies that still sell ephedra products, on the other hand, were vocal in their opposition to the proposed new FDA regulations, noting that the herb was being unfairly targeted compared to conventional pseudoephedrine-based over-the-counter products.

The recommended warning label for products that contain ephedra/ma huang (though not Mormon tea), originally developed by the AHPA and later adopted by the NNFA, reads: "Seek advice from a health care practitioner prior to use if you are pregnant or nursing, or if you have high blood pressure, heart or thyroid disease, diabetes, difficulty in urination due to prostate enlargement, or if

taking an MAO inhibitor or any other prescription drug. Reduce or discontinue use if nervousness, tremor, sleeplessness, loss of appetite, or nausea occur. Do not exceed recommended dose. Not for children under 18. *Keep out of reach of children.*" The AHPA has put ephedra on its restricted use list, meaning that members' ephedra products are required to carry the label warning.

This label warning is similar to those found on ephedra-alkaloid-containing over-the-counter products.

Major herbal educational associations, including the ABC and HRF, also agree with the policy of regulating ephedra through restrictions on suggested dosage and total daily use as well as requiring full label warnings. Mark Blumenthal, executive director of the ABC, says bluntly that the sale of ephedra "in products substituting for illicit street drugs cannot be condoned" and that the FDA already has adequate authority to act against these "aberrations" and that "it should do so." The NNFA has also come out against the sale of "street drug knockoffs."

One reason that the FDA is not pushing for an immediate ban on all ephedra products may be that it realizes how difficult it would be to prove that ephedra, when used responsibly at low doses and sold with proper warnings, is actually unsafe. The herb has been used for thousands of years with much success. Over the past sixty years, millions of people have used over-the-counter remedies containing ephedra-based alkaloids. In over-the-counter medicinal products, single recommended doses of pseudoephedrine average 30 to 60 mg and total daily intakes up to 240 mg. Single recommended doses of ephedrine average 25 mg and total daily intakes up to 125 mg. Regulations that seek to ban natural ephedra products but leave unregulated ephedra-alkaloid-containing over-the-counter remedies obviously have to do some twists and turns. According to Robert McCaleb, president of the HRF, Texas at one point proposed regulations that sought "to prevent the sale of even low-dose natural products containing these stimulant ingredients, while protecting the products of the pharmaceutical industry."

McCaleb has also pointed out the difficulty of making blanket restrictions against products that contain both ephedra alkaloids and caffeine. He notes, "It is common for ephedrine and caffeine to be consumed together. For example, like many other Americans, most asthmatics who use OTC products like Primatene also drink coffee, tea, or cola. People taking cold remedies containing ephedra alkaloids also routinely consume caffeinated beverages." If it is the combination of these two alkaloids that is so dangerous, he notes, shouldn't any law also require warnings on all ephedra-alkaloid-containing medicines and all caffeinated beverages? Wouldn't this be necessary to warn the unsuspecting parent who's giving a child Sudafed and allowing her to drink a Coke as well?

While ephedra has taken most of the heat for adverse reactions from ephedrine/caffeine combinations, it should be noted that some of the same symptoms (rapid heart rate, shaking, headache, shortness of breath) that have been blamed on it are also consistent with an overdose of the more socially approved drug caffeine. As the *HerbalGram*-sponsored test of natural-high products demonstrated, at least one product ("herbal ecstacy") apparently has higher levels of caffeine than ephedrine.

"In a society that is enamored with increasingly exotic varieties of coffee, the ma huang issue takes on a particular irony," noted Blumenthal and Penny King in an extensive 1995 examination of ephedra in *HerbalGram*. "Yes, ma huang and its ephedra alkaloids are generally more potent [central nervous system] stimulants than coffee and caffeine. Yes, ma huang and its alkaloids do have more generally agreed-upon contraindications than coffee and caffeine. But this is a question of degree. When viewed dispassionately, coffee and caffeine probably should be sold with some responsible label warnings. . . . [Caffeine] is highly subject to abuse, producing hypertension, insomnia, irritability, and addiction in untold millions of Americans. . . . This comparison ought to provide some perspective and balance to the ma huang debate."

Or, as a lawyer for three ephedra-based natural-high products put it in response to New York's attempted crackdown, "This is the alcohol, nicotine, and caffeine crowd going, 'This is the only way to party, no other way to party should be legitimate.'"

HOW SAFE ARE EPHEDRA PRODUCTS?

Ephedra is a potent stimulant and it can cause side effects. In average dosages, such as 15 to

25 mg of total alkaloids, these are usually minor. Adverse effects may include those typical of stimulants: insomnia, nervousness, headaches, dizziness, hand tremors, increased blood pressure, rapid heartbeat, and nausea.

In high doses, or extreme overdoses, ephedra may in some cases be life-threatening. Certainly, someone with high blood pressure or a heart condition who takes a 400 mg dose of ephedrine, for example, increases the risk of suffering a heart attack or stroke. A 1991 review of the pharmacology and psychoactive alkaloids from ephedra cautioned that "toxic psychosis" was reported as a side effect with "the daily dose of ephedrine prior to the psychotic episode varying within wide limits, the average being 510 mg." Long-term ephedra use may weaken the heart, adrenal glands, and other organs.

As with other potent nervous system stimulants, ephedrine-based stimulants are sometimes abused. How quickly tolerance to ephedra's stimulant effects builds up with continued prolonged use is a matter of dispute. Most medical texts, including the AMA's *Drug Evaluations* and *Goodman and Gilman's The Pharmacological Basis of Therapeutics,* state that tolerance to ephedra's effects develops quickly, necessitating larger and larger doses. Naturopath Michael Murray, on the other hand, notes that "according to the American Pharmaceutical Association, 'There is far more discussion of ephedrine tachyphylaxis (rapid decrease in effectiveness) or tolerance than is evidenced as a significant problem in the scientific literature.'"

Ephedra products should be avoided by those with heart disease, hypertension, thyroid disease, and diabetes. People who are taking MAO inhibitors, women who are pregnant or lactating, and anyone under age eighteen should also not use them. Combining ephedra with substances that block certain types of neurotransmitter receptors in nerve cells (so-called alpha-2 blockers, such as the alkaloid yohimbine from yohimbé) can cause a potentially dangerous increase in blood pressure. Consult with a health professional if you intend to take ephedra for more than seven days consecutively.

Ephedra and ephedrine are on the "banned drug list" of both the National Collegiate Athletic Association and the United States Olympic Committee. (Both groups also prohibit high blood levels of caffeine, approximately equal to consuming 750 mg of caffeine in one sitting.) Renowned Argentinean soccer player Diego Maradona was kicked out of the competition in the latter rounds of the 1994 World Cup because in postgame urine tests he tested positive for a number of ephedrine compounds. Taking ephedra can possibly cause a positive test result on a drug test for amphetamine use.

- -

IS EPHEDRA RIGHT FOR YOU?

- -

Some people are better candidates for benign if not beneficial use of ephedra than others. Certainly anyone with the health conditions just mentioned or with a history of abuse of stimulant drugs should not use ephedra. Herbal writer Subhuti Dharmananda, Ph.D., notes that ma huang tends to divert energy and bloodflow from the body's core and its internal organs to its surface. When the digestive system is in good health, this diverting action doesn't cause any particular problem. But, he says, if your system is weak, "it can't tolerate the depletion of energy from the center. Instead of a feeling of strength and vitality, one feels jittery, and perhaps tired." Therefore, people who are weak, nervous, suffer from sleep problems, or subsist on an unhealthful diet are not likely to benefit from ma huang.

He says, "Persons who are underweight, recovering from illness, or who have been under a lot of emotional stress often find that ma huang makes them feel worse. One can hardly blame the herb. It is doing what it is supposed to do." These people need a tonic herb, such as ginseng, to build energy over the long term. The ideal candidate for ephedra is someone with a strong constitution, an efficient digestive system, and good overall health. "Since most members of fitness centers are strong and respond well to ma huang, it has a great reputation there. However, those with more sedentary lifestyles who are seeking an alternative to their daily coffee consumption need to take stock of their condition before relying on [ephedra] as an alternative," Dharmananda says.

It is also worth mentioning that in China ephedra was traditionally used not so much on its own but in combination with other herbs. For example, someone with a cold might combine decongestant ephedra with an expectorant herb such as licorice. Herbalists say that licorice, as well as nutrients such as vitamin B complex, vitamin C, and zinc, can nourish the adrenal glands and help to counter the stress on the organ caused by ephedra use.

If you want to use ephedra to promote weight loss, it's unlikely to be helpful if you already have a high metabolic rate.

TAKING EPHEDRA / MA HUANG

The dosage suggestions below should yield an average total ephedra alkaloid content of 15 mg, and an ephedrine content of 12 mg, putting the effects somewhere in the vicinity of drinking a cup of tea. Although higher than the FDA-mandated 8-mg-ephedrine-per-dose limit, this dosage is consistent with ephedrine dosages in over-the-counter remedies for approved FDA uses and with long-term medical and traditional use of ephedrine.

As a single herb, ephedra is sold dried and in capsules, concentrated drops, tinctures, and extracts. Read labels closely to determine total alkaloid content, ephedrine content, and suggested doses. In general:

- For the powdered herb containing 2.5 percent total alkaloids, a suggested dose is 600 mg.
- Use one tablespoon of the whole herb (with an approximate total alkaloid content of 1.25 percent) to brew a cup of ephedra tea containing some 15 mg of total alkaloids.

Mix the dried herb in the water, bring to a boil, and simmer for ten to fifteen minutes.

- Extracts are often standardized for an alkaloid (mostly ephedrine) content of 6 to 8 percent. To yield 15 mg of alkaloids, take 215 mg of a 7 percent alkaloid content extract.

- Tinctures, liquid extracts, and concentrated drops vary widely in alkaloid content. Adjust for the desired alkaloid content if the dose is standardized per dropper, or follow label recommendations.

Guarana, Maté, and Kola Nut

◎

EXOTIC CAFFEINATED HERBS

A naturally occurring substance found in more than one hundred plants, caffeine is the most popular mind-altering drug in the world. Caffeine's stimulating effects may have been discovered by Stone Age people 600,000 years ago, when they are thought to have chewed caffeine-containing leaves, seeds, or fruits to extend endurance and ward off hunger. Today, the vast majority of the caffeine ingested worldwide each year is extracted by adding hot water to either coffee or tea, which together account for an estimated 97 percent of caffeine consumption. Approximately half of adult Americans drink at least two cups of coffee per day, with tea and caffeinated soft drinks increasing in popularity. A small amount of caffeine consumption can also be attributed to over-the-counter drugs and to chocolate, derived from seeds (called cacao or cocoa beans) of the tropical cacao tree (*Theobroma cacao*). Yet a trio of exotic caffeinated herbs—guarana, maté, and kola nut—are more popular than coffee and tea in some parts of the world and recently have begun to appear in herbal products commonly available in health food stores. Variations in caffeine content, the presence of other compounds, and different traditional uses for these herbs provide a number of reasons for considering their advantages and disadvantages as alternatives to coffee, tea, and chocolate.

Before discussing these three herbs, let's take a closer look at the much-maligned group of compounds that accounts for most of their effects, beneficial and adverse.

CAFFEINE AND ITS CHEMICAL RELATIVES

Caffeine, which was first isolated from coffee in 1820, is the most prominent in a group of related alkaloids known as xanthines. Xanthine is a basic compound that occurs in animal and plant tissue. Caffeine and other xanthines, such as theophylline and theobromine, resemble each other in structure and have similar effects on the body. Scientists distinguish among these important xanthines in part by the number of methyl groups attached (methyl is a carbon and hydrogen atom compound). Thus, caffeine is a trimethylxanthine, a xanthine compound with three methyl groups. Theophylline and theobromine are both dimethylxanthines with two methyl groups; they differ from each other in how the methyl groups are structurally arranged.

Caffeine is readily absorbed into the bloodstream from the stomach and small intestine and circulated to tissues throughout the body. Scientists are still trying to understand fully caffeine's exact mechanisms of action within the body. One of caffeine's most direct effects is on the cellular level, where it interferes with the activity of adenosine, a compound that acts to maintain a steady state of bodily arousal. By flattening out the body's adenosine speed bumps, caffeine allows the body to slip into high gear. Caffeine also has important indirect stimulant effects on the body that are thought to involve dopamine, acetylcholine, and other neurotransmitters. Perhaps most prominently, caffeine causes the adrenal glands to release adrenaline and noradrenaline into the bloodstream. These hormones stimulate the nervous system, brain, lungs, and other organs, reaching a peak effect approximately thirty to sixty minutes after caffeine is consumed orally.

Caffeine's effect on the central nervous system results in a delay in the onset of sleep. It leads to an improvement in alertness and concentration, and for many people a greater ability to sustain mental effort. Caffeine speeds up some types of reaction time, improving performance in certain physical tasks such as driving. Caffeine stimulates skeletal muscles, boosts the heart's pumping action, and temporarily increases blood pressure, potentially benefiting physical endurance and sports activity. Caffeine stimulates the kidneys to produce more urine, the stomach to produce more stomach acid, and the bowels to move.

Caffeine does not accumulate in body fat. Rather, it is metabolized in the liver, with adults normally being able to break down half of a caffeine dose within approximately six hours. Caffeine's metabolites are excreted into the urine by the kidneys and eliminated from the body. Because some of these metabolites themselves, however, may have mind-altering effects, the stimulation from caffeine may last twelve hours or longer in many cases. Infants under the age of six months may take days to process a single dose of caffeine; tobacco smokers, on the other hand, process caffeine about twice as quickly as nonsmoking adults.

Theophylline was first isolated from tea in 1885. Theophylline also stimulates the central nervous system, possibly to an even greater degree than does caffeine. Theophylline boosts heart rate and increases urine production. More so than caffeine, it also relaxes smooth muscles, especially bronchial muscles in the windpipe. Theophylline's ability to dilate and open breathing passages, loosen phlegm, and expand lung capacity makes it a useful drug to relieve the symptoms of an asthma attack. Theophylline has long been used in a number of conventional asthma drugs, such as Bronk-aid and Bronkotabs, often in combination with ephedrine or other compounds with similar effects, or with calming drugs to prevent common side effects such as nervousness, insomnia, appetite loss, and rapid heart rate. A single therapeutic dose of theophylline may range from 100 to 300 mg. The prevalence of stimulatory side effects and the relatively slim margin of safety recently has caused physicians in the United States to curb their enthusiasm for theophylline as an asthma remedy. Theophylline, however, does not occur in rich enough concentrations in plants to have noticeable effects on the body. It occurs in highest amounts in tea, yet herbal authority Varro Tyler estimates in *Herbs of Choice* that "consumption of 55 pounds (25 kg) of tea would be required to equal one 100 mg tablet of theophylline."

Theobromine is much less potent than caffeine and theophylline in its ability to stimulate the central nervous system, relax smooth muscle, and promote the flow of urine. Researchers estimate that it has one-seventh to one-tenth the stimulant effect of theophylline and caffeine. Theobromine thus has few therapeutic applications but is sometimes used instead of caffeine for certain medical conditions such as angina pectoris, a recurrent pain in the chest from a sudden decrease in the blood supply to the heart. Among the richest plant sources of theobromine is cacao beans, which contain low levels of caffeine but 1.5 to 3.0 percent theobromine. Theobromine occurs only in small amounts in kola nuts and tea and not at all in coffee. Because some chocolate products have seven to ten times as much theobromine as caffeine, its effects can nevertheless be significant. For example, a cup of cocoa may have 15 mg of caffeine but an additional 150 mg of theobromine, resulting in a total stimulant effect equivalent to a dose of 30 to 35 mg of caffeine. A two-ounce chocolate bar may have 50 mg of caffeine and 300 mg of theobromine, the dosage equivalent of 80 to 90 mg of caffeine. (Chocolate's mildly mind-altering effects may not be due solely to xanthines; a recent study found that chemicals in chocolate may bind to the same bliss-associated receptors in the brain that are targeted by the THC in marijuana.)

Although caffeine-containing herbs may have been used for hundreds of thousands of years, caffeine consumption has skyrocketed in recent centuries. Ethnobotanist Terence McKenna and others have pointed out that caffeine is the quintessential drug of the Enlightenment and the Industrial Revolution. "Their stimulant properties made caffeine in coffee and its close cousin theobromine in tea the ideal drugs for the Industrial Revolution: they provided an energy lift, enabling people to keep working at repetitious tasks that demanded concentration. Indeed, the tea and coffee break is the only drug ritual that has never been criticized by those who profit from the modern industrial state," McKenna notes in *Food of the Gods*. The three most prominent caffeine-containing drugs—coffee, tea, and chocolate—reached Europe around the same time (circa 1500 to 1600) and relatively quickly became widely accepted mind-altering substances. Prior to that, coffee drinking occurred primarily in Arabia and tea drinking in Asia. Asians preferred a tea-brewing method, moreover, that kept caffeine levels fairly low (see the discussion of green tea in chapter 2).

Studies on caffeine's effects on learning, memory, and cognition suggest that its reputation as an ideal mental stimulant is overstated. Some studies have confirmed that caffeine can improve such functions as short-term recall, reading speed, and auditory reaction time. The results, however, have not been uniform. A 1989 study, for example, found that doses of 125 and 250 mg of caffeine caused no significant differences in tests for recall or response time, but the higher dose seriously impaired performance of a numerical test. "Caffeine may have a deleterious effect on the rapid processing of ambiguous or confusing stimuli," the researchers concluded. A 1986 test in which college students were administered 100 mg of caffeine found that those who took the drug recalled fewer words than did control subjects. In general, studies suggest that the more complex the mental function, whether it be reading comprehension or high-level mathematics, the less likely caffeine will benefit performance.

Even so, the methylxanthines' effects on the mind and body hold an undeniable appeal for many people. They provide a feeling of increased energy and well-being, at least temporarily. They tend to lift the spirits and dispel lethargy and fatigue. The increase in the ability to focus for long hours on mental tasks is a property embraced by generations of students. Xanthine-containing herbs make you feel as if you can run farther and cycle longer, and to a certain extent that feeling is supported by a genuine physiological effect. Caffeine can improve ability to pay attention and prolong waking hours. It does not, however, sober up a drunk individual.

Individuals' reactions to caffeine and other methylxanthines vary considerably. Caffeine does not promote increased vigor and enhanced mood in everyone, and certain people are more susceptible than others to caffeine's potential side effects, even at relatively low dosages. For example, some people seem to tolerate 500 mg or more of caffeine per day without adverse effects such as restlessness, anxiety, tremors, and insomnia, while others experience these symptoms from as little as 50 to 100 mg. Excess caffeine can also cause a variety of other symptoms, including abdominal pain and nausea or aggravated ulcers (from an excess of stomach acid), twitching of skeletal muscles, high blood pressure, and heart palpitations. Extremely high doses (on the order of 3 to 5 g) of caffeine can cause convulsions or even, in very rare cases, death from heart attack. Consuming more than about 350 to 400 mg of caffeine per day can lead over time to at least three of the characteristics of a physical addiction—craving; the development of a tolerance to increased dosages; and withdrawal symptoms such as headache, fatigue, and irritability when caffeine is withheld. Another factor usually associated with physical addiction—an impaired ability to function in society—is less prevalent (and, perhaps, actually countervailed, in the sense that caffeine promotes adaptation to the increased speed and efficiency of modern industrial society). Psychological addiction to caffeine is not uncommon.

The long-term health effects from daily caffeine consumption remain controversial. Numerous studies have been conducted that have reported mostly—though not exclusively—

negative results on caffeine's effects on the risk of heart disease (some studies do show coffee raises blood cholesterol levels and increases the risk of heart attack), colon and bladder cancer, kidney disease, osteoporosis, and birth defects. Caffeine has been more definitively tied to worsening premenstrual syndrome, panic disorder, fertility, and birth weight. Caffeine use is associated with consumption of other addictive drugs, such as nicotine and alcohol. Nutritional deficiencies can be a concern when the caffeine-induced increase in urine flow causes vitamins and minerals to be flushed out of the body. A few studies do actually suggest health benefits, such as a recent one that showed a reduced suicide rate among some regular caffeine users. The consensus among most health authorities is that moderate caffeine consumption among adults, such as 50 to 150 mg per day, is relatively safe and innocuous. There is also general agreement that users should avoid consuming more than 300 mg of caffeine per day, which is only slightly in excess of average American consumption of 250 mg per day. (Per capita caffeine consumption is about twice as high in Scandinavian countries such as Finland and Sweden, where coffee drinking is a national pastime.) There is growing concern over the widespread acceptance of caffeine consumption, primarily from soft drinks and chocolate, among children. The recent introduction to the U.S. market of caffeinated bottled water also highlights the continuing popularity of the stimulant.

GUARANA: BRAZIL'S POTENT BERRY

Guarana is derived from a perennial plant (*Paullinia cupana* var. *sorbilis*) in the soapberry family. Also known as Brazilian chocolate and Brazilian cocoa, guarana is native to the jungles surrounding the central Amazon River basin in Brazil. In the wild the plant is a woody, climbing vine that yields bunches of reddish, grape-size fruit. Scientists have determined that the seed kernels from these fruits have higher caffeine levels (ranging from 2.7 to 5.8 percent dried weight) than coffee or tea. Sweet, colalike, guarana-based soft drinks were introduced in Brazil some eighty years ago and are now widely popular there, and in recent years guarana-based dietary supplements have begun to make inroads in the North American health food industry.

Indian tribes native to the Amazonian River basin were drinking guarana beverages when the first Europeans arrived in the sixteenth century. Native Indian tribes in the Amazon still prepare guarana in the traditional way. They open up the segmented fruit and remove the seeds, usually one to three per fruit. With their hard, dark brown coating, the seeds resemble small horse chestnuts. Indians cut off and discard the coating and soak the seed kernels in water. The kernels are then dried by laying them out in the sun or roasting them on a clay griddle. Pounding with a pestle in a mortar crushes the seeds into a powder. During the pounding stage, Indians add small amounts of water intermittently and sometimes cassava flour, so that the final result is a dense, doughy paste. This is kneaded like bread dough to remove any air pockets. The dough is then rolled into a sausage-shaped tube about six inches long and slowly fired or smoked for up to two months, until it takes on a hard consistency. Finally, it is ready to make into a guarana drink. Indians grate or scrape about a half-teaspoon of powder off the end of the stick, add the light brown powder to hot or cold water, sweeten, and drink.

Native tribes are thought to have developed this elaborate process for a number of reasons. Thus processed, guarana resists becoming moldy, a problem with the ground powder in the humid jungle. Also, the guarana rods store and travel well. Indians use guarana for prolonged fasting and take the sticks along on extended voyages, sometimes subsisting on little more than their guarana drink and what can be foraged along the way. Indians sometimes also just nibble off the end of the guarana rod. Guarana is a traditional social stimulant, aphrodisiac, and appetite suppressant. As an herbal medicine it was relied upon to treat diarrhea, fever, headaches, and other ailments. Many tribes also drink it on a daily basis as an overall system strengthener and digestive tonic, because of its purported ability to prevent disease and maintain wellness.

The first outsider to write about guarana was a Jesuit missionary to the Amazon in 1669. White miners, settlers, and others who came to the Amazon often adopted guarana drinking. The German naturalist K. F. P. von Martius inspired the earliest scientific research into guarana in the beginning of the nineteenth century. He studied guarana in the field during an expedition to South America from 1817 to 1820, gave it its Latin name, and sent specimens back to Europe for laboratory analysis. In 1826 his brother isolated an alkaloid and dubbed it guaranine, not realizing it was the same as caffeine. Modern scientists and herbalists usually refer to guarana's active compound as caffeine. When the labels for some herbal-upper products refer to guarana's active ingredient only as guaranine, the intent may be to mislead consumers who might otherwise want to avoid the better-known caffeine.

Researchers have also determined that guarana contains other alkaloids, including the xanthines theophylline and theobromine. Caffeine is, however, the dominant xanthine—a 1994 study of guarana powder found that 92 percent of the xanthine content was caffeine, 5 percent theobromine, and 3 percent theophylline. Guarana also has relatively high levels—5 to 6 percent—of tannins (explaining its astringent action on the digestive system); starch and gum; an essential oil; and perhaps most significantly trace amounts of a saponin known as timbonine. Saponins are complex plant compounds, typically found in plants such as soapbark, best known for their ability to produce a soapy lather. Certain saponin-rich plants such as ginseng, however, may also have important system-strengthening or tonic properties (see chapter 3).

"Future research may well show that various saponins also play an important part in [guarana's] pharmacology, particularly with regard to its long-term influence as a general tonic and prophylactic," stated guarana researcher Anthony Richard Henman in his comprehensive 1982 study of guarana. "In recent years, however, claims have been made for guarana's suitability as a tea and coffee substitute, particularly for those suffering from cardiovascular afflictions, and this could be related to the counterbalance given to the stimulant alkaloids in the drug by the saponins which are so well represented in the plant family which includes guarana (the Sapindaceae)." Unfortunately, Henman notes, what research has been done on guarana has focused on its alkaloids: "This would seem to be a grave oversight, particularly in the light of recent research into the therapeutic properties of ginseng and other Old World stimulants, which have demonstrated clearly that the pharmacological activity of such plants is due mainly to their saponin contents. Both guarana's popular reputation and my own subjective perception of its effects would support the proposal of a special category for this plant, with its effects being perceived to lie somewhere between those of the classic caffeinated beverages and those of the Oriental 'somatensics' [such as] ginseng."

Henman also praises guarana as "an ideal crop for supplementing the incomes of small peasant farmers in the Amazon basin." He notes that among its attractions are that it can be planted and grown as a fast-growing perennial shrub in the midst of other crops rather than requiring further forest clearance; natives need little technical assistance to cultivate and harvest it; it lends itself to small-scale hand-processing; the final product has a high value per unit of weight; and the worldwide demand for guarana is currently greater than the supply. Also, caffeine can be derived from the whole plant, not just the seed kernels. The seed husks and even the leaves, which contain up to 1.2 percent caffeine, are also potential sources of caffeine. Indeed, guarana did develop into an export crop for its caffeine content in the 1920s, though it has since been supplanted by synthetic caffeine and caffeine derived from coffee and tea production.

FROM SOFT DRINKS TO HERBAL UPPERS

Today, approximately three-quarters of the annual guarana crop is not prepared traditionally and consumed locally but rather is highly processed into extracts and concentrates to provide flavor and caffeine for the South American soft drink industry. Colalike guarana sodas have been termed the national drink of Brazil, where they account for approximately 15 to 20 percent of the soft drink market (second only to colas). Guarana sodas share with North American colas only a passing connection to the original herb—colas have little if any kola nut anymore, and guarana sodas have vanishing amounts of real guarana. Brazil had to pass a law in 1944 requiring a minimum amount (0.6 percent, later reduced to 0.3 percent) of certain ingredients for soft drinks to merit the name guarana, orange, or whatever. Comparisons of the estimated annual guarana crop with annual guarana soft drink production indicate that even this small amount of guarana is lacking in many of the sodas. Like colas in the United States, some guarana-based soft drinks in Brazil have additional flavors and are caffeine-free.

Soft drink manufacturers are eager to establish guarana-based sodas in the United States, the world's largest soft drink market (Mexico is second and Brazil is third) and one in which caffeinated drinks dominate, accounting for at least 80 percent of all soft drink sales. In 1995, PepsiCo began test marketing a guarana-flavored soft drink, Josta, in Houston, Seattle, and other cities. Josta contains 55 mg of caffeine per twelve ounces, slightly more than the 40 to 45 mg of most colas. PepsiCo's promotional campaign for Josta is aimed at the youth market and contains veiled references ("enhancing the most primal joys of life") to guarana's reputation as an aphrodisiac. A PepsiCo spokesperson has described early test results as encouraging, and it is likely that Coca-Cola, which like PepsiCo is a major player in the Brazilian soft drink industry (Coca-Cola has been selling its Guarana Tai soft drink in Brazil for more than two decades), will be test marketing guarana-based soft drinks in North America in the near future.

A tiny but growing portion of the annual guarana crop is also being diverted to the health food market in the United States, Europe, and Japan, where it has become a popular constituent in the herbal uppers category because of its high caffeine content. Products with names like Hit Energy, Zoom, Energy Elixir, and Super Pep promise customers instant energy, alertness, and heightened perception. Guarana is also being used in natural-high products with names such as "herbal ecstacy" that are typically potent combinations of caffeine and ephedrine (see chapter 4). Health food stores in Europe even carry guarana energy bars and chewing gum. Guarana has a reputation for lifting mood and increasing stamina without causing the edginess of similar amounts of coffee.

Unfortunately, the guarana products appearing on health food store shelves are unlikely to match traditional guarana in quality and healthfulness, according to Henman's comprehensive analysis in the *Journal of Ethnopharmacology*. Guarana processing plants grind the seeds at high temperatures, causing oxidation of certain compounds and resulting in a commercial powder that is bitter tasting and more likely to irritate the gastrointestinal system. Henman says that in his experience, the traditional stick preparation yields a product that is relatively mild in light of the high caffeine content. One explanation may be that naturally occurring fats and oils in the seeds slow digestion. "It seems likely, therefore, that the stimulant properties are absorbed very slowly through the intestinal tract, with the effect of a single dose often being noticeable for a full six hours, or twice as long as that of an average cup of tea or coffee," he says. It should be noted, however, that a 1992 study found no significant differences in the rate of the release of caffeine from capsules of guarana and capsules containing an equivalent amount of caffeine. The study also found no difference in the rate of caffeine absorption (measured using in vitro rat intestines) between a guarana suspension and a solution containing an equivalent amount of caffeine.

Should herbal producers in the near

future decide to focus on providing a high-quality guarana supplement, it could begin to transcend its reputation as merely a heavy-duty caffeine source.

Another South American plant related to guarana is yoco (*Paullinia yoco*), which is unusual in that natives of southern Colombia brew a stimulating drink not from its leaves or seeds but from its bark. Stems can also be chewed for an energy boost. Studies done in the 1920s determined that yoco bark contains up to 2.7 percent caffeine. Yoco seems to be commercially unavailable in North America, though at least one company sells yoco plants by mail order.

TAKING GUARANA

A few herbal producers offer guarana whole, ground, cut and powdered, or in capsules. The labels for capsule products may or may not state the caffeine or guaranine content, which can be important for determining the dose that is right for you. For example, a 1,000 mg capsule that contains 4 percent caffeine represents a 40 mg dose of caffeine.

MATÉ: THE STIMULATING TEA OF PARAGUAY

This exotic caffeinated herb is derived from the leaves of a small South American evergreen tree (*Ilex paraguariensis*) in the holly family. Maté is also known as Paraguayan tea and

in Spanish as yerba maté, *yerba* meaning plant or herb and *maté* referring not only to the tea but to the vessel from which it is drunk as well as the tree itself. Maté is native to the lowland forests of Paraguay, northern Argentina, and southern Brazil. South American Indian tribes have long brewed the leaves and twigs into a light green, smoky-flavored tea that they drink to prevent fatigue, suppress the appetite during periods of fasting, and treat headaches, arthritis, and other ailments. Maté has recently begun to make inroads north of the equator—the popular Morning Thunder tea produced by Celestial Seasonings contains maté, as does Traditional Medicinals' Mucho Maté.

The traditional preparation methods natives use for maté bear some resemblance to those used to make Chinese tea. Leaves or leafy branches are picked and then dried, either by being hung over a fire or being spread out on large pans for slow heating. The quality of the final product is partly determined by the age of the leaves—young leaf buds are prized—and the degree of drying or roasting. The dried leaves may be kept coarse or crushed into a powder. Native South Americans often brew maté in the same vessel from which they drink it, a small, hollowed-out gourd that is often richly decorated. They add burnt sugar and lemon to make a traditional drink called *chimarrao,* which is sucked up scalding hot through a *bombilla,* a sort of straw with a bulblike strainer on the end to filter the tea.

Native South American Indians taught the early Spanish settlers how to brew maté. Jesuit missionaries in Paraguay made the initial attempts to cultivate maté in the seventeenth century, leading to another popular name for this herb: Jesuit's tea. The French botanist Auguste de Saint Hilaire studied the plant and gave it its scientific name in 1822. At the time maté was the stimulant of choice not only in southeastern South America but in parts of Chile, Peru, and Brazil as well. Later in the nineteenth century South American elites and immigrant Europeans began to turn to imported Chinese tea and African coffee, shrinking the base for maté and making it more a drink of natives and the common people. As coffee cultivation took hold in Brazil, maté drinking declined there, and per capita consumption is now only a pound or so a year. Remnants of the early Jesuit plantations still exist (Spanish-Portuguese forces expelled the Jesuits in 1767), though maté is also widely wildcrafted. Environmentalists point to maté as a forest product that can be harvested in a sustainable way without causing harm to it or to the natural ecology of the area.

In Uruguay, Paraguay, and Argentina maté has managed to withstand the challenge from imported Chinese and Indian tea. In recent years, per capita consumption of maté in these countries has been about fifteen pounds, roughly equivalent to per capita coffee consumption in average coffee-drinking countries such as Switzerland and France.

Among maté's constituents are tannins, an essential oil, vitamins and minerals, and alkaloids including from 0.6 to 2.2 percent caffeine by weight, with the average probably being slightly less than 1 percent. Thus it is relatively weak as a source of caffeine compared to coffee, tea, and guarana, with one cup providing only 15 to 25 mg of caffeine. Drinking maté results in the familiar increase in alertness, concentration, and mental focus. Some have noted that maté's effects are particularly stimulating to the mind as opposed to the body, making it useful for long hours of study or intense intellectual effort.

Excessive consumption of maté can lead to "a feeling of exhaustion," as the nineteenth-century German authority on psychoactive plants Baron Ernst von Bibra noted a century ago, as well as overstimulation, insomnia, and dehydration (from its diuretic action). Large doses may cause nausea. Epidemiologists have noticed an association between maté drinking and an increased risk of cancer of the esophagus. Researchers are unsure, however, what part other factors, including the extremely hot temperature of the beverage that some maté drinkers prefer, as well as tobacco and alcohol consumption, may play in the increased cancer risk.

MATÉ'S CAFFEINATED COUSINS

Botanists have identified two additional holly species related to maté that also contain caffeine. One is yaupon, a rare North American shrub or small tree whose Latin name, *Ilex vomitoria,* gives a clue to its traditional use. The Cherokees drank a tea made from yaupon's caffeine-containing leaves as part of ceremonial rights that included induced vomiting. Yaupon leaves themselves, however, are not emetic. Other Indian tribes north of the Rio Grande may also have used yaupon medicinally or to induce visions and evoke ecstasy. The only caffeine-containing plant native to North America, yaupon is not commercially available as an herb, although nurseries in the South may carry yaupon holly trees. At approximately 0.1 percent, the caffeine content of yaupon leaves is relatively low.

A second holly species, guayusa (*Ilex guayusa*), like maté, is native to South America, especially the eastern Andean foothills of Ecuador and Colombia. It was briefly a plant of commerce between South America and Europe during the early 1700s, due to the Jesuits promoting it (mistakenly) as a cure for venereal disease. After the Jesuits' abandoned guayusa plantations were reclaimed by the jungle, the plant became virtually unknown to the outside world for two centuries. Native South Americans continued to use it, however, mostly for ritual purposes.

Scientists have determined that the leaves of one strain of guayusa are the richest plant source yet identified for caffeine, containing up to 7.6 percent of the alkaloid. The strong tea natives brew from guayusa has also been used as a stimulant, a headache remedy, and, like yaupon, a ceremonial purgative. Some South American natives also add guayusa leaves to another psychoactive plant preparation termed *ayahuasca* or *yajé*. A principal (if not the only) ingredient in these potions is bark from *Banisteriopsis caapi,* the hallucinogenic "vine of the soul" that is a major visionary herb in South America. Ayahuasca is a bitter drink that makes some people sleepy, so traditional use sometimes involves combining it with stimulants such as tobacco or guayusa that help to neutralize the taste somewhat and

keep users awake to experience fully ayahuasca's hallucinatory effects.

TAKING MATÉ

Bagged teas such as Morning Thunder and Mucho Maté are the most popular maté products in health food stores. You can also find maté in bulk leaves, cut and sifted, and liquid extracts. An average dose is one cup of brewed tea or one dropperful of the liquid extract.

KOLA NUT: THE BETTER HALF OF COCA-COLA

The kola nut is a seed kernel from a tree (*Cola nitida, C. vera,* and other species) that is native to the tropical rain forests of West Africa and is cultivated there and in the Caribbean, South America, India, and Indonesia. The plant is in the same family as the cacao tree and, like cacao, kola nuts contain caffeine (about 1 to 3.5 percent by weight; averaging 1.5 to 2.0 percent) and theobromine (less than 1 percent), as well as tannin and an essential oil. The methylxanthines in kola nut no doubt account for its ability to boost mood, stimulate the central nervous system, and promote urine flow.

Kola nut, also known as bissy nut, has long been chewed by traditional peoples of Africa for its stimulating properties, much like some Asian and South Pacific populations chew betel nut. (The term "betel nut" is actually shorthand for a combination of the betel nut, which is the kernel or seed of the fruit of the tropical betel palm tree, *Areca catechu,* the mineral lime, and up to a half-dozen or so additional herbs.) Kola nuts come six or more to a pod and are slightly smaller than chestnuts. Natives cut open the leathery pods, remove the seeds, cut off the seeds' outer coating, and chew the inner white or reddish cotyledon. "Traditionally cola does not seem to have been infused to make a beverage, but more recently the toasted and ground nut has been used as a coffee substitute," notes anthropologist Richard Rudgley, author of *Essential Substances: A Cultural History of Intoxicants in Society.* In Africa, dried kola nuts also once had additional traditional social and ritual uses, serving as money and symbolic tokens.

Kola is, of course, the cola in Coca-Cola. For the first dozen or so years after its founding in 1892, the Coca-Cola Company included in its formula not only kola extract (and sugar, water, caffeine, flavorings, and other ingredients) but also significant levels of cocaine from coca extract. The cocaine has long since been removed, and Coke's exact ingredients are a company secret, but Coca-Cola may still contain tiny amounts of kola and coca extracts. Most modern cola-flavored soft drinks no longer use real kola nut either for flavor or for caffeine (the caffeine is synthetic, or derived from coffee or tea production). Caffeine content in colas is usually 35 to 55 mg per 12 ounces, although the new breed of extra-caffeinated colas has higher levels (Jolt, for example, has 72 mg of caffeine per 12 ounces).

Scientists have not conducted many studies on kola nut. As the authors of a 1978 study noted, "Except for a generalization that its effects are probably due to its caffeine content, no attempts have been made to quantify its specific actions." These researchers did find that low doses of kola nut given to cats caused an increase in blood pressure, while high doses led to a fall in blood pressure. A 1990 Bulgarian study found a similar dose-dependent action. Mice fed one dose (5 milligrams of the herb per kilogram of body weight, or 5 mg/kg) of kola nut extract showed a significant increase in locomotor activity while those fed a higher dose (10 mg/kg) exhibited signs of a depressive effect on locomotor activity. These results suggest that more is not necessarily better if you are seeking stimulation from kola nut.

Kola has a traditional reputation as an aphrodisiac and impotence remedy. Modern herbalists occasionally make use of its stimulating and mood-boosting properties to help treat people suffering from mild depression, especially if it is accompanied by weakness and exhaustion. Kola nut drinkers say that it has a more dramatic physical impact on the body than does tea, sometimes causing tingles or energy rushing up the spine and increased skin sensitivity.

TAKING KOLA

Kola nut is not widely available as a single herb. In the supplement industry it is most commonly used in energizing formulas that may also contain other caffeine sources as well as ephedra, or in "nervines" (tonic formulas to strengthen and nourish the nervous system) with other herbs such as oats (*Avena sativa*), gotu kola (*Centella asiatica*), and damiana (*Turnera diffusa, T. aphrodisiaca*). A few companies do offer kola nut cut and sifted, powdered, and in concentrated drops. The powder can be brewed into a bitter tea (add a tablespoon to a cup of water, bring to a near boil, reduce heat and simmer for five minutes, strain, and sweeten). An average dose of the concentrated drops is ½ to 1 dropperful.

Phenylalanine and Tyrosine

⊚

THE STIMULATING AMINOS

Most people know of amino acids as the building blocks of protein molecules. The body makes proteins from twenty amino acids, eight of which (isoleucine, leucine, lysine, methionine, phenylalanine, threonine, tryptophan, and valine) are "essential"—they must be obtained through diet or supplements. Two of these essential amino acids, phenylalanine and tryptophan, as well as a few of the "nonessential" ones (produced by the body) such as tyrosine, glutamine, and GABA, have additional roles in the body that are associated with subtle effects on the mind. Through mechanisms such as stimulating the production of mind-altering neurotransmitters (including serotonin, dopamine, and noradrenaline) in the brain and controlling the synthesis of hormones, these amino acids can affect mood, energy levels, sexual desire, and memory and learning.

With one major exception (tryptophan; see chapter 16), amino acid supplements are widely available and inexpensive in North America. Some have garnered significant scientific attention in recent years, though the unfortunate health disaster resulting from a batch of contaminated tryptophan being sold in the late 1980s has also caused increased regulatory pressure and skepticism about all amino acids from some health authorities. Overall, because the mind-altering aminos work with the body's own biochemical pathways, they are relatively safe and effective alternatives to conventional stimulants, relaxants, and smart drugs. But like most other mind-altering substances, they are best used occasionally rather than on a daily basis indefinitely. Taking high doses of single amino acid supplements for an extended period of time may cause an imbalance in, or affect the function of, other amino acids. In addition, too much protein in the form of mixtures of amino acid supplements may be toxic over the long term to the liver and kidneys.

When using single amino acids for their mind-altering properties, it is best to take them by themselves (that is, not with other amino acids) and on an empty stomach. This is necessary because amino acids, when they are combined together as in protein foods, may compete with each other for transport to and uptake by the brain. The relaxant effects of some, such as tryptophan and GABA, are then neutralized by the stimulant effects of others, such as phenylalanine and tyrosine.

PHENYLALANINE: THE RAVERS' FAVORITE

Phenylalanine is probably the most popular mind-altering amino, now that tryptophan has been banned. Phenylalanine is a common ingredient in powdered energy formulas with names like Blast and Energize. Frequently, it is phenylalanine-containing drinks that are promoted at so-called smart bars and at raves, the music-fueled, all-night parties popular among urban youths, as alternatives to alcohol (though phenylalanine is not an inebriant like alcohol). Many people buy phenylalanine supplements at health food stores to brighten their mood and increase their alertness.

As an amino acid in nature, phenylalanine is found in common protein foods, including poultry, meats, soybeans, fish, dairy products, nuts, and seeds. Another common dietary source is the synthetic sweetener aspartame (NutraSweet), which is a compound of phenylalanine and aspartic acid, another potentially stimulating amino acid. Such sources supply the average person with an estimated 500 to 2,000 mg of phenylalanine from diet alone.

Like other nutrient amino acids, phenylalanine comes in three forms, known as L-phenylalanine, D-phenylalanine, and DL-phenylalanine (also known as DLPA). The prefixes L and D stand for *levo,* from the Latin for left, and *dextro,* from the Latin for right. The directions refer to minor differences in the molecular structure, as evidenced by light refraction. The L-form of amino acids is usually more biologically active than the D-form, and the prefixes are sometimes omitted entirely. This is the custom we'll follow with respect to tyrosine and tryptophan, which are L-aminos. With phenylalanine, however, the L-, D-, and DL-forms produce slight variations in effect. L-phenylalanine is predominantly a nervous system and sexual stimulant, mood and cognition enhancer, and appetite suppressant. While D-phenylalanine also apparently has antidepressant and memory-boosting properties, it is taken primarily to control chronic pain. DLPA, which is half L-phenylalanine and half D-phenylalanine, combines these two sets of effects. Interestingly, the phenylalanine in animal protein is mostly L, while that in plants is mostly D.

Phenylalanine is one of the amino acids that is able to cross the blood-brain barrier. With the help of necessary enzymes and essential cofactors, phenylalanine is transformed in a series of steps into the amino acids tyrosine and dopa and then into three important neurotransmitters: dopamine, noradrenaline, and adrenaline. These neurotransmitters have various actions in the body that relate to brain, nervous system, and thyroid function, as well as to mood, sexual desire, blood pressure, and more. For example, within a certain range increases in noradrenaline are known to brighten mood. Phenylalanine may have a lesser effect on dopamine, which has been tied to increased arousal and enhancement in sexual desire.

D-phenylalanine in particular has been shown to promote the action in the brain of the small protein molecules known as endorphins and enkephalins. Endorphins are endogenous (produced within the body) morphines, natural opiates that reduce pain and promote mild euphoria. In addition to having analgesic and mood-boosting properties, enkephalins also stimulate motivation. The endorphins and enkephalins block the transmission of pain at specific sites or nerve receptors in the brain. (Morphine acts at the same sites.) D-phenylalanine is thought to work by inhibiting the enzymes that normally break down endorphins and enkephalins. This allows endorphins and enkephalins to stay active longer, thus enhancing mood and preventing the perception of pain.

The pain-relieving properties of D-phenylalanine and DLPA have been tested with positive results in a number of animal and human studies. For example, in a 1979 study done on mice, researcher Seymour Ehrenpreis and colleagues found that D-phenylalanine was an effective analgesic. Subsequent research on humans has confirmed that D-phenylalanine and DLPA can relieve pain without causing either significant adverse effects or any tolerance (in contrast to prescription painkillers, which are often addictive). Health practitioners who have used D-phenylalanine or DLPA for pain relief report that it works well for back pain, arthritis, migraine headache, and other

conditions. It may be necessary to take the supplement for two to four weeks for the peak effects to be noticed. D-phenylalanine also seems to enhance the pain-relieving effects of acupuncture.

If the body has sufficient levels of vitamin B_6, it can also use L-phenylalanine to make the intriguing compound phenylethylamine (PEA). Though it is still only partially understood, PEA in the brain may act as a neurotransmitter with stimulating and mood-boosting effects. In a 1986 study, scientists noted that a high percentage of depressed subjects, who had low levels of a PEA-related substance in their urine, enjoyed improved moods after supplementing their diet with 1 to 4 grams of L-phenylalanine plus vitamin B_6. In many subjects the mood-brightening effects were evident almost immediately, while others responded after a week. Other studies using depressed subjects have also shown positive results from daily doses of either D-phenylalanine or DLPA. A noted 1979 study on twenty-seven subjects determined that DLPA was comparable in its mood-boosting effects to the conventional tricyclic antidepressant drug imipramine (Tofranil).

Phenylalanine is relatively benign and is certainly safe enough to deserve its current status as a dietary supplement. The L-form can, however, cause side effects typical of nervous system stimulants, such as high blood pressure, agitation, anxiety, and insomnia. If this is a problem, reducing the dosage, using DLPA, or taking supplements only once in the morning may work. People with high blood pressure should definitely be wary of using L-phenylalanine or DLPA. On occasion people report headaches or nausea from taking phenylalanine.

Certain people should avoid all forms of phenylalanine supplements. Women who are pregnant or lactating should not take phenylalanine or should at least check with their health practitioner first. Because tyrosine helps to produce melanin, the pigment that colors skin and hair, phenylalanine and tyrosine should be avoided by anyone suffering from malignant melanoma. Phenylalanine should not be used by anyone taking MAO inhibitor antidepressants—combining phenylalanine and MAO inhibitors can lead to dangerously high blood pressure. Children, anyone with psychosis, and those suffering from the condition known as phenylketonuria, a genetic disorder of phenylalanine metabolism, should also not take phenylalanine supplements.

Taking Phenylalanine

Phenylalanine typically comes in a powder and in capsules that range from 250 to 1,000 mg. DLPA capsules are often 375 to 450 mg; also look for products with names such as PhenCal. As mentioned, phenylalanine is also a common ingredient in powdered "brainfood" and energy-drink formulas. Some of these products also contain caffeine. Since the stimulant properties of phenylalanine and caffeine seem to enhance each other, check labels carefully to gauge the product's strength. For example, a well-known pick-me-up formula contains 600 mg of phenylalanine and 80 mg of caffeine, along with some vitamins, minerals, and other ingredients. You'll want to make sure your reentry parachutes are in working condition before imbibing.

An average stimulating and mood-boosting dose of L-phenylalanine is 375 to 500 mg, or 750 to 1,000 mg of DLPA. Most often this is taken first thing in the morning when the stomach is empty, at least twenty to thirty minutes before breakfast. On an empty stomach the effects are usually felt within an hour or so. Alternatively, you can take phenylalanine between breakfast and lunch. You can enhance the effects of phenylalanine and promote its conversion to noradrenaline by taking it along with 25 to 50 mg of B_6 or vitamin B complex plus 250 to 500 mg of vitamin C.

TYROSINE: IMPROVING ENERGY AND MOOD

Though tyrosine is found in most protein foods, nutritionists consider it a nonessential amino acid because it is derived in the body from phenylalanine. Whether orally consumed or produced in the body from phenylalanine, tyrosine readily crosses the blood-brain barrier and helps the brain to synthesize the neurotransmitters dopamine, noradrenaline, and adrenaline. Tyrosine also stimulates the thyroid to synthesize hormones that help to regulate the body's metabolism.

The effects from consuming tyrosine are similar to those from taking phenylalanine, since phenylalanine breaks down in the body into tyrosine. People take tyrosine to increase energy levels, boost overall metabolism, enhance alertness and mood, bolster sexual desire, and improve motivation and memory. Some evidence indicates tyrosine can also help to control appetite, although if weight loss is your goal, phenylalanine is the better choice since its action in the gut may be independent of tyrosine synthesis. (Phenylalanine promotes the secretion of cholecystokinin, a hormone that may help control appetite by indirectly aiding digestion.) D-phenylalanine or DLPA are also preferable to tyrosine for pain relief.

Some people report better results from using phenylalanine, and others from using tyrosine. Phenylalanine may be better absorbed by most people and produce fewer headaches; many users find that tyrosine is less potent as a nervous system stimulant compared to phenylalanine. Tyrosine may be less likely to increase blood pressure as well. If one amino doesn't work for you, try the other. If your chronic low mood is a result of low serotonin levels rather than noradrenaline, tryptophan or 5-HTP may be more effective than tyrosine.

Tyrosine's most promising role therapeutically is in the control of anxiety and stress and the treatment of some forms of depression, including serious conditions such as manic-depressive illness. Researchers say that some depressed people, especially if they have low blood levels of tyrosine, may benefit from taking tyrosine. A 1983 study demonstrated that 300 mg of tyrosine per day was similar in effectiveness to conventional antidepressants, which have much more serious adverse side effects compared to tyrosine. The mood-enhancing action of tyrosine (as well as that of some antidepressant drugs) is thought to relate

in part to its ability to increase brain levels of noradrenaline. Anecdotal evidence and a limited number of clinical studies also indicate that tyrosine may be useful for helping to alleviate the fatigue, mild depression, and irritability of premenstrual syndrome; to detoxify the body from cocaine and other drugs; and to aid in the treatment of narcolepsy. Because of its role in the formation of dopamine, tyrosine is also being considered as a treatment for Parkinson's disease, the neurological condition characterized by stiffness and muscle tremor.

The potential adverse effects cited above for phenylalanine also apply to tyrosine, with the exception of the warning to phenylketonurics, since tyrosine can't transform back into phenylalanine. Thus, proceed with caution if you suffer from insomnia or high blood pressure, and don't take tyrosine at all if you are pregnant or lactating, a child, taking MAO inhibitors, suffer from psychosis, or have malignant melanoma. Some users report mild gastric upset when they have taken tyrosine on an empty stomach, which is the recommended course for enhancing its effectiveness.

Taking Tyrosine

Tyrosine is most commonly found in 500 mg capsules, though some producers offer powdered and sublingual forms. Like phenylalanine, it is most effective when it is taken before breakfast on an empty stomach, which reduces the possibility that other amino acid supplements or the amino acids in protein foods will compete with tyrosine for transport into the brain. Most people take tyrosine early in the day to avoid possible insomnia from taking it later.

Therapeutic doses of tyrosine, such as for some forms of depression, may be 2 to 4 g up to three times daily. Many health authorities recommend, however, that you work closely with a physician or a knowledgeable nutritionist or naturopath if you intend to take more than 2 to 3 g of tyrosine or use it more than occasionally. Small doses are sometimes more effective in any case—when you take large amounts of tyrosine, the brain may adjust by inhibiting the action of an enzyme necessary for tyrosine to be transformed into neurotransmitters. For occasional use as an energizer and mood enhancer, try starting with 250 to 500 mg before breakfast (or 50 to 100 mg sublingually). Take with 25 mg of vitamin B_6 or B complex, plus 250 to 500 mg of vitamin C. If no effects are noticed, work your way up to 750 mg of tyrosine twice a day, before breakfast and lunch, or try phenylalanine.

PART THREE

Mood Brighteners

St. John's Wort

◉

TONIC FOR THE NERVES

St. John's wort has a rich tradition of thera-peutic uses, but a much more limited his-tory of scientific research. Nevertheless it is a promising herb for helping to alleviate feelings of sadness, anxiety, and mental and nervous exhaustion. Though it doesn't have immedi-ate and prominent mind-altering effects, many people have found that it works over time to relieve depression, soothe the nerves, and boost the spirit.

St. John's wort is a yellow-flowering peren-nial shrub (*Hypericum perforatum*) native to Europe and western Asia. It spreads easily and is considered a weed in some areas, including parts of North America and Australia, where it has been introduced from Europe. Those who are aware of the plant's potential uses, how-ever, regard it as anything but a weed. Herbal-ists from the time of ancient Greece through the Middle Ages used St. John's wort to treat diarrhea, menstrual disorders, fevers, and other conditions. They also employed the

herb topically, to relieve the pain of burns and promote the healing of wounds.

St. John's wort has also long been recog-nized as having an affinity for the human spirit and a potential role in the treatment of ner-vous conditions. Its ability to protect people from harm is suggested by the name, accord-ing to various interpretations. Wort is Old English for plant, and St. John's may refer to an early European folk belief that, if the herb is gathered on St. John's Day (June 24) or slipped under one's pillow on St. John's Eve, it magically shields the person against witchcraft and evil spirits. The genus name *Hypericum* is also revealing: it is said by some to come from the Greek roots *hyper* for "over" and *eikon* for "image" or "apparition," referring to the plant's ability to ward off evil spirits. The ori-gin of *perforatum* is less disputed and more mundane: the leaves have patches that look like perforations when held up to the sun.

St. John's wort has long been used to help

treat nervous system disorders, especially conditions such as melancholy, hypochondria, and depression. Like wild oats and other traditional nerve tonics, it helps to restore emotional stability and nervous system strength. Nerve tonics promote greater energy over the long term rather than immediate stimulation, as do caffeine and ephedrine, while in the short term nerve tonics often have a calming effect. According to Simon Mills in *Out of the Earth*, "This combination of restorative and relaxant effect is not contradictory, and underlies [St. John's wort's] recommendation for the treatment of a number of such conditions where tension and exhaustion combine."

These traditional uses for St. John's wort have begun to gain important confirmation in well-designed clinical trials. St. John's wort shows promise in the treatment of chronic fatigue syndrome and seasonal affective disorder (the depression that comes on during the winter in northern latitudes). Moreover, just within the past few years a number of double-blind, placebo-controlled studies have found that St. John's wort extracts offer impressive results in alleviating symptoms of the type of mild to moderate depression that afflicts tens of millions of Americans.

For example, a study published in 1994 was conducted on 105 men and women, ranging in age from twenty to sixty-four, suffering from mild to moderate depression of short duration. After four weeks, 67 percent of those who took 300 mg of a St. John's wort extract three times daily showed a positive response, compared to 28 percent of those who took a placebo. Tests showed improvements in categories relating to depressive mood, difficulties in falling asleep, emotional anxiety, and feelings of guilt. The authors noted that St. John's wort's effect was similar to conventional antidepressants yet did not cause any undesirable side effects. They emphasized that the herb is recommended for mild to moderate depression or temporary depressive mood, not for serious depression.

In an extensive 1995 review of recent scientific studies done on St. John's wort, German professor and phytomedical researcher Hans Reuter noted that scientists have published some two dozen controlled clinical trials on the effects of alcohol extracts of St. John's wort on mood and emotion. In aggregate, these studies used almost 1,600 human subjects, primarily taking dosages of 300 to 900 mg of extract per day for at least four weeks. (A particular standardized extract product, known to scientists as LI 160 and packaged in Europe under the brand name Jarsin, was the most commonly used formulation.) According to Reuter:

The clinical effectiveness of Hypericum *was clearly demonstrated in three of four comparative studies with placebo. The reported responder rates have been found to be equivalent to those achieved with standard synthetic substances [i.e., prescription antidepressants]. It is generally accepted that* Hypericum *is effective in the treatment of outpatients with mild to moderate depression. Besides effectiveness, therapy with* Hypericum *is also characterized by an excellent tolerability. Thus in a drug monitoring study with 3,250 patients, side effects, usually mild, were observed in only 2.5 percent of cases.*

Reuter's findings were corroborated by a formal meta-analysis of St. John's wort studies that was published in the *British Medical Journal* in 1996. A team of German and American researchers combined the results from twenty-three randomized clinical trials that tested 1,757 subjects with mild to moderately severe depression. Fifteen of the studies compared St. John's wort's effectiveness to a placebo, and eight trials compared the herb to conventional antidepressant drugs. The meta-analysis determined that St. John's wort is much more effective than a placebo and provokes response rates (64 percent of the subjects in the five trials that provided comparative data) that are similar to or even slightly better than conventional antidepressants (59 percent). The researchers also determined that St. John's wort was better tolerated than conventional antidepressants, with one in five subjects reporting side effects from taking St. John's wort compared to more than one in three from conventional antidepressants.

The growing evidence for St. John's wort's beneficial effects on mood has even attracted the attention of the federal government. Three components of the National Institutes of Health (the Office of Alternative Medicine, the National Institute of Mental Health, and the Office of Dietary Supplements) recently announced a major collaborative effort to fund research on St. John's wort for the treatment of depression.

People who take St. John's wort report a variety of benefits, including less weakness and tiredness, better sleep patterns with longer periods of deep sleep, fewer headaches, a more positive self-image, reduced levels of fear and anxiety, and increased appetite. Some even report an improvement in short-term memory. St. John's wort's antidepressive action is not accompanied by prominent sedative effects, nor does the herb cause adverse interactions with alcohol. The German Commission E, the government body whose monographs on herbs regulate their use as prescription and over-the-counter medicines in that country, recognizes St. John's wort preparations as safe and effective for light depressive states, anxiety, and nervous restlessness. German physicians are convinced of the herb's value for these conditions—they write an estimated three million prescriptions for St. John's wort–containing products annually and are much more likely to recommend it than they are Prozac.

ANSWERS NEEDED ON COMPOUNDS AND ACTIONS

The compounds in St. John's wort responsible for its mood-brightening effects are a matter of dispute. Herbal preparations are derived from the plant's stems, leaves, and especially its yellow flowers, which often have dark dots. These are special oil glands that contain the reddish pigment hypericin and related compounds, which have been found in few other plants. The fresh plant has low levels (usually 0.1 to 0.3 percent) of hypericin, concentrated in the flowers but also found in the leaves, plus a number of other compounds, including flavonoids, tannins, and essential oils. A noted 1984 study by researcher O. Suzuki and colleagues linked hypericin to inhibition of monoamine oxidase (MAO), increased neurotransmitter action, and an improvement in mood. (MAO is an enzyme that breaks down neurotransmitters, including serotonin and noradrenaline, that have mood-brightening effects. A large class of antidepressants are MAO inhibitors, which work by allowing the mood-brightening neurotransmitters to stay active longer in nerve synapses in the brain.)

Subsequent studies done in 1989 and 1990, however, have cast doubt on the theory that the herb's effects on mood can be attributed only to hypericin. According to herbalist Christopher Hobbs, "Work in recent years, including some human trials, has shown that the whole-plant extract of St. John's wort is more effective than extracts that just focus on the hypericin." Researchers are now trying to determine whether various flavonoids and xanthones in St. John's wort's are crucial for its effects on mood.

Not only the compounds but their mechanism of action is in dispute. It is possible that these compounds, alone or in combination with hypericin, are MAO inhibitors. Or the mechanism might be unrelated to MAO action. Some recent research found that inhibition of MAO occurred only when high concentrations of the herb were present, such as would be induced by doses much higher than are typically administered therapeutically. St. John's wort may mimic Prozac by working mainly through an effect on serotonin. Other possible antidepressant mechanisms relate to St. John's wort's potential to alter dopamine or nor-

adrenaline activity and to increase melatonin levels in the body. "Though there are some suggestions concerning the mode of action of *Hypericum* as an antidepressive, the real mode of action remains uncertain. Nevertheless clinical studies have proven its effectiveness in the treatment of mild depressive states," Reuter states. Other researchers have speculated that St. John's wort's notable lack of toxicity is related to its ability to act on relatively subtle levels through multiple channels in the body.

TAKING ST. JOHN'S WORT

Questions about how St. John's wort causes its effects are important. If the herb does work predominantly through inhibition of MAO, it is possible that it could share with MAO inhibitors the unwanted side effect of dangerously increasing blood pressure after the person takes certain drugs or consumes foods (such as cheese and red wine) rich in tyramine. This "cheese effect" has not been observed in persons taking St. John's wort, but until the herb's mode of action is clarified it may be prudent to avoid eating tyramine-rich foods when taking St. John's wort. The full list of foods, beverages, and medications (including many common over-the-counter remedies, such as nasal decongestants, and the amino acid tryptophan) that should be avoided when taking MAO inhibitors is extensive; see the *Physicians' Desk Reference* or talk to your doctor. Most natural health practitioners consider St. John's wort only a weak MAO inhibitor, but they recommend working with a knowledgeable herbalist or naturopath if you intend to take high doses of St. John's wort for extended periods of time for its antidepressant properties.

A minuscule percentage of people taking high daily doses of St. John's wort may experience photosensitivity, which is increased skin reactivity to light from the sun. This phenomenon has been widely noted in cows and other livestock (one of the reasons that many ranchers consider the plant a weed), though there are only a very few isolated cases of fair-skinned people reporting hives or sunburn associated with extended exposure to the sun and St. John's wort intake.

The most common side effects from taking St. John's wort include nausea, stomachache, lack of appetite, tiredness, restlessness, dizziness, itchiness, and allergic reactions such as rash.

St. John's wort should not be taken by pregnant or breast-feeding women or by anyone taking prescription antidepressant drugs. Switching from a prescription antidepressant to St. John's wort should be done only with the help of a medical professional.

The herb is usually sold dried and in concentrated drops, tinctures, and extracts. A few companies combine it with other nerve tonics such as gotu kola and oats in products with names like Phyto Proz Supreme and Depress-Shun, or with calming nutrients in products such as 5-HTP SeroTonic. A typical dose of St. John's wort is 250 to 500 mg of the powdered herb two to three times daily, or 1 to 2 dropperfuls twice daily of tincture or concentrated drops. Formulations based on the standardized extracts used in Europe (and in most of the medical studies done on St. John's wort) are also beginning to become available in North America; look for products with names like HyperiCalm. An average dose of a standardized extract containing 0.3 percent hypericin is 200 to 300 mg two to three times daily. This dose may need to be taken for three to six weeks before the herb's full mood-lifting action is evident.

Rose, Jasmine, and Neroli

◎

THE UPLIFTING ESSENTIAL OILS

Essential oils are concentrated liquids derived from the leaves, roots, flowers, or other parts of various aromatic plants. Making up only a small percentage, ranging from 0.01 to 10 percent, of these plants' mass, essential oils nevertheless often account for much of their therapeutic, cosmetic, and culinary potential. Essential oils are thought to play crucial roles in protecting plants from disease, parasites, and predators, and these complex compounds can also serve humanity in a variety of ways. Indeed, herbalists and traditional healers have been using aromatic herbs to heal the body or alter mind and emotions for thousands of years, from well before the advent of methods such as steam distillation for isolating plants' essential oils.

Some seven hundred plants are sufficiently aromatic for the essential oil to be extracted, although in practice there are perhaps fifty or so common essential oils that account for all but a tiny percentage of total use. Most essential oils are clear or pale in color and are volatile—easily evaporated and dispersed into the air. They are typically derived by steam-distilling large amounts of plants and are sold in small quantities of an ounce or less. Compared to a tea made from the dried herb or even to an herbal liquid extract, essential oils are extremely concentrated. Because essential oils are so potent, only a few drops at a time are used to produce the desired effects. See the sections at the end of this chapter on "Potent But Generally Safe" and "Taking Essential Oils" before attempting to use them.

The practice of using essential oils for therapeutic purposes has come to be known as aromatherapy, even though this name is somewhat misleading. Certainly, many people use essential oils by inhaling their aromas. After essential oil molecules evaporate into the air, they are inhaled through the nostrils and dissolved in the mucous membrane lining the roof of the nasal cavity. Special receptor cells in olfactory nerve twigs are stimulated, though the exact mechanism of this crucial step in the smelling process is still unclear. Smell sensations are then transferred, in the form of nerve impulses, to the two olfactory bulbs sitting above the bone in the roof of the nose. The olfactory bulbs lie at the end of olfactory nerves, which are connected to the smell centers of the brain. A crucial part of the brain that is stimulated is the limbic system, an area in the center of the brain that is thought to be ancient in evolutionary terms. It is here that the brain mediates not only our sense of smell but also functions relating to mood, memory, emotions, and even sexual desire, possibly through the release of neurotransmitters, such as acetylcholine and dopamine, that can result in sedation, stimulation, and other mind-altering effects. This whole process is exceedingly sensitive. The human nose can detect some compounds in essential oils even when they are found in the air at a concentration of only a few parts per billion—a half-dozen molecules is enough to create a smell the nose can detect.

The name aromatherapy suggests, however, that this aroma route is the only effect essential oils have. This is clearly not the case, when you consider how much of the current practice involves the use of essential oils applied to the body during massage (diluted first in a carrier oil), as a component of a topical cream, or added to the bath. Various studies have confirmed that substances, including essential oils, applied to the skin make their way into the bloodstream and to the brain. Because the user can also smell the essential oil during such topical applications, the body is absorbing molecules both through the olfactory system and through the skin.

Aromatherapists, like practitioners in most other healing practices, have different ideas and approaches to the field. Some are more oriented toward holism and spirituality, willing to refer to an essential oil as a plant's "soul" or "vital energy." Holistic aromatherapists often try to make a perfect match between an individual's unique condition and the diverse properties of an essential oil. Other practitioners see the need for more scientific research into oils' chemical constituents and how they affect the body on the biomolecular level. The approaches are not necessarily mutually exclusive. It is difficult to isolate a person's reaction to an odor from his or her expectations and previous experiences with it, which no doubt can affect mind, mood, and emotions. Scientific studies must be done, however, to determine physical pathways and to demonstrate how most if not all people react to certain essential oils or their compounds. Even though the mechanisms by which essential oils act on the mind and body are only partially understood at this time, it is not too early for the average person to begin to benefit from these potent substances.

The recognition that essential oils in the air can quickly reach the brain through the olfactory system and affect mood, behavior, and mental function has spread from scientists to businesspeople. Some companies have even begun to experiment with adding scents to office air systems to increase workers' productivity and mental sharpness. Though such efforts have a somewhat disturbing Big Brother aspect to them, there is no reason not to choose your own essential oils for their mild mind-altering effects.

The effects of essential oils are highly individual. The same fragrance can generate different moods and emotions in different people. If a fragrance doesn't appeal to you or does not have the desired effect, try another. Experiment to see what works for you.

Boosting Mood and Sensuality

The most popular essential oils for enhancing mood and increasing sexual desire seem to be three derived from flowers with exceedingly exquisite scents: Rose, Jasmine, and Neroli. Their scents come at a cost, however—these essential oils are considered rare and precious. They are among the most expensive essential oils on the market, often retailing for five times or greater the cost of other oils. For example, most essential oils retail in the neighborhood of $10 to $20 for a 10-milliliter or one-third-ounce bottle. Rose, Jasmine, and Neroli are typically sold in smaller sizes. Expect to pay, for example, approximately $10 to $15 for a 1 ml bottle of Neroli; $15 to $25 for 1 ml of Jasmine; and $20 to $40 for 1 ml of Rose. Methods of extraction, the plant's origin, whether the plant was wildcrafted or grown organically, and a host of other factors cause the wide variation in prices.

The high cost tempts marginal producers to adulterate or dilute their product. If it is not expensive it is probably adulterated or mislabeled, though it does not necessarily follow that all expensive oils are therefore genuine.

Take extra assurances to find reliable sources of high-quality products.

A more economical alternative is to use one of the combination products, which go by names like Euphoria and Sensuality, that some essential oil producers are now marketing. These massage oils, bath oils, scented candles, and the like usually contain small amounts of the expensive oils such as Rose and Jasmine, and larger amounts of other less costly oils such as Ylang Ylang, derived from the flowers of a tree (*Cananga odorata* var. *genuina*) native to Southeast Asia, and Rosemary (see chapter 12) that may also have some mood-boosting properties.

ROSE: THE LOVE OIL

The Greek poet Sappho termed the rose "the queen of flowers" circa 580 B.C.E. and it remains to this day a prominent symbol of love, romance, and beauty. Its redolent bouquet has been prized for use in perfumes, and the stunning beauty of its blossoms has made it a garden favorite almost worldwide. The plant's medicinal properties have not survived the test of time, though a few herbalists still use rose tea to treat digestive problems, nervous tension, and other conditions.

Despite its extremely high cost, Rose is a favorite essential oil for many people. Like Jasmine, the pale yellow-green essential oil uplifts the spirit and brightens mood. "The rose procures us one thing above all: a feeling of well-being, even of happiness, and the individual under its influence will develop an amiable tolerance," noted aromatherapy pioneer Marguerite Maury. Many aromatherapists recommend essential oil of Rose for anxiety, insomnia, and stress-related conditions. Inhaling Rose breeds confidence. Women may respond better to Rose than men, especially women suffering from lack of appetite and the kind of nervous debility and overall tiredness that used to be a prominent condition called neurasthenia. Rose's sensual aroma can also put a spark back into those who are experiencing a lack of libido.

The high cost of Rose essential oil has caused producers to market synthetic rose oils, some of which are promoted using the euphemistic term "nature identical." The perfume industry uses most of the synthetic rose oil, but it is occasionally sold as a less expensive version of the natural essential oil. Synthetic oils are, however, a pale imitation of natural ones, even when the oils are relatively simple ones with a limited number of compounds. Natural Rose oil, with its unique combination of at least four hundred separate chemical constituents, is a masterwork of art compared to the chicken scrawl modern chemists can concoct in their labs.

The *Rosa* genus has only a few hundred species, but growers can readily hybridize roses, a process that has been going on for so long that there are now thousands of types of roses, mainly modern hybrids developed for their dramatic sizes and colors. It is a few of the ancient traditional species and their cultivars, however, that are the most exquisitely scented and thus the most widely cultivated for their essential oil. Chief among these are damask rose (*Rosa damascena*) and cabbage rose (*R. centifolia;* also known as Provence rose), both probably native to the Middle East but now grown in Europe, China, and elsewhere.

JASMINE: EXQUISITE EUPHORIA

Jasmine is an olive family genus containing hundreds of species of shrubs and vines with fragrant flowers. The plants most often cultivated for use in perfumes and aromatherapy are woody climbers with star-shaped white flowers: common jasmine (*Jasminum officinale*) and royal or Spanish jasmine (*J. grandiflorum*). Though native to Asia and the Middle East, jasmine is now cultivated in France and other countries around the Mediterranean, including some in North Africa. Jasmine is widely used in perfumes, cosmetics, and some foods and beverages. The Chinese add it to green tea as a flavoring.

The traditional healers of India and China used jasmine to treat skin conditions and digestive upsets, but the herb's most popular uses then and now revolve around the uplifting effects associated with its exquisite scent. Jasmine "produces a feeling of optimism, confidence and euphoria. It is most useful in cases where there is apathy, indifference or listlessness," states aromatherapist Robert Tisserand, author of *The Art of Aromatherapy*. Jasmine improves the mood of those suffering from anxiety or depression and helps to counter the effects of nervous exhaustion. The essential oil also has a reputation as an aphrodisiac, another traditional use in Asia. Both men and women find that the sensual aroma of Jasmine boosts the libido and promotes intimacy and lovemaking.

At one time the highest quality Jasmine essential oil was steam-distilled from the flowers. Because the flowers yield so little essential oil (upward of a quarter-million flowers may be needed to make a single ounce of the essential oil), steam distillation is rarely used for Jasmine anymore. Most if not all of the Jasmine on the market today is in the form of an orange-brown *absolute,* which is an aromatic extract made up primarily of the essential oil but also containing wax and other nonvolatile compounds. The principal method for obtaining an absolute is to extract the plant's aromatic compounds with a solvent such as hexane, remove the solvent with alcohol, and evaporate the alcohol. The small amounts of waxy residues that can't be totally removed make absolutes thicker and more viscous than pure essential oils, or even semisolid. Unfortunately, absolutes may also contain traces of the (often toxic) solvent used in the initial extraction process. The absolute also won't have the same identity and ratio of chemical constituents found in the essential oil. The upshot is that many aromatherapists contend that absolutes should be used only in fragrances, not in remedies that are meant to be inhaled or applied to the body for their therapeutic effects.

Although the conventional absolute process is faster and cheaper than steam distillation, Jasmine absolute, like the essential oil, is still considered rare and precious. Even more expensive is Jasmine absolute derived from another process—enfleurage—that is more natural than solvent extraction. *Enfleurage* is the French term meaning "impregnating with flowers." Instead of using steam distillation, producers lay vast amounts of jasmine flowers out on trays filled with a fat or a carrier oil. Over time the fat or carrier oil draws the essential oil out of the blossoms, requiring the depleted flowers to be repeatedly replaced with fresh ones. When the fat or carrier oil is finally saturated with essential oil, the essential oil is extracted using alcohol. (Because some nonvolatile compounds are extracted as well, the result is technically an absolute rather than an essential oil.)

Compared to the conventional solvent-extraction process, the enfleurage process takes much more time and results in a lower yield. The finished product is extremely expensive, costing more than Jasmine absolute and sometimes even more than Rose essential oil. (Rose is also often sold as a less costly absolute.) While only a select few producers (see Resources) offer Jasmine as an enfleurage, its purity and lack of any trace solvents make it a better choice for experiencing Jasmine's subtle mind-altering effects.

NEROLI: ORANGE BLOSSOM SPECIAL

Neroli is a pale yellow essential oil, darkening upon being left standing, with a slightly sweet, citruslike aroma. The citrus component of the fragrance is no accident: Neroli is steam-distilled from the small, fragrant white flowers of an evergreen tree known as the bitter orange or sour orange tree (*Citrus aurantium; C. bigaradia*). Thus, Neroli is also known as

Orange Blossom oil and Neroli Bigarade oil. Bitter orange trees are native to Asia but now grow widely in the Mediterranean area, California, and elsewhere. The essential oil is used to flavor some foods and as a fragrance in colognes and perfumes. Orange flower water, a by-product of the essential oil distillation, is a traditional product used medicinally to aid digestion or induce sleep, and as a culinary ingredient in North African recipes. Neroli oil should be distinguished from Niaouli, an essential oil derived from the bark and leaves of an Australian tree.

Neroli oil is named after a late-seventeenth-century princess of Nerole, near Rome. Like many aristocratic Italians and French of the time, the Princess was enamored of the art of perfumery that was sweeping Europe. She used the essential oil of the bitter orange tree blossoms so enthusiastically on and around her that it became known by her name. Later, in Spain, Neroli oil became intimately associated with prostitutes, perhaps because they recognized its potential aphrodisiac properties. Men in the area came to assume that Neroli-scented women were women of the evening.

Today, Neroli is still recognized as a sensuous oil with the ability to increase a dormant libido. It is also used to brighten mood, reduce stress- and tension-related complaints, and lift nervous depression. Some people find that it calms nerves and relaxes muscles effectively enough to promote sleep. A few find that Neroli goes beyond merely reducing anxiety and smoothing mood swings to actually bring on mild euphoria. In 1992, a controlled study in which Neroli was applied topically by foot massage to patients recovering from cardiac surgery found that subjects experienced significant reductions in anxiety, tension, and pain.

POTENT BUT GENERALLY SAFE

When they're used correctly, essential oils are among the least toxic natural substances. Because they are so concentrated, however, if they are misused they can be extremely toxic. Typically, only a few drops of an essential oil are necessary to cause the desired effect. As little as a teaspoonful of certain oils may be fatal if taken internally. Some essential oils (Hyssop and Sage, for example) also have certain compounds that, if used repeatedly even in small amounts for long periods of time, could lead to cancer. More commonly, the adverse effects are annoying but not serious, such as dizziness, nausea, and headache.

Here are the most basic safety guidelines for using essential oils:

- Don't take essential oils orally. Some oils can be taken safely in tiny oral doses, but you should do this only when working closely with an experienced aromatherapist.
- Don't use essential oils if you are pregnant. Some oils, including Basil and Rosemary (see chapter 12), are more problematic than others during pregnancy, but the safest route is to avoid all of them.
- Don't use essential oils if you are prone to epileptic seizures or have any other kind of seizure disorder, suffer from severely high or low blood pressure, have asthma, or are undergoing treatment for cancer.

- Essential oils should be diluted with a carrier oil before they are applied to the skin. Tiny amounts of a few essential oils, such as Lavender applied to a cooled burn or a smidgen of Rose dabbed on as a perfume, are safe to use "neat" or undiluted on small sections of the skin. But always dilute for wider application, and then you'll want to . . .
- Patch-test. Some people are sensitive to certain essential oils, which can cause allergic reactions or photosensitivity. Put a drop of the oil to be tested on a cotton swab and wipe a little on the inside of the arm. Cover with a bandage and take a look twenty-four hours later. If there are any signs of redness or itching, don't use that oil.
- Avoid getting essential oils in the eyes.
- Keep essential oils out of the reach of children. When you use essential oils on children, reduce the dosage by one-half or more.
- Use essential oils on an occasional or as-needed rather than everyday basis. Overusing oils may cause them to have an effect that is opposite to that intended. For example, frequent use of Basil may cause it to have a mentally dulling rather than stimulating effect.
- Discontinue using any product that causes dizziness or other adverse side effects.

PROTECTING YOUR INVESTMENT

Essential oils will last a year or longer without degrading if you take some special precautions. Leave a dropper bottle open only long enough to remove the drops you need. Essential oils evaporate easily and are affected by oxidation when exposed to air. Glass is less reactive than plastic and is preferable for storing mixtures of essential oils and a carrier oil, for example. When using an essential oil dropper, prevent it from coming in contact with anything as the oil drops. Keep essential oils tightly capped and in a cool, dark, dry place (bathroom cabinets are generally disqualified on the last count).

TAKING ESSENTIAL OILS

Essential oils are usually sold in small, dark-glass bottles with drop dispensers. Sizes range from 1 milliliter up to an ounce (30 ml). Most retailers and mail-order suppliers stock fifty to one hundred of the most common oils, plus, as mentioned, a dizzying array of suggestively named formulations, including oil combinations, massage oils, bath oils, soaps, and more. Aromatherapy producers have also invented many new gadgets for using essential oils in recent years, such as "Aroma Fitness" kits (different scents to be diffused during stages of your workout); diffusers that switch on for five minutes and then off for twenty-five; diffusers to hang in the car or around your neck; aromatherapy air coolers that add scent to cooled, humidified air; and vaporizers with controls for intensity of scent and time of dispersion. Most specialized catalogs have a better selection of such products than the average natural food store.

The most common ways to make use of essential oils for the purposes of stimulation and mood enhancement are to diffuse them into the air for inhalation, to apply them during massage, and to add them to bath water.

Inhalation

Any number of methods can be used:

- Place a few drops of an essential oil on a tissue, handkerchief, or clean cloth, bring it up to your nose, and inhale deeply.
- Vaporize the oil to disperse it into the room. A simple method is to mix two to three drops of essential oil with water in a small bowl and put the bowl on a working radiator to allow the oil gradually to be evaporated into the room. A variety of commercial products are available as well, including lightbulb rings, clay bowls that sit above candles, and electric vaporizers with small fans.
- Spritz the room. Put 8 to 10 drops of oil in a water-filled spray bottle or plant mister, gently agitate it, and spray a fine mist into the room.
- Inhale oil-enriched steam. Add 5 to 7 drops of essential oil to a bowl or pot of hot but not scalding water. Drape a towel over your head and around the bowl. Hold your face about twelve inches above the water for a few minutes, breathing deeply to capture the steam as it rises. This method works especially well for situations that call for relatively large doses of aromatherapy, such as when an essential oil is being used therapeutically to help clear sinus congestion or soothe a throat irritation (add Eucalyptus for these purposes). A side benefit is the cleansing effect this type of "head sauna" has on facial skin. You can also buy electric steam inhalers designed with a soft hood over which you place your mouth and nose.

Massage

Working an oil into the skin promotes penetration and circulation of the active compounds. A full-body massage using an essential oil–scented massage oil can be wonderfully relaxing, stimulating, or sensual, depending upon the oil, the masseuse, and so forth. You can also use an "essential massage oil" on your own feet, legs, arms, and abdomen to work out stress and tension, or just do the neck and shoulders of a friend or coworker. Remember, give and ye shall receive. . . .

Always dilute essential oils with a carrier oil for use as a massage oil. A 1 to 3 percent solution of essential oil in carrier oil is ideal. Approximate that ratio by mixing 3 to 5 drops of essential oil per tablespoon of carrier oil. For a carrier oil, use a high-quality vegetable oil such as almond, safflower, sunflower, avocado, or jojoba. Wheat germ oil also works well and is naturally high in vitamin E, which acts as a preservative.

Bath

Adding essential oils to the bath is a way of combining the two principal means of absorption: through the skin and inhaled. The oils dispersed in the bathwater come in contact with the skin. At the same time, especially if the bathwater is hot, the oil will evaporate off the surface of the water and allow you to inhale some, stimulating those parts of the brain as in inhaling steam.

Add three drops of essential oil to a full tub of water. Stroke the water a few times before getting in to disperse the oil. If your skin doesn't begin to react with tingles, you can add up to three more drops. Another method, suggested by aromatherapist Daniéle Ryman, is to mix three drops of essential oil in a capful of mild shampoo, and pour the mixture under the running water. "This will help the oils disperse in the water rather than sit in a film on the top," Ryman says. Pull the shower curtain or close the bathroom door to keep the fragrant steam enclosed.

Because Peppermint (see chapter 12) can be irritating to many people's skin, don't use it in a bath.

PART FOUR

Brain Boosters

Vasopressin, Deprenyl, Piracetam, and Hydergine

⊚

THE CLASSIC SMART DRUGS

The term *smart drug* refers to a relatively new and hard-to-classify category of medicinal substances. Many of the smart drugs have therapeutic effects for conditions that afflict elderly people, such as Parkinson's disease and Alzheimer's disease. In the United States, a few of the drugs considered smart, such as deprenyl and Hydergine, have received FDA approval for use in the treatment of these aging-related conditions, since studies have generally shown positive effects on subjects' memory, attention, and mood. The FDA has not, however, recognized any smart drug as effective for the purpose of improving brain function in normal and healthy persons. In this regard it is at odds with regulatory authorities in Europe and elsewhere, where nontherapeutic use of smart drugs has become more medically accepted in recent years.

Dozens of smart drugs are now available to those who want to increase their memory, concentration, and learning ability. Because of how these substances work, many have desirable "side effects," such as the ability to brighten mood and create a sense of well-being if not euphoria; to stimulate the nervous system and increase alertness; and to enhance libido and sexual response. Here we'll look at only four of the most popular smart drugs (vasopressin, deprenyl, piracetam, and Hydergine) with these additional prominent mind-altering effects. These four are also among those smart drugs that have the most scientific research to back up their claims and the best safety records. Nevertheless, it is necessary to emphasize that, with the exception of piracetam (which is not on the market at all in the United States), these are prescription drugs, not over-the-counter substances as are others dealt with in this book. Those who prefer not to experiment with these smart drugs may wish to try the brain-boosting nutrients such as choline, DMAE, and pyroglutamate (see chapter 10) or the herb ginkgo (see chapter 11).

Vasopressin is a natural brain hormone. It is released by the pituitary gland and, like the endorphins and several other pituitary hormones, is structurally a peptide, or protein fragment. Like melatonin, the vasopressin that is naturally found in nerve cells throughout the brain and spinal cord is the same substance (with, as we'll see, a minor molecular modification) that is now being taken as a drug. Much as melatonin is becoming known as the sleep hormone, vasopressin is gaining recognition as the memory hormone.

From Diabetes to Amnesia

Being a hormone, vasopressin has varied effects, with the following three being among the most prominent:

■ Vasopressin causes vasoconstriction, or narrowing of small blood vessels, with an accompanying increase in blood pressure. This "pressor" function is responsible for the hormone's name. It now appears, however, that the effect is relatively temporary and minor (except in high intravenous doses) and

that *vasopressin* is something of a misnomer. According to the *Physicians' Desk Reference* (PDR), "Cardiovascular pressor effects with [a synthetic vasopressin nasal solution] are minimal or absent when it is administered as a nasal spray in therapeutic doses." The *PDR* estimates the ratio of vasopressin's pressor to antidiuretic (water-retaining) activity in the range of 1:1000. *Goodman and Gilman's The Pharmacological Basis of Therapeutics* states, "Despite its unfortunately chosen name, vasopressin should not be employed as a pressor agent." Vasopressin is still occasionally used surgically to help stop internal bleeding after an operation.

■ Vasopressin prompts the kidneys to keep more of the body's water stored in the blood rather than transfer it to the urine for excretion. Thus, an alternative medical name for vasopressin is *antidiuretic hormone*. This water-retaining function is responsible for the hormone's primary accepted medical use, in the treatment of the rare condition diabetes insipidus. People who have this disorder lack vasopressin in the body, usually because their pituitary gland is just not producing enough of the hormone. They lose tremendous amounts of bodily water through urination and are always thirsty. Dehydration is common. Taken as a drug, vasopressin effectively regulates the body's water levels and prevents the symptoms of the disease.

■ Vasopressin affects the brain and central nervous system in a way that promotes memory, improves attention and concentration, and enhances learning. This is the function that has caused vasopressin to become one of the most popular smart drugs. Unfortunately for consumers, the FDA does not recognize this function of vasopressin and consequently the vast majority of physicians won't prescribe it for cognition-related purposes. When vasopressin is sniffed as a nasal spray, the usual route of administration, its effects are often felt within five to ten seconds. People report that lost memories are recalled and information that is being read or heard is more easily retained. Some users experience increased energy and alertness, a brightening of mood or greater self-confidence, and even an intensification of orgasm during sex. Typically the effects last for about an hour or two.

How vasopressin promotes memory is still being studied, but apparently the mechanism is related to the hormone's ability to help capture information that arrives at the brain in the form of electrical impulses. As smart-drug authorities Michael Hutchison and John Morgenthaler describe the process, vasopressin is involved in "picking out and chunking together related bits of information from the stream of consciousness, integrating these chunks into coherent structures, and then 'imprinting' these images or concepts into long-term memory by transforming electrical impulses into complex proteins that contain memories and are stored away in the brain. The act of remembering the stored information is also mediated by vasopressin."

A number of scientific studies have been done in the past two decades that confirm the memory- and cognition-enhancing function of vasopressin, both on animal and human subjects. Vasopressin has been shown to help pre-vent amnesia when researchers try to induce it, and to reverse it among those subjects who already have it, whether due to head injuries or aging. Animals taught to avoid a stimulus will maintain the new behavior longer when administered vasopressin. Small doses of vasopressin in normal, healthy humans improve their ability to recall sequences of words, speed reaction time, and promote memory retention and retrieval. A 1984 double-blind study on forty-eight healthy males, young and old, concluded that the results "strengthen recent claims that vasopressin facilitates cognitive performance in normal humans."

The body's natural vasopressin levels can be adversely affected by taking certain other drugs. On the one hand, stimulants such as amphetamines and cocaine cause the release of vasopressin. The danger is that constant use of such drugs can deplete the body's supply of vasopressin and lead to the kind of spaciness and depression typical of stimulant abusers. On the other hand, taking marijuana and alcohol tends to suppress production and release of vasopressin. Overuse of these substances is also known to impact brain functions tied to vasopressin, such as memory and recall. Anecdotal reports from marijuana users confirm that vasopressin somehow mediates their high. They say that a few whiffs of vasopressin at the tail end of a marijuana experience can clarify the mind and even dissipate the high. Depression itself may affect bodily levels of vasopressin—researchers have found that some depressed persons have lowered levels of the hormone in their cerebrospinal fluid (as do those suffering from Alzheimer's disease).

Studies have suggested that melatonin stimulates vasopressin release.

A Promising Safety Record

Vasopressin appears to be safe, especially for a prescription drug. One caveat is that the substance did not come into commercial use until around 1970 and long-term safety data is still generally lacking. Major side effects have not been identified. The most common minor side effects, which occur infrequently, include runny nose, nasal congestion, headache, nausea, abdominal cramps, heartburn, and increased bowel movements. Because vasopressin can narrow blood vessels, it should be avoided by people with high blood pressure, heart disease, circulatory problems, or angina pains. Anyone with kidney disease or epilepsy should also avoid it. Because the body retains more water when taking vasopressin, it is not a good idea to accompany excessive use of the drug with excessive intake of water. You could develop the rare condition of water intoxication. Though no problems have been reported in pregnant or breast-feeding women, reproductive studies have not yet been carried out, so these women should also not use vasopressin.

No fatalities from overdose have been reported—the *PDR* says that the lethal dose of vasopressin spray has not been established, but that the intravenous LD50 (lethal dose 50, the point at which 50 percent of laboratory subjects are killed by a substance) for vasopressin in rats is 7,266 mg per kilogram of body weight. Lethal doses vary among animal species, and translating to humans is guesswork at best, but this represents roughly a one-pound dose of the drug for a 150-pound person. By this scenario, if you wanted to commit suicide by injecting vasopressin, you'd have to be extremely wealthy—a 5 ml bottle that contains approximately 1 mg of vasopressin costs about $20, so your lethal dose would set you back about $10 million. The *PDR* also notes that there have been no reports of drug abuse or dependence on vasopressin.

Vasopressin can be derived naturally (extracted from the pituitaries of pigs) or, more commonly, synthesized in the lab. Either way it is chemically identical to the human hormone. The most popular type of commercial vasopressin is a vasopressin compound known as lysine-vasopressin. This is generically known as lypressin; prominent trade brands are Diapid and Syntopressin from Sandoz Pharmaceuticals. Another type is arginine-vasopressin, or argipressin. The additive compounds, lysine and arginine, are amino acids; a 1982 study found that the effects of the two types of vasopressin are similar. Smart-drug author and pharmacist Ross Pelton discounts manufacturers' claims that one type or the other is more potent or causes fewer side effects than simple vasopressin. "A third explanation may make more sense," he notes. "The drug companies are making synthetic analogs of vasopressin so that they can have a specific product to patent and market."

Vasopressin is a prescription drug in the United States. See Resources for information on obtaining it from foreign sources without a prescription.

Taking Vasopressin

Vasopressin comes in only two forms: an injectable liquid (obviously not appropriate for home use) and a nasal spray. It is not available in the form of capsules or tablets for oral consumption because when vasopressin is eaten, protein-decomposing enzymes in the gut inactivate it before it can have any effect. As a nasal spray, vasopressin bypasses the intestinal tract by being absorbed into the mucous membranes of the nose and then transported directly to the brain.

The tiny nasal spray bottles of vasopressin typically hold 5 to 10 ml of the concentrated liquid, at a cost of $20 to $40. Dosages are measured in international units (IU) or in "posterior pituitary units" (also known as pressors) per milliliter. Proper dosing technique calls for sitting or standing in an erect position with both the nasal spray bottle and the head held upright. A single spray into a nostril typically delivers a dose of two pressor units. (Vasopressin should never be inhaled into the lungs, as this can cause shortness of breath.) An average daily use for medical purposes, which should not be exceeded for smart-drug use, is one nasal whiff into each nostril three to four times per day, amounting to 12 to 16 units per day. At that rate a 5 ml bottle represents approximately a three-week supply of vasopressin. Most people who use vasopressin for cognitive purposes ingest more like 4 to 6 units per day.

Inhaling more than two or three sprays into a nostril at one time will probably just waste your drug, since excess that drips into the throat ends up being inactivated in the digestive tract.

Vasopressin should be stored in the refrigerator (not the freezer) if you're not using it daily, though you need to allow it to warm to room temperature before you inhale it.

DEPRENYL: BOOSTING MIND, MOOD, AND LONGEVITY

Deprenyl is a drug with structural resemblances to amphetamine and to phenylalanine, the stimulating amino acid (see chapter 6). It was developed by a Hungarian researcher in the 1950s as a derivative of phenethylamine (PEA; also known as phenylethylamine), itself a product in the metabolism of phenylalanine. A naturally occurring compound found in various animal tissues, PEA may have mood-boosting and other neurotransmitterlike properties in the body. PEA is also found in high concentrations in certain plants, such as cacao, leading to much speculation about its possible connection to the romantic, lovey feelings associated with heavy consumption of chocolate. On the other hand, chemist Alexander Shulgin's experiments with PEA have found that, at least when it is taken orally in doses up to 1,600 mg, it has no mind-altering effects. No such debate is associated with the marked pharmacologic effects caused by taking oral doses of the drug deprenyl.

Deprenyl has been the subject of hundreds of medical studies in recent years, the bulk of them testing its effects as an adjunct in the treatment of Parkinson's disease and, to a lesser extent, Alzheimer's. Parkinson's is a degenerative brain disorder characterized by muscle weakness, trembling, and eventually dementia. It has been closely correlated with a deficiency in the neurotransmitter dopamine. Deprenyl has shown considerable promise as a treatment for Parkinson's, leading the FDA in 1989 to approve its use against the disease. Deprenyl may not only delay the onset of Parkinsonian symptoms but may also lead to improvements in patients' memory, attention span, and energy levels, without causing tolerance or significant side effects.

In Europe and elsewhere, deprenyl is also recognized as an effective mind-altering smart drug for healthy people. Many people take low dosages of deprenyl on a daily basis to elevate mood, boost energy levels, and stimulate sexuality. Regular deprenyl users often report that it improves their verbal memory or other aspects of cognitive function. Some say that it makes them more assertive, ambitious, confident, and capable of coping. Older men in particular find that deprenyl increases their libido and improves sexual performance.

Even those users who don't experience such dramatic effects often continue to take deprenyl because of its promise as an aid to increased longevity. Deprenyl acts as an antioxidant to protect brain cells from free radical damage, and one animal study published in 1989 found that deprenyl extended rats' maximum life span by almost 40 percent. Other animal studies have found that deprenyl also extends average life span. Of course, long-term studies on humans have not been con-

ducted and deprenyl's effects on longevity remain speculative.

A Unique Dopamine Protector

Much of deprenyl's mood-boosting and sex-enhancing properties are due to its effect on certain neurotransmitters in the brain, particularly dopamine and noradrenaline. Researchers have determined that deprenyl has a protective effect on a section of the midbrain, the substantia nigra, rich in dopamine-producing nerve cells. Deprenyl also has an apparently unique effect on the enzyme monoamine oxidase (MAO), which is widely distributed throughout the body. MAO breaks down dopamine and other neurotransmitters. MAO levels in the brain tend to rise as people grow older; dopamine levels tend to fall. By selectively inhibiting this action of MAO, as well as directly stimulating the brain to produce more dopamine, MAO inhibitors such as deprenyl improve mood, increase alertness and energy levels, and enhance sex drive.

Deprenyl appears to be unique among MAO inhibitors, however, in that it targets MAO-B, one of the two main types of MAO enzymes. Other MAO inhibitors, such as the antidepressant phenelzine (Nardil), work by inhibiting MAO-A. Unfortunately, inhibiting MAO-A can activate too many neurotransmitters, leading to symptoms such as nervousness. Taking MAO-A inhibitors can also cause some people to experience a dangerous side effect—a sudden rise in blood pressure—after eating certain common foods and beverages (especially aged cheese and red wine) that are rich in the chemical tyramine. By inhibiting mainly MAO-B, the type of MAO that is predominant in the brain, deprenyl avoids this "cheese reaction." So far, deprenyl is the only widely prescribed MAO inhibitor that has this desirable ability to selectively inhibit MAO-B.

Researchers note that deprenyl's effects on the body have not been fully explained yet, and the drug appears to exhibit mechanisms of action that are independent of its inhibition of MAO-B. Deprenyl is thought to interfere with dopamine reuptake at the synapse, for example, again allowing dopamine to stay active longer and produce its mood-brightening effects. Deprenyl also metabolizes in the liver into forms of amphetamine, which can stimulate the central nervous system. How much of deprenyl's effects are due to the action of metabolites is unclear.

Deprenyl resembles vasopressin in its safety record—most indications are that it is safe, and not a single death from overdose has been reported. It is true, however, that human experience with the substance is relatively limited and long-term studies are lacking. At low smart-drug dosages (1 to 10 mg, depending on age), deprenyl causes few side effects. At higher doses (above 10 mg daily), deprenyl has been known to cause speediness, anxiety, dizziness, nausea, nightmares, and insomnia. Although "cheese reactions" have not been reported in deprenyl patients, taking more than 10 mg per day may possibly cause deprenyl to act like other MAO inhibitors, leading to a hazardous increase in blood pressure. (Reactions are almost unheard-of at doses in the range of 10 to 20 mg, but may

occur at doses of 30 to 60 mg per day, levels sometimes used for treating severe depression. A 1991 study of ten patients with major depression suggests, however, that such high doses of deprenyl are unnecessary if it is used in conjunction with phenylalanine.) High doses of deprenyl thus should be avoided or accompanied by strict dietary prohibitions. Since there is no indication that high dosages make deprenyl work any better as a mood booster and stimulant for normal, healthy people, suggested dosages should not be exceeded.

Those who should not take deprenyl include anyone taking selective serotonin reuptake inhibitors such as fluoxetine (Prozac), tricyclic antidepressants such as amitriptyline (Elavil) and desipramine (Norpramin), or other MAO inhibitors. Women who are pregnant or breast-feeding and children should also not take deprenyl. Taking deprenyl at the same time as central nervous system stimulants such as caffeine may result in overstimulation.

Tablet Versus Liquid

Deprenyl is a generic name, as is selegiline and selegiline hydrochloride. Trade names for deprenyl include Eldepryl, Jumex, and Movergan. Eldepryl is the most popular prescription form of deprenyl in the United States, particularly for its FDA-approved use against Parkinson's disease. Those who are taking deprenyl as a smart drug, however, generally prefer not to use Eldepryl. One reason is that Eldepryl comes only in 5 mg tablets, and many people want to calibrate deprenyl dosages into one-milligram increments (see dosage suggestions below). Cutting tablets into pieces is difficult and time-consuming, compared to liquid forms of deprenyl that can be dose-divided more conveniently. Another reason is that in recent years the manufacturer of Eldepryl, Somerset Pharmaceuticals of Tampa, Florida, has alienated many smart-drug users of deprenyl by initiating lawsuits against various companies that distribute liquid forms of deprenyl. Lawyers for Somerset have even sent letters to liquid deprenyl consumers requesting that they "refrain from making any additional purchases" of liquid deprenyl and "complete the enclosed information sheet" about past purchases, noting that Somerset is asking for voluntary cooperation but reserves the right to compel the information through subpoena, court order, or deposition. Smart-drug users, who by necessity must be willing to buck the medical and regulatory establishments to obtain these substances, not unexpectedly reacted negatively to this letter. The influential *Smart Drug News* said in an editorial that many of its readers were "personally enraged by the content of the letter" and that henceforth the newsletter would no longer recommend Eldepryl. Rather, it would encourage readers to use the liquid deprenyl, contending that "the legal and regulatory endorsement of Eldepryl-brand deprenyl by FDA is scientifically and medically irrelevant." Liquid deprenyl is likely to be better absorbed than the pill, in any case.

A popular source for liquid deprenyl is Discovery Experimental & Development, a Florida-based company that obtains the product from a Mexican manufacturer. Discovery has tried unsuccessfully to get FDA approval for liquid deprenyl. See Resources for information on how to order liquid deprenyl and other smart drugs.

Taking Deprenyl

Some people notice positive effects on mood and energy from taking a single dose of deprenyl, though it is not uncommon for full results to become evident only after many months of daily ingestion. As a smart drug deprenyl is usually taken in doses that are adjusted for age, as follows. One drop of the liquid deprenyl supplies one milligram of deprenyl. Daily dosages of 6 mg and higher should be divided in half and taken twice daily, in the morning and the early afternoon. Single doses are best taken in the morning. For best results store liquid deprenyl in the refrigerator.

AGE	DOSAGE
30–35	1 mg twice a week
35–40	1 mg every other day
40–45	1 mg every day
45–50	2 mg every day
50–55	3 mg every day
55–60	4 mg every day
60–65	5 mg every day
65–70	6 mg every day
70–75	8 mg every day
75–80	9 mg every day
80 and over	10 mg every day

Though it came into clinical use only in the late 1960s, piracetam is the granddaddy of a whole class of related smart drugs. Observers of the worldwide smart-drug scene estimate that greater numbers of normal, healthy people take piracetam for its brain-boosting effects than any other smart drug. Piracetam is also the compound that inspired the name *nootropic,* coined by pharmacologist Cornelius Giurgea. With almost thirty years of international use behind it and a multitude of scientific studies (done mainly in Europe) exploring its effects, piracetam's popularity is rapidly expanding even in places like the United States, where it is neither sold by pharmacists nor recognized as therapeutically useful by the medical establishment. Many of those who have looked beyond the official dismissals of piracetam, however, see a safe and promising substance.

Piracetam is a pyrrolidone compound with ties to two naturally occurring amino acids. It is a derivative of GABA (see chapter 16) and is similar in its chemical structure to pyroglutamate. Taken orally, piracetam enhances mental performance in various ways. Studies done on animals, people with aging-related conditions, and healthy humans have generally shown positive results in aspects of learning and information processing. Some types of memory and recall often improve with daily use of piracetam. Many people report en-

hanced alertness and attention span. Studies have demonstrated that piracetam can improve reaction time under conditions of low oxygen availability, prevent age-related driving performance decline, and enhance verbal skills. Some regular users even contend that piracetam somehow "superconnects" the two hemispheres of the brain, resulting not only in a significant improvement in verbal memory but enhanced feelings of creativity and intuition.

Piracetam may provide beneficial effects on the brain even when administered before birth. In the mid-1980s Italian scientists conducted research on the offspring of mice that were fed a piracetam-related compound from the beginning of pregnancy through birth. According to a study published in 1988, the researchers found that the newborns outperformed control mice in various learning- and memory-related tests. The smart-drug mice also interacted more with their environment and displayed more self-grooming. The effects were long-lasting and still in evidence among mature offspring.

A number of skiers and mountain climbers have begun to take piracetam because of its apparent ability to protect the brain from the adverse effects of low-oxygen levels. Airline flight crews and frequent flyers may benefit as well—pressurized cabins often have lower oxygen levels than are normally found at sea level. Studies have confirmed that piracetam can help prevent hypoxia, a deficiency of oxygen getting to bodily tissues. For example, in a double-blind study published in 1988, researchers exposed healthy male subjects in their late twenties and early thirties to air with an oxygen content of 10.5 percent, almost half as "thin" as air at sea level (which is approximately 20 percent oxygen). Subjects given 1,600 or 2,400 mg of piracetam were able to maintain normal mental functioning, as determined by tests that measured such factors as reaction time and decision making, as well as normal breathing rates. Subjects exposed to the low-oxygen air and given placebos, however, experienced notable declines in their mental performance. A 1995 study done on eighteen healthy volunteers who were exposed to a similar low-oxygen condition also found that piracetam protected the brain from adverse effects, in this case as measured by electroencephalographic mapping. A 1991 study done on trained rats found that those that were administered piracetam were significantly less affected by subsequent exposure to low-oxygen conditions than were those treated with saline.

Researchers have tested the ability of piracetam and other nootropics to help treat people with head injuries, Alzheimer's disease, epilepsy, age-related memory disorders, vertigo, movement disorders such as myoclonus, and other conditions. While some such patients clearly do benefit, sometimes more dramatically than do normal, healthy subjects, other patients don't. Researchers are unsure why, and so far have not been able to predict which of those among a group of subjects are most likely to be helped by piracetam.

Research into piracetam's potential effectiveness for improving the performance of children with learning disorders has also provided both positive and negative results. Some

children seem to improve, others improve but the effect is not long-lasting, and still others are unaffected by piracetam. A double-blind, placebo-controlled study done in 1987 on 225 children suffering from the reading disability dyslexia did find that piracetam can help them read faster with greater comprehension and increase their verbal memory. At least two other studies on piracetam and dyslexia have also reported increased reading speed or other positive results. A recent study done on sixty-six young children with aphasia, a language disorder often caused by a problem in a particular area of the brain, found that after six weeks 4.8 g per day of piracetam promoted the effectiveness of intensive speech therapy as a treatment for the condition.

A number of parents who have children suffering from Down's syndrome also say that piracetam promotes cognitive improvements. While acknowledging that the drug "appears to be safe," and "it is certainly possible that there might be some beneficial effect," the National Down Syndrome Congress does not recommend piracetam's use until controlled scientific studies are done on piracetam for Down's syndrome.

Mind-Turning Mechanisms

Scientists have proposed a number of mechanisms for how piracetam and related nootropics can affect the mind. A 1991 study done on mice determined that piracetam has a potentially restorative or stimulating effect on the parts of the nervous system most affected by the neurotransmitter acetylcholine, crucial for proper cognition, memory, and learning.

Other studies have suggested that piracetam increases either the levels, the activity, or the receptors of neurotransmitters. Researchers have also shown that piracetam can have a positive effect on blood circulation, membrane fluidity, glucose metabolism, and oxygen use in the brain. Piracetam apparently helps the brain synthesize new proteins, possibly the mechanism by which new information is stored as memory. Piracetam has also been shown to increase the production of adenosine triphosphate (ATP), the body's principal energy-carrying compound, and to protect the brain from damage by certain free radicals. By promoting the action of certain enzymes in cells, piracetam has been shown to reduce adverse effects of lipofuscin, a fatty pigment that builds up with aging and can interfere with proper brain and nerve function. In the final analysis, however, piracetam's primary mechanism of action within the body remains a mystery.

Piracetam's overall safety has been confirmed by both human and animal studies. The substance seems to be totally lacking in toxicity, whether in single doses many times larger than the average dose or when taken in mega-doses for extended periods of time. As much as 10 to 20 g of piracetam per day, for example, have been safely used in the treatment of certain types of seizures. Researchers who have tried to establish an LD50 for piracetam have failed—no amount seems to cause fatalities in laboratory animals.

A small percentage of piracetam users report that it causes speediness, anxiety, insomnia, and similar side effects, especially if taken at the same time as stimulants. Some users may experience nausea, diarrhea, and gastro-intestinal problems. Reducing the dosage will often alleviate the side effects—few people have any ill effects from less than 2.4 g daily. Anyone with severe kidney failure and persons taking anticoagulant drugs such as Coumadin (warfarin) should not use piracetam; also avoid during pregnancy and breast-feeding.

Beyond Nootropil

Piracetam is the generic name for this compound. The most widely recognized trade name is Nootropil, the name given by its developer, Union Chemical Belge of Brussels, Belgium. Since the expiration of the worldwide Nootropil patent in 1985, Hoffman-La Roche, Ciba-Geigy, and numerous other North American and European pharmaceutical companies have begun to market piracetam, or closely related compounds with similar molecular structures, under a bewildering variety of names: Normabrain, Dinagen, Cerebroforte, Gabacet, and so forth. Among the newly developed analogs and related compounds are oxiracetam (Neuractiv) and pramiracetam (Neupramir), both of which are derived from the same base substance as piracetam. Oxiracetam and pramiracetam are considered to be somewhat more potent than piracetam. Average dosages are lower, so if you purchase these products make sure to follow the suggested use guidelines.

Despite its apparent safety and effectiveness piracetam is not available by prescription or over-the-counter in the United States, where it has no FDA-approved uses. Piracetam can be purchased from foreign sources. In many countries it is available as an over-the-counter substance.

Some substances that are chemically related to piracetam are available as nutrients in the United States. Pyroglutamate, which seems to function much as piracetam does to boost memory and learning, is not restricted by the FDA. It is available in various forms, such as arginine pyroglutamate.

Taking Piracetam

Piracetam typically comes in 400, 800, or 1,200 mg tablets or capsules; it is also available as a liquid. The most commonly recommended daily dose for enhanced mental function is 1,600 to 2,400 mg per day, in three divided doses.

Piracetam's effects are usually noticeable within an hour, although daily use allows piracetam gradually to reach peak levels in the brain. For increased effect, many people combine piracetam with choline, DMAE, or other nutrients that enhance acetylcholine production. Piracetam and ginkgo have been shown to work well in combination. Combining piracetam with Hydergine or other smart drugs may increase their effects as well. Learn to recognize one drug's effects and dosage levels before adding additional ones to your regimen. Also start with low doses of any additional drug to avoid overstimulation or other side effects.

HYDERGINE: LSD'S BRAINY COUSIN

Hydergine is a semisynthetic drug based on the structure of three alkaloid compounds found in ergot. Ergot is a purplish, grainlike mass produced by a fungus (*Claviceps purpurea*) that grows naturally as a parasite on the kernels of rye and other cereals. Hydergine is the trade name bestowed on the substance by its developer, Sandoz; the generic name is ergoloid mesylates. Among the most widely used prescription drugs in the world, only within the past decade has Hydergine begun to gain recognition in North America as an all-star smart drug. Studies have shown that it has the remarkable ability to safely boost the supply of blood and oxygen to the brain, increase brain cell metabolism, prevent damage to brain cells from the action of free radicals, and enhance memory and intelligence.

Ergot: A Chemical Treasure House

Hydergine's unusual properties can be traced to its natural parent substance, ergot. Ergot has long been a dangerous and toxic substance to those who have ingested large amounts of it unknowingly, usually by eating bread made from contaminated grain. Written descriptions of ergot poisoning go back at least to the Middle Ages and, with less certitude, to 600 B.C.E. Historians now believe that ergot-infested rye was the cause of numerous wide-scale poisonings in Europe and elsewhere from the Middle Ages through the seventeenth century, when ergot was identified as the cause. (Isolated serious outbreaks have continued, however—most recently an episode that occurred in Russia in 1926.) Eating ergot-infested rye can cause people to develop gangrenous limbs or suffer from convulsions, possibly with psychoticlike complications. Certain French and German folk names for ergot, which translate to "drunken rye" and "mad grain," indicate an early awareness that the substance had mind-altering properties. Ergot has even been sited as a possible factor in such episodes of mass hysteria as witch burnings and as the active ingredient in the sacred hallucinogenic drink consumed in the mysterious annual religious rites held in the Greek city of Eleusis until the fourth century.

Herbalists of the late Middle Ages, however, recognized a therapeutic side to this unusual substance. At least since the late 1500s, wise-woman healers and midwives have known that small doses of ergot could serve as a means for stimulating uterine contractions, whether to abort the fetus or to precipitate a difficult childbirth. The medical profession did not acknowledge this use of ergot for another two centuries, when in 1808 a report on ergot's ability to quicken childbirth appeared in a New York medical publication. As its medical use spread physicians quickly began to realize that ergot was difficult to use, however, and that in significant numbers of cases it caused stillbirths or harm to the newborn. By the late 1820s its only recognized safe use was as a remedy to control post-delivery bleeding.

The problem was that natural ergot is complex and variable in its action, and doctors could not easily control the dose of the drug they administered. The answer was to isolate and purify ergot's active compounds, but researchers who attempted to do this discovered that the substance was agonizingly unstable and troublesome to work with. Ergot is now known to contain some thirty alkaloids; it also varies in its constituents depending upon local conditions of its growth and other fac-

tors. Success eluded medical researchers until the first two decades of the twentieth century. By the early 1930s researchers had isolated a number of ergot alkaloids that showed promise as treatments in obstetrics, migraine, and nervous disorders. It was then that ergot research was lucky enough to attract the attention of Albert Hofmann, a young Swiss biochemist working for Sandoz. Though he didn't know it at the time, he was to commit much of the rest of his life to researching ergot compounds.

Among Hofmann's pioneering innovations in ergot derivative drugs was LSD-25. He first formulated this controversial hallucinogen in 1938, "with the intention of obtaining a circulatory and respiratory stimulant," he says in his autobiographical account, *LSD: My Problem Child.* Unaware of the new compound's mind-altering effects, Hofmann shelved it as pharmacologically unpromising and didn't discover its hallucinogenic properties until 1943. According to Hofmann's account, during the intervening five years he focused on determining the exact chemical structure of ergotoxine, a substance first isolated in 1907. Hofmann suspected ergotoxine was not homogenous but rather a mixture of alkaloids. Hofmann says:

The solution of the ergotoxine problem was not merely scientifically interesting, but also had great practical significance. A valuable remedy arose from it. The three hydrogenated ergotoxine alkaloids that I produced in the course of these investigations . . . displayed medicinally useful properties during testing by Professor Rothlin in the pharmacological department. From these three substances, the pharmaceutical preparation Hydergine was developed, a medicament for improvement of peripheral circulation and cerebral function in the control of geriatric disorders. Hydergine has proven to be an effective remedy in geriatrics for these indications. Today [circa late 1970s] it is Sandoz's most important pharmaceutical product.

Scientists now know that ergot contains what has been called a "veritable treasure house of pharmacological constituents," including compounds not found in any other source. Indeed, there are some who think that Hofmann's formulation of Hydergine will, like a nondescript turtle that eventually outpaces a Day-Glo hare, someday be recognized as a more significant discovery than that of LSD. By the early 1950s Hydergine was in production and on its way to achieving importance quite a bit beyond the field of geriatrics. European physicians now consider it an invaluable remedy for a number of conditions relating to reduced oxygen supply to the body. For example, it is administered to victims of heart attacks and strokes, near drowning, drug overdose, and altitude sickness. (A cruel but revealing study done on cats deprived them of oxygen and blood to the brain. Those that received doses of Hydergine still showed normal brain function after 45 minutes, whereas untreated cats were basically brain-dead after 15 minutes.) Hydergine is widely used in emergency rooms, and in some countries is even routinely given to patients scheduled for surgery. Furthermore, since the early 1980s Hydergine has been embraced by normal, healthy people as the premier smart drug of our time, a potent yet nontoxic brain booster and mood enhancer. While Hydergine's popu-larity in North America remains limited, in recent years it has ranked among the top ten most popular drugs in the world, accounting for upward of half a billion dollars in annual sales.

Positive Effects on Brain Function

Hydergine's only FDA-approved use in the United States is for a relatively limited set of conditions related to senility, dementia, cerebral insufficiency (lack of blood flow to the brain), and Alzheimer's disease. For patients of these mostly geriatric-related conditions it offers symptomatic relief of declines in cognitive skills, mood, self-care, and motivation. Normal and healthy users of Hydergine report similar effects: an improvement in alertness and concentration, enhanced abilities to learn and remember, and an overall brightening of mood. Some users report almost immediate benefits, while others say that the full effects take a few weeks to become apparent.

Researchers have by now conducted a number of well-controlled double-blind studies on the impaired elderly taking Hydergine; most of these support positive short-term effects on brain function and mood. Hydergine has been shown to stimulate recent memory, improve reaction time, and lead to greater mental clarity. Fewer studies have been done that have demonstrated long-term benefits for normal, healthy persons, though those studies that have not confirmed dramatic improvements in mental function have also not found any long-term toxicity. For example, referring to a long-term study published in 1986, Ward Dean, M.D., a coauthor of *Smart Drugs II,* remarks, "The study was terminated after seven years because of the excess number of subjects in the *placebo* group (the group *not* taking Hydergine) who became too ill to continue the study."

Exactly how Hydergine accomplishes its effects is still being determined. It is known that its ability to act as a potent antioxidant in the brain protects cells from harm. According to a number of studies, including a 1988 report in *Gerontology,* Hydergine may help slow the accumulation in the brain of lipofuscin. Researchers also believe that Hydergine promotes the growth of new brain cell dendrites, the fiberlike connections between neurons that play a key role in learning and nervous system function. Hydergine has been shown to affect brain waves and neurotransmitter levels. The various and diverse positive actions Hydergine has on the body has led Pelton to conclude that basically the drug "slows down the aging process."

Hydergine's safety is well established. No fatalities have been reported in the almost fifty years of its use. Rats administered an extremely high daily dose (186 mg per kilogram of body weight, approximately 2,000 times the average human dose) for twenty-six weeks showed no evidence of ill effects on organs or blood chemistry. Among human users, those side effects that have been observed, even from taking relatively high daily doses (12 to 15 mg) for extended periods of time, have been minor: nausea, headache, gastric disturbances, and irritation under the tongue (from sublingual use). Users report that these effects occur only rarely, though starting off with too high an initial dose (more than 6 mg, for example) does increase the potential for nausea. Hydergine has one of the shortest listings in the entire *PDR* under contraindications, precautions, and adverse reactions, categories that for many drugs require whole columns of print. The only people who should definitely avoid Hydergine are those who suffer from psychosis.

Hydergine is often taken in combination with piracetam, for their synergistic effects. Reducing the dosage of each is recommended, particularly during the initial stages.

Because Sandoz Pharmaceuticals' patent on Hydergine has expired, competing generic products are now on the market. Ergoloid mesylates (also known as dihydrogenated ergot alkaloids) is, however, a complex compound, requiring a series of steps to modify the three ergot alkaloids it is derived from and balance them in the required ratio. Until recently, there was some question as to whether the generics (which often cost substantially less than Hydergine) had duplicated exactly the Hydergine formula. The products do now appear to be standardized. Bioavailability tests that were done on the generic ergoloid mesylates tablets produced by one large drug manufacturer did find an equivalency to Hydergine; the FDA considers the generics equal to Hydergine. Hydergine nevertheless remains the most popular formulation of ergoloid mesylates.

Taking Hydergine

Hydergine is most commonly found in tablets ranging in size from 1 to 4.5 mg. It also comes in a liquid, liquid-filled capsules, and in sublingual tablets, all of which may be better absorbed than the tablets. A common starting dose for people new to Hydergine is 1 to 2 mg per day. In the United States, the highest recommended dose approved by the FDA is 3 mg per day. A number of the Hydergine studies that showed cognitive benefits, however, administered dosages higher than 3 mg per day.

The average suggested dosage in Europe is often 6 to 9 mg per day. Many Hydergine users in the United States level off at 4.5 to 6 mg per day, in three divided doses. Although this is higher than the FDA-approved dose, the data suggests that it is still a very safe level of consumption.

other sites in the nervous system. It acts along pathways that result in a slowing of heartbeat, stimulation of the sweat glands, and increased secretions in the mouth and lungs. Acetylcholine plays a prominent role in sexual response, carrying messages to nerves in the penis that affect muscles and arteries involved with erection. Women may also experience decreased sexual activity when acetylcholine is less active in the body. Perhaps most significantly from our perspective is that acetylcholine transmits messages between neurons in the brain that affect aspects of memory, thinking, mood and emotions, and intellect. When these neurons are deprived of adequate acetylcholine as a neurotransmitter, the result may be memory loss, depression and mood disorders, and possibly even Alzheimer's disease or other serious neurological conditions over the long term.

Pharmaceutical companies have developed medications that can affect some of these processes. For example, certain drugs can inhibit or protect the enzyme that breaks acetylcholine down, or block receptor cells from receiving or using acetylcholine. The objective may be to prolong or neutralize some of acetylcholine's actions, depending on the person's condition. Acetylcholine itself has so many varied effects on the body that it is not very useful as a single-bullet therapeutic agent.

Aging can also affect how acetylcholine is used in the body. As with other neurotransmitters, acetylcholine levels in the brain tend to fall with advancing age, as free radical activity takes its toll and the processes of transporting choline to the brain and producing acetylcholine in the brain become less efficient. Some elderly people may have lost more than half of their ability to produce acetylcholine.

What can you do about this? Well, acetylcholine is manufactured from choline or from the related compound di-methyl-amino-ethanol (DMAE) in the body. Choline consumption can affect blood levels, which partly determine how much choline is in the brain and how much acetylcholine is released into the central nervous system. Thus one way to boost the action of the cholinergic nervous system, and gain more of the benefits of acetylcholine's actions as a neurotransmitter, is to take supplemental amounts of either of these substances. Indeed, many people are now doing just this. Athletes who take choline-based supplements say that they experience greater energy and less fatigue. Many people who use choline, DMAE, or the amino acid brain booster pyroglutamate as smart drugs notice a brightening of mood or fewer mood swings, greater alertness and ability to concentrate, and enhanced short-term memory.

CHOLINE: THE MEMORY NUTRIENT

Researchers in the mid-nineteenth century discovered, isolated, and synthesized choline. Its most important functions, however, were not begun to be recognized for seventy years. In the early 1930s, researchers performed an experiment on dogs that had had their pancreases removed. The animals developed fatty accumulations in the liver that eventually

Choline, DMAE, and Pyroglutamate

◉

FOOD FOR THE BRAIN

The human nervous system is so complex that it makes even the most sophisticated computer-robot seem a Lego contraption by comparison. Though an oversimplification, it helps to understand the nervous system by dividing it into parts responsible for certain actions. One way that doctors do this is by reference to certain neurotransmitters, the chemicals that transmit messages at nerve endings, such as between nerve cells (*neurons*) or between nerve cells and muscle cells. Some parts and functions of the nervous system are more controlled by one neurotransmitter than another. For example, the "adrenergic" nervous system is largely affected by adrenaline, the stimulating hormone and neurotransmitter secreted from the adrenal glands in higher amounts when the body is faced with a "fight-or flight" circumstance, and the related noradrenaline.

Another useful classification is the cholinergic nervous system, which refers to functions most controlled by the neurotransmitter acetylcholine. Acetylcholine is the neurotransmitter at all nerve-muscle cells. It plays an essential role in the process that allows skeletal muscles to contract, helping to control movement and coordination and providing the body with proper muscle tone. In normal, healthy people acetylcholine levels may affect stamina and energy levels. When the body malfunctions in a way that prevents acetylcholine from transferring the right messages from nerves to muscles in certain tissues, diseases can begin to develop that are marked by twitching and other signs of loss of muscle control, such as Parkinson's disease and myasthenia gravis.

Acetylcholine can also be found at many

caused them to die. The scientists determined that feeding the dogs choline-containing substances could prevent the fatty liver condition. At least for certain animals, it became apparent that choline-containing compounds are crucial for promoting the utilization of fat.

Beginning in the 1950s, researchers also began to demonstrate the important functions of acetylcholine as a neurotransmitter. Because people with Alzheimer's disease have been shown to have reduced levels of acetylcholine (and other neurotransmitters) in the brain, a number of studies have focused on the potential for choline-based supplements to affect the disease. Some of the findings have been promising. Animal and human studies have shown that in certain circumstances increased choline consumption can elevate choline levels in the blood and then the brain, with brain acetylcholine levels eventually rising as well. Researchers found that some Alzheimer's patients who take choline supplements report a brightening of mood and show better results on memory tests.

Ultimately, however, the choline-Alzheimer's link proved to be disappointing, at least in terms of curing the condition. Clearly, just taking lots of choline cannot reverse Alzheimer's. The mechanism is complex, and acetylcholine function is probably only one factor. It is also possible that Alzheimer's may be related to a falloff in the body's ability to use choline, so that by the time Alzheimer's develops choline supplementation is too late. In a recent study published in the *Journal of the American Medical Association,* researchers described how they gave choline supplements to two groups of volunteers, one made up of twenty- to

forty-year-olds, and the other of sixty- to eighty-five-year-olds. Levels of choline-containing compounds in the brain increased by approximately 60 percent for the young group, but by only 16 percent in the elderly. Choline levels in other parts of the body did not differ between the groups.

It is likely that adequate choline consumption throughout life has a positive role in helping to prevent memory deficits and the onset of Alzheimer's. Studies have also begun to confirm that normal, healthy people can benefit from optimal choline consumption. Choline has been shown to improve students' ability to recall long lists or sequences of words and to reduce memory problems. For example, in a 1994 study researchers gave forty-one healthy people the equivalent of about 500 mg of choline daily. After five weeks those who took the nutrient experienced almost half as many memory lapses as subjects taking a placebo. Studies such as this one have caused choline to become known as the "memory nutrient."

The Many Faces of Choline

Most of the choline we take into our bodies is not free choline but choline combined with other compounds. Most prominently, choline is a component of lecithin, a fatty acid widely distributed in both plants and animals. Lecithin in the body is broken down before it is converted into acetylcholine.

(The scientific term for lecithin is *phosphatidyl choline.* Many supplement manufacturers and others also use the term lecithin more loosely, to refer to products that include phosphatidyl choline as well as other fats and substances, such as the amino acid serine. A convention that will be used here is to employ the technical term phosphatidyl choline to refer to "pure lecithin," and lecithin to refer to the commercial mixtures that may contain as little as 5 percent of phosphatidyl choline.)

Basically phosphatidyl choline is a combination of choline with fatty acids, the oily alcohol glycerol, and a fatty form of the mineral phosphorus. Phosphatidyl choline is thus a phospholipid, a type of structural fat that is soluble in both fat and water. Phospholipids such as phosphatidyl choline and inositol have a number of important functions in the body, including helping to regulate cholesterol levels, transporting fats to cells and aiding in the metabolism of fats, and protecting myelin, a fatty material that forms a protective sheath around some nerve fibers. The membranes of cells in the brain and elsewhere in the body contain various phospholipids, including phosphatidyl choline. The phosphatidyl choline in brain cells is more easily transported across the blood-brain barrier than is free choline. When choline is pulled out of cell membranes in the brain for conversion to acetylcholine, however, the cell is left in a weakened state. Consuming enough dietary phosphatidyl choline, and consequently having choline available in sufficient quantities in the blood, is a more healthful long-term strategy for maintaining proper neurotransmitter levels.

An Essential Nutrient?

Nutritional researchers have accepted choline as an essential nutrient—a vitamin—for certain animals, such as rats and guinea pigs, for many years. Numerous studies have demonstrated that these animals routinely develop liver disorders, kidney malfunctions, and other health problems when choline is removed from their diet. Most recently, a 1995 study linked low choline intake to liver cancer in rats. Choline's status as an essential nutrient for humans, however, has been the subject of much debate among nutritional researchers. Until the early 1990s, a number of authorities said that choline did not qualify as a vitamin, basically because deficiencies had not been proven in humans and because some choline is synthesized in the body (from either of two amino acids, methionine and serine). In recent years, however, studies have begun to indicate that humans suffer significant health problems when they fail to consume adequate dietary choline. A major study headed by noted researcher Steven Zeisel, M.D., Ph.D., of the University of North Carolina and published in 1991 found that humans fed a choline-deficient diet do develop liver disorders (particularly "fatty liver") and other adverse health conditions. Deficiencies in choline may also lead to problems in cellular membranes and nerves' myelin sheaths. Many nutritionists now consider choline to be a B-complex vitamin. The Food and Nutrition Board of the National Academy of Sciences, which sets RDAs, has yet to concur. The Board did recently announce that it is considering an RDA for choline.

Choline may be especially essential for newborns and infants. One of the most famous animal studies was conducted by Columbia University researchers on rats in 1988. They fed pregnant rats extra choline, and also administered supplemental doses to newborn rats. Compared to nonsupplemented rats, these choline babies were expert maze runners, apparently remembering their pathways much more efficiently than those rats that had not received choline supplements. The choline-fed rats also apparently retained their enhanced memories throughout their lives, even when they were fully grown.

This study takes on added importance when you consider that human breast milk is an especially rich source of choline, providing higher levels of the nutrient than either formula (though all FDA-approved infant formulas contain choline) or cows' milk. Also, there is evidence that average choline consumption for adults is falling in industrialized countries. This is because many of the best sources of dietary choline are foods that are not only high in phosphatidyl choline but high in saturated fat: peanuts, organ meats, egg yolks. Egg yolks contain 8 to 9 percent phosphatidyl choline—the word *lecithin* is derived from the Greek *lekithos* for egg yolk. Vegetarian sources of dietary choline, such as cauliflower and some of the leafy green vegetables, provide lower levels of the nutrient. Soy foods are a relatively rich source of dietary choline.

One researcher wrote, in response to Zeisel's study, "Very many Americans now unwittingly put themselves on lifetime low-choline diets by abjuring dietary cholesterol: By an unfortunate coincidence, the cholesterol-rich foods that they avoid (e.g., egg yolks, liver) also happen to be the major sources of dietary choline. Perhaps many of us are a little choline-deficient much of the time."

Prolonged and rigorous exercise can also lead to reduced blood levels of choline.

The food industry adds lecithin to products ranging from mayonnaise to chocolate, as an emulsifier (an agent used to help liquids hold together that normally don't dissolve in each other or mix well), thickener, or stabilizer. Processed foods, however, do not have high enough levels of phosphatidyl choline to be dietarily significant.

Estimates of the average dietary intake of choline by Americans vary, but most fall in the range of 500 to 750 mg per day. Suggested optimal requirements also vary, but it is likely that the body needs at least 1,000 mg or more of choline every day just to prevent a marginal deficiency in the nutrient.

An Enviable Safety Record

Lecithin, phosphatidyl choline, and choline are safe and nontoxic at normal levels of supplementation, including those dosages suggested in "Taking Choline," beginning page 128. According to the *Physicians' Desk Reference,* "No major side effects have been reported in connection with consumption of large quantities of phosphatidyl choline or commercially available (less pure) lecithin." The Food and Drug Administration has reported that taking up to 13.5 g of lecithin per day is safe.

Minor side effects from taking lecithin, phosphatidyl choline, and choline infrequently occur at average doses but are not uncommon when much higher doses are taken. These may include nausea, muscle stiffness (especially in the neck and shoulders) and muscle-tension headaches, upset stomach, intestinal cramps, and diarrhea. Some people experience overstimulation in the form of restlessness or insomnia.

You would have to take extremely high doses of pure choline for the substance to be life-threatening. *Goodman and Gilman's The Pharmacological Basis of Therapeutics* estimates the oral LD50 dose for humans to be 200 to 400 g of choline, approximately one hundred times what is considered the high range of supplemental doses. Megadoses that are in the range of ten times average are sometimes used therapeutically, such as in the treatment of manic depression and other serious psychiatric disorders. Anyone wishing to take such high levels should work closely with a physician. High doses of choline can be countereffective and actually cause depression in some people.

Others who should avoid supplementing choline include anyone with ulcers (since choline can increase stomach acid), epilepsy, a history of depression, or Parkinson's disease. People who are taking anticholinergic drugs, which are meant to benefit certain conditions (such as motion sickness) by blocking the effects of acetylcholine, should obviously not supplement choline.

Taking Choline

The following summarizes the essential factors related to the three main forms of supplemental choline: lecithin, phosphatidyl choline, and choline.

Lecithin

Pros: Because it is less potent than choline supplements, lecithin is less likely to cause side effects. Compared to choline, lecithin contains fatty acids with potentially beneficial effects on the liver.

Cons: With their high levels of fats, lecithin supplements have a considerable tendency to become rancid (refrigerate after opening and discard if the taste is bitter or acrid). The large doses necessary to obtain significant choline can also add to fat intake, a possible health concern if you are already eating a high-fat diet (one teaspoon of lecithin granules contains about two grams of fat). Required doses of lecithin are so high that most people can't stay committed to taking lecithin supplements.

Choline potency: High-quality lecithin products may now contain 20 percent or so phosphatidyl choline, though many are still in the 5 to 10 percent range. Choline itself constitutes only 13 percent of phosphatidyl choline.

Forms: Lecithin comes in a powder, granules (which can be sprinkled on cereal or dissolved in juice or other liquids), oil-filled capsules, and a liquid.

Dose: An average daily dose that is 10 percent phosphatidyl choline is 5 g, or two to three teaspoons (yielding 500 mg phosphatidyl choline and 65 mg choline) to 10 g, or four to six teaspoons (yielding 1,000 mg phosphatidyl choline and 130 mg choline).

Phosphatidyl Choline

Pros: Phosphatidyl choline is a more concentrated source of choline compared to lecithin. Like lecithin, phosphatidyl choline contains fatty acids with potentially beneficial effects on the liver.

Cons: Phosphatidyl choline adds some fat to the diet; supplements can become rancid.

Choline potency: The percentage of phosphatidyl choline in phosphatidyl choline products varies from 20 to 100 percent. Some popular products are designated "pc55" because they contain 55 percent phosphatidyl choline.

Forms: Phosphatidyl choline typically comes in capsules and powders.

Dose: An average daily dose of pc55 is two 500 mg capsules (yielding 550 mg phosphatidyl choline and thus 72 mg choline) to four 500 mg capsules (yielding 1,100 mg phosphatidyl choline and thus 144 mg choline).

CHOLINE

Pros: Compared to the multigram doses of lecithin, much lower amounts of choline (and fats) can be taken in convenient capsule form. Supplements don't easily become rancid.

Cons: Some people who take higher than average doses of choline develop a fishy smell to their body and breath. This is due to undigested choline reaching the large intestine, where bacteria metabolize it into the fishy-smelling compound trimethylamine. Dividing doses (consuming lesser amounts a number of times per day rather than a large dose all at once) or taking lower amounts avoids this side effect for most people.

Choline potency: Three common forms of choline have varying potency. Choline bitartrate is 42 percent choline. Choline chloride, usually the form used in liquid products, is 75 percent choline. Choline dihydrogencitrate, often a powder, is 36 percent choline.

Forms: Choline is available in powders, tablets, capsules, and liquids.

Dose: An average daily dose of choline bitartrate is 250 mg (yielding 105 mg of choline) to 500 mg (yielding 210 mg of choline).

Because of the slightly different actions that lecithin and phosphatidyl choline have compared to choline, some people are now taking both types of supplements. However you take your choline, it is a good idea to take it along with 25 to 50 mg of vitamin B_5 or B complex to improve choline's brain-boosting effects. Older people may benefit by taking slightly higher levels of choline supplements.

A convenient and increasingly popular way to consume choline is to take any of the many combination products now on the market. Nutrient producers often combine choline with vitamin B complex and other nutrients. Choline is also found in combination supplements that go by names like Memory Upgrade, Choline Cocktail, Choline Cooler, Memory Boost, and Memory Fuel. The choline content of these capsule products vary, and some include stimulants such as caffeine; check labels closely.

DMAE: THE CHOLINE SUBSTITUTE

DMAE, the abbreviation for di-methyl-amino-ethanol, is a compound that is structurally and chemically similar to choline. Actually, choline could be referred to as TMAE, since its extra methyl group makes the chemical name sometimes used for it tri-methyl-amino-ethanol. Like choline, DMAE occurs naturally in the body, both as a precursor and a metabolite of choline. DMAE is also found in tiny amounts in certain foods, particularly fish such as sardines. When it is consumed in food or taken in the form of a supplement, DMAE acts as a choline substitute. An early study on DMAE characterized it as a possible precursor of brain acetylcholine, and a number of other studies have confirmed that taking DMAE prompts the body to synthesize more choline. This causes an increase in blood levels and eventually brain levels of choline. By boosting choline concentrations, DMAE promotes the same acetylcholine-related behavioral effects, such as an increase in memory and brain function. DMAE also plays a role in the protection of cellular membranes and may have antioxidant properties that can help reduce deposits of the harmful pigment lipofuscin in the skin and brain.

As a supplement, DMAE is often used instead of, or in conjunction with, choline. One advantage DMAE has compared to choline is that DMAE transports more readily across the blood-brain barrier. Lacking phosphatidyl choline's bulky fatty acids, DMAE also beats it across the blood-brain barrier. Thus you can take lower doses of DMAE and gain similar benefits.

DMAE's brain-boosting action is frequently accompanied by a mild but noticeable stimulation of the central nervous system. The effect is not as profound as the fast-acting nervous system stimulants such as caffeine and ephedrine, but rather builds slowly over the course of weeks or months. In this regard it might be compared to the action of ginkgo or some of the tonic herbs. Over time, people notice that DMAE increases alertness and vigilance, boosts energy levels, and elevates mood. Many people now take it every day to prevent fatigue and aid concentration; some say it increases their ability to handle multiple tasks simultaneously and to learn new material. A few report intensified dreams. Because of positive effects on average life span and maximum life expectancy demonstrated on a strain of mice in a study done in 1973, some people are also taking DMAE as a potential longevity aid, though most researchers consider longevity-related claims for DMAE still unproven.

Deaner and Deanol

DMAE is sometimes used in the treatment of the central nervous system disorder tardive dyskinesia, but otherwise its current therapeutic applications are limited. From the 1950s until 1983, Riker Laboratories had FDA approval to market a DMAE-based prescription drug, trademarked Deaner (also known as deanol). Except for an attached acid, DMAE is chemically identical to Deaner, and equivalent doses of the substances have similar effects on the body. Doctors prescribed Deaner primarily for children who suffered from certain types of learning disabilities associated with behavioral problems and hyperactivity—what is now known as attention deficit disorder (ADD) and attention deficit hyperactivity disorder (ADHD). Deaner seemed to work well for many children as a less-toxic alternative to central nervous system stimulants such as amphetamine and methylphenidate (Ritalin), which can cause nausea, headache, weight loss, and other adverse side effects. Children taking DMAE seemed to fidget less and to be better able to concentrate on their work and to succeed academically.

A number of the studies indicating that Deaner helped to increase attention span and reduce the behavioral problems associated with hyperactivity had been done in the late 1950s. In the early 1980s the FDA decided that Riker needed to update Deaner's safety and efficacy research. The agency asked Riker to sponsor a new round of scientific studies to reconfirm Deaner's potential usefulness for learning disorders and thus maintain the drug's "approved-use" status. Riker apparently looked at the fact that a series of studies on DMAE and Deaner published in the late 1970s had raised questions about the compound's role as an acetylcholine precursor and Alzheimer's treatment; that the company would have to spend millions of dollars to conduct the required research over a number of years; and that the drug has a relatively small market and limited profit potential. In 1983 Riker decided to withdraw the drug from the U.S. market rather than proceed with the testing.

Deaner and other deanol products are still sold in other countries and can be mail-ordered to the United States (see "Ordering Supplements and Smart Drugs from Foreign Sources" in Resources). Many people also find DMAE to be similar in its effects to its chemical cousin, the smart-drug centrophenoxine (Lucidryl). Like Deaner, Lucidryl is not sold in the United States, so it presents the same purchasing disadvantages compared to DMAE: higher cost and the uncertainties of foreign mail order. One potential advantage drugs such as deanol and centrophenoxine may have compared to DMAE is more highly regulated production processes, though DMAE purchased from reputable sources should be high quality.

DMAE causes few side effects and has not demonstrated any long-term toxicity. The most common side effects are similar to those caused by stimulants: anxiety, nervousness, increased blood pressure, and insomnia. In a minority of people DMAE may also cause headaches, leg cramps, and muscle tension. High daily doses are more likely to cause adverse effects, though some people seem to be sensitive to DMAE and feel overstimulated even from average doses. DMAE is not addictive, though a few people have reported experiencing a loss of physical and mental energy when they've suddenly stopped taking it. To be on the safe side, pregnant or breast-feeding women, anyone who suffers from convulsions, epilepsy, or seizure disorders, and people with manic-depressive illness should avoid using DMAE.

DMAE is often used in combination with other nutrients, particularly choline and the B-complex vitamins pantothenic acid (B_5) and PABA, but also smart drugs such as piracetam (see chapter 9), amino acids such as phenyl-alanine and tyrosine (see chapter 6), and herbs such as ginkgo (see chapter 11). Lower average doses of DMAE are suggested if you are also taking any form of supplemental choline or any of the pharmaceutical smart drugs covered in chapter 9. Nutrient producers offer a range of DMAE-containing combination products with names like Mental Edge, Memory Mate, Extension I.Q., and Thinker's Edge.

Taking DMAE

It is necessary to examine product labels closely to determine the exact DMAE content of a DMAE supplement. The most common form of DMAE is DMAE bitartrate, which contains 37 percent DMAE and 63 percent tartaric acid. A typical capsule product labeled "100 mg DMAE" is usually 37 mg DMAE and 63 mg tartaric acid. The 100 mg bitartrate capsules are the most common DMAE product, though you can find capsules containing as much as 500 mg of DMAE bitartrate. DMAE also comes in powders and liquids.

DMAE's effects seem to vary considerably from one person to another. It is best to start with a low dose and increase it only if you need to and you experience no adverse effects. With advancing age, the body's acetylcholine levels are naturally lower, so dosage may be age-dependent. An average daily dose for those new to DMAE is 100 mg of DMAE bitartrate, providing 37 mg of DMAE. Those in the forty-to-sixty age range may find that 200 mg of DMAE bitartrate (74 mg of DMAE) works well, while the elderly may need 300 mg, providing 111 mg of DMAE. Some people work their way up to much higher doses, such as 250 to 350 mg of pure DMAE, and report increased alertness, energy levels, and ability to concentrate, while others find such high levels too stimulating.

The full brain-boosting effects of DMAE may not be apparent until after several weeks of daily use. A technique to "kick in the effects" of DMAE is to take a so-called attack dose of 400 to 500 mg for the first day or two of DMAE use, and then to cut back the dosage. This does increase the risk of side effects.

PYROGLUTAMATE: THE AMINO SMART DRUG

Pyroglutamate is an amino acid found in meats, vegetables, and fruits. From these and other foods (or as a supplement) pyroglutamate is absorbed into the bloodstream and becomes concentrated in the cerebrospinal fluid. Pyroglutamate also crosses the blood-brain barrier and is naturally present in large amounts in the brain. There it functions as a piracetamlike nootropic. These substances' similarity in function is due to a close chemical resemblance—both pyroglutamate and piracetam are pyrrolidone compounds. People who have taken pyroglutamate often report that they notice an increase in alertness and concentration and an improvement in memory and overall mental performance without any adverse reactions.

Pyroglutamate has not been as extensively studied as piracetam. A few studies, however, have shown brain-boosting effects on animals and humans. For example, in a 1988 study researchers showed that a pyroglutamate compound improved memory and learning capacities in old rats. Also, a 1990 double-blind, placebo-controlled study done on forty elderly humans found that after two months subjects with age-related memory decline who took pyroglutamic acid experienced an improvement in some verbal memory functions. Another human study, done in 1985, determined that pyroglutamate can reduce alcohol-induced memory deficits. Italian researchers who have studied pyroglutamate have also found that it can benefit persons suffering from depression and low mood.

Part of pyroglutamate's brain-boosting property may be due to an effect on acetylcholine levels. A 1984 study done on guinea pigs showed that pyroglutamic acid increased the brain's release of acetylcholine and GABA, and a 1987 study done on rats also found that a pyroglutamate compound boosted brain acetylcholine levels and had some "cognition-enhancing properties."

The big advantage that pyroglutamate enjoys over piracetam is that, as a naturally occurring amino acid, pyroglutamate is regulated by the U.S. government as a nutritional supplement rather than a drug. This is in spite of the fact that in high doses pyroglutamate has arguably druglike effects. Because the FDA has not approved any medical uses for piracetam, it is not sold in the United States and interested users must purchase it from for-eign mail-order sources. Pyroglutamate is not widely available in North American natural foods stores, but it can be found; it can also be mail-ordered.

Pyroglutamate may have other compounds attached to it and is sold under a variety of names, including pyroglutamic acid, pyrrolidon carboxylic acid (PCA), and arginine pyroglutamate. Pyroglutamate is also included in some brain-boosting nutritional formulations, with names such as Higher Mind, 4-Thought, Deep Thought, and Memory Boost.

Taking Pyroglutamate

Pyroglutamate and its close relatives come in tablets and capsules (usually 500 or 1,000 mg) and in powders from a number of smart drug and amino acid producers (see Resources). An average dose is 500 mg once or twice daily. For increased effect, combine with choline, DMAE, or other nutrients that enhance acetylcholine production.

Ginkgo

◉

THE MIND AND MOOD HERB

Ginkgo is currently one of the most popular medicines of any type, herbal or otherwise, in much of Europe, especially France and Germany. It is also rapidly gaining widespread acceptance in North America. People who suffer from a variety of conditions, as well as many normal, healthy people, are starting to take ginkgo regularly to promote better brain function, boost energy levels, and smooth out everyday mood swings. The elderly in particular find that ginkgo can help to slow down memory loss and improve mental performance. Thankfully, ginkgo increases concentration and alertness without providing the sudden jolt to the central nervous system typical of caffeine and potent stimulants. Rather, ginkgo manages to prevent fatigue while promoting a long-term increase in energy.

Like green tea, ginkgo also offers some important health benefits beyond its effects on mind and mood that make it particularly attractive as a natural substance. Ginkgo acts as an antioxidant to neutralize certain free rad-

icals, harmful molecules that can increase the risk of disease. Ginkgo dilates blood vessels and increases blood circulation, not only to the brain but to the ears (where it can help prevent hearing loss), to the extremities (where it can prevent vascular diseases such as claudication, from a narrowing of the arteries of the legs due to atherosclerosis), and to the sex organs (where it can prevent impotence and improve sexual function). Studies have shown that ginkgo extracts can inhibit platelet-activating factor (PAF), a bodily substance that affects the ability of blood particles to stick together and is suspected of playing a crucial role in some of the most common diseases of modern society, such as asthma, stroke, and heart disease. Ginkgo protects the body from aging-related brain dysfunctions and quite possibly as well from aging-related vision problems, such as macular degeneration.

Combine these positive benefits with a remarkable safety record—ginkgo appears to be among the least toxic medical substances known—and it is no surprise that more and more people are turning to this herb for its healthful effects.

Few plants have been as successful as the ginkgo tree in surviving the changing conditions on earth over the past 150 to 200 million years. Around the end of the Jurassic period, when the dinosaurs were at their zenith and the first small mammals that would eventually evolve into humans made an appearance, *Ginkgo biloba* trees (also known as maidenhair trees, from some European's myopic association of the tree with the maidenhair fern) were dropping their distinctive fan-shaped leaves and creating a fossil record. Obviously something in the tree's unique chemistry has helped it to become a "living fossil." Not only has the species (which is the oldest living tree species, and the only living member of its genus, family, and order) survived almost unchanged for millions of years, but individual ginkgo trees have lived a millennium or longer. Actually, the plant's closest brush with extinction may have come just recently, when at the end of the last ice age ginkgos were wiped out everywhere except in a few remote parts of Asia.

That the species managed to hold on is a boon for humanity, for ginkgo has proven to be a valuable herb in the estimated five thousand years of its medicinal use. Herbalists in ancient China regarded ginkgo as a digestive aid and a remedy for various conditions, including intestinal worms and bladder disor-

ders. Practitioners of the ancient medicine of India were also familiar with ginkgo and used it in formulas meant to promote longevity. Ginkgo trees were introduced to Japan about a thousand years ago—and a few of these ancient imports may still be living today.

The tree and the herb seem to have been unknown to Europeans until the early eighteenth century. The first Westerner to describe ginkgo was the peripatetic German doctor Engelbert Kaempfer (1651–1716). In the early 1690s he spent two years in Japan collecting information on various natural sciences. In a work published in 1712, he mentioned the Japanese *ginkyo* tree. This name was perhaps a misspelling or transliteration of the original Chinese word *yinkuo,* for "hill apricot" (a reference to the tree's fruit). Ginkgo trees are thought to have been first introduced as exotics to Europe around 1730 and to England in the mid-1750s. Linnaeus gave the Latin name *Ginkgo biloba* to the plant in 1771—*biloba* because the leaves look vaguely like the human brain, being bi-lobed. The first ginkgo tree did not arrive in North America until shortly after the Revolutionary War, when one was introduced as an ornamental to a garden near Philadelphia.

Although ginkgo trees have been known to Westerners for almost three centuries, the herb has not been accepted as a potentially therapeutic substance until relatively recently. An important advance was the identification in the 1930s of flavonoids in the leaves. Another breakthrough came only within the past twenty-five years, when European plant scientists developed a potent leaf extract. The slow progress of ginkgo's transition from

Eastern to Western medicine may have been due in part to the fact that practitioners of traditional Chinese medicine valued ginkgo fruits, which grow on female trees, and the nuts inside the fruits, more than they did the leaf. The Chinese used these other parts of the ginkgo tree (often in combination with other herbs) to help treat conditions ranging from coughs to vaginal infections. The Chinese as well as the Japanese also make culinary use of ginkgo fruits and nuts. Ginkgo fruits, however, are very pungent, if not rancid, smelling. Westerners generally find them offensive. Also, the fruits contain a chemical substance that can cause a rash if it comes in contact with the skin. In Europe as well as North America, the fruitless male trees were favored to the females in gardens and for use as shade trees to line streets, and this disdain for ginkgo fruit may have delayed the medical recognition of the herb.

Ginkgo leaf preparations, it should be noted, were not unknown to the ancient Chinese. One ancient record apparently acknowledges the leaves' ability to "benefit the brain." The ancient Chinese also recommended ginkgo leaf tea as an asthma remedy.

Today's ginkgo preparations represent a synthesis of traditional East and high-tech West. Almost all of the ginkgo preparations used in studies and sold in natural foods stores are standardized extracts, derived from the dried green leaves in a process developed by German researchers. The raw material comes not only from Far East sources but from the United States—a large South Carolina ginkgo plantation sends ginkgo leaves to Europe for processing into standardized extracts. Human-

ity has been both a bane and a boon to the ginkgo tree. Encroachment of the species' native habitat has probably rendered the tree extinct as a truly wild plant but medicinal acceptance—and the tree's longevity, ability to resist insects, and overall vigor as an urban shade tree—has ensured a viable future for the ginkgo.

Plant scientists adjust ginkgo extracts so that typically the final herbal product has a potency of 24 percent of certain flavonoid compounds known as "flavoglycosides." (Product labels may also refer to these flavonoid compounds as "flavone glycosides" or "ginkgo-heterosides.") In addition, producers typically standardize extract products for 6 percent of certain complex terpene compounds, such as bilobalide and one or more of the ginkgolides (identified as ginkgolide A, B, C, and M), that are apparently found nowhere else in the plant kingdom. Scientists have recently managed to synthetically reproduce the ginkgolides, and some studies now focus on the potential therapeutic effects of the individual ginkgo compounds. The multicomponent standardized extract, however, is thought to be more active than any of its single compounds. In addition to its standardized components, ginkgo is known to contain organic acids, carotenoids, sterols, and other compounds. A 1996 study, in fact, found that a "nonginkgolide non-flavonoid fraction" was the ginkgo compound with the most dramatic effect on the function of the corpus cavernosa, two cylindrical bodies of spongy tissue in the penis that cause an erection when engorged with blood. This fraction may thereby play an important role in one of the mechanisms responsible for ginkgo's mild prosexual effects and its potential in helping to prevent or treat impotence.

Standardized ginkgo leaf extracts are now common drugs worldwide, where total annual sales are estimated to be in excess of one billion dollars. In Europe, some products are sold by prescription while others are over-the-counter. Among the most respected standardized ginkgo products is the one known as EGb 761, which was developed by the W. Schwabe Company of Germany. This formula, which is sold as Rökan in France and as Tebonin in Germany, is the one most often used in clinical studies of ginkgo.

MANY POSITIVE EFFECTS

Standardized ginkgo extracts have been extensively researched in the past twenty years, with published studies now numbering in the many hundreds worldwide. Researchers say that ginkgo extracts' ability to stimulate circulation in the brain and ears may help prevent dizziness, hearing loss, headache, and tinnitus. Studies indicate ginkgo has potential use in the treatment of impotence, varicose veins and other circulatory conditions, and Alzheimer's disease. Ginkgo has also been found to delay the deterioration of cognitive function and improve short-term memory. In a 1992 article published in the respected British medical journal *The Lancet,* researchers determined that, of eight clinical trials for cerebral insufficiency (lack of blood flow to the brain, which has been tied to memory loss, hearing prob-

lems, and other conditions) that were judged to be well controlled, seven showed positive effects for ginkgo.

A similar article, published in an issue of a French medical journal in 1986 that devoted a number of articles to ginkgo research, concluded that ginkgo extract "seems to be effective in patients with vascular disorders, in all types of dementia, and even in patients suffering from cognitive disorders secondary to depression, because of its beneficial effects on mood." Another study in the same journal described the results of a double-blind, placebo-controlled trial done on healthy young women. Researcher Ian Hindmarch found that ginkgo extract significantly improved the volunteers' short-term memory. "These results differentiate *Ginkgo biloba* extract from sedative and stimulant drugs and suggest a specific effect on memory processes," he concluded.

The authors of a 1989 study on the effects of ginkgo extract on patients suffering from Parkinson's disease noted that "the efficacy of the *Ginkgo biloba* extract was not only found clinically or in standardized ratings but also documented by objective data, obtained by a computerized EEG method." They concluded that ginkgo "seems to be a substance with a broad spectrum of influence." A 1985 study published in a German journal found that ginkgo was responsible for a clear improvement in mental alertness and reaction time among elderly subjects who showed higher-than-average levels of mental deterioration for their age. In a 1994 study of forty patients with Alzheimer-type senile dementia, researchers documented significant improvements in memory, attention, and other aspects of mental and psychomotor performance among the subjects who took 80 mg of a ginkgo extract three times daily. Improvements were noticeable after one month and continued to occur until the end of the three-month trial. A 1995 study that was double-blind and placebo-controlled determined that men and women in their fifties, sixties, and seventies who were suffering from age-associated memory impairment (AAMI) became quicker at processing auditory information after taking a ginkgo extract daily for two months. Numerous other well-designed studies have confirmed that ginkgo can help improve aspects of AAMI.

Ginkgo's ability to improve mood and brain function has been tied to various actions on the body. Researchers have found that ginkgo improves blood flow in both arteries and veins, including the tiniest capillaries far from the heart. Ginkgo's stimulating effect on blood circulation in the brain helps to deliver more oxygen to brain cells, protecting the organ from adverse effects of oxygen deficiency. Ginkgo also helps the brain obtain and use greater amounts of its primary fuel, glucose. Ginkgo promotes the body's production of the compound adenosine triphosphate, which is necessary for energy at the cellular level. As a potent antioxidant, ginkgo scavenges free radicals (especially the superoxide radical) that could otherwise damage cell membranes and impair brain function. Ginkgo is also thought to increase nerve transmission, protect serotonin and acetylcholine function, and promote brain waves of a frequency associated with alertness. Most recently, a 1996

study done on rats found that a ginkgo extract could inhibit monoamine oxidase (MAO), the enzyme that breaks down neurotransmitters in the brain. MAO inhibitors can thus elevate mood and reduce anxiety. (Human studies are unlikely to show that ginkgo is potent enough as an MAO inhibitor to cause the adverse effects sometimes associated with conventional MAO inhibitors; see the discussion of MAO inhibition in the section on St. John's wort's action in chapter 7.)

AN ADMIRABLE SAFETY RECORD

Ginkgo extracts have been thoroughly tested for safety and found to be nontoxic even at doses well beyond average. Long-term use has not been shown to cause any major side effects, nor have any adverse impacts on the liver or kidney. The aforementioned 1992 analysis in *The Lancet* found no serious side effects in any trial, as well as no known drug interactions. One study of more than 8,500 patients who took ginkgo for six months revealed the astonishingly low rate of 0.4 percent of the subjects reporting minor side effects, mostly mild upset stomach. In another study of almost 3,000 patients taking ginkgo extract, 3.7 percent experienced minor gastric upset. Ginkgo caused no lasting adverse effects when subjects discontinued its use.

If you want to harvest the leaves (a good time is in the early fall, just as they begin to turn from green to yellow in color) to make your own extract or leaf tea, find the fruitless male trees (which are more common in North America anyway) or avoid directly touching the fruits, which can cause irritation.

TAKING GINKGO

Ginkgo comes in tablets, capsules, concentrated drops, tinctures, and extracts. A popular brand-name ginkgo product in North America is Ginkgold, the same formulation developed by Schwabe and used in many of the clinical studies. Most of the major North American herbal producers offer a similar if not exactly identical standardized extract product. Ginkgo is readily available in health food and natural foods stores, and even pharmacies in North America. Ginkgo is also an ingredient in many brain-boosting herbal and nutrient combination formulas with names like Higher Mind and Brain Alert.

An average dose is 40 mg three times daily of a standardized extract containing a minimum 24 percent flavonoids. People over age fifty may consider taking 60 mg three times daily for extra protection against the adverse effects of aging.

Most people find that they need to take ginkgo every day for a number of months before full effects are felt, though some people report benefits within two to three weeks. Ginkgo researchers have reported that results are more obvious and lasting the longer the treatment is continued. It is safe and probably most effective when taken on a daily basis indefinitely.

Peppermint, Basil, and Rosemary

⊚

STIMULATING ESSENTIAL OILS FOR MIND AND BODY

Three plants in the Lamiaceae or mint family are among those that aromatherapists most often recommend to energize the body and maximize mental performance: Peppermint, Basil, and Rosemary. Much of the evidence for these oils' stimulating effects is anecdotal and folkloric, yet a few scientific studies have begun to link common compounds with potentially mind-altering effects. For example, a 1994 study published in *Chemical Senses* tested the effects of inhaling cineole on healthy human subjects. Cineole is a liquid compound found in high amounts in the essential oil of Eucalyptus but also in Peppermint, Basil, and Rosemary. Researchers found that cineole caused an increase in blood flow to various regions of the brain.

Another study published in the same journal later in 1994 was among the first to assess the effect of odor specifically on learning. Volunteers were given maze-solving problems while wearing either a floral-scented or an unscented mask. Researchers found that subjects who considered the floral smell pleasant learned to complete the tasks 17 percent faster on average with the scented mask on compared to when they wore the unscented mask. The researchers concluded, "These findings imply that future studies may validate the use of odors as adjuvants to learning and education, as well as rehabilitation."

Peppermint, Basil, and Rosemary are widely available as single oils, or you can purchase combination products that typically include one or more of these essential oils plus a few others known for their stimulating effects. Look for products with names like Concentrate, Focus, Creativity, Mental Power, Clear Mind, Clarity, Inspiration, and Brain-Dead. Many of these are available as oils and aromatic mists for diffusing, and lotions for massage or other topical application. Some are also available as a smelling salt for direct inhalation.

See chapter 8 for background information on essential oils, including the best ways to store and to take them.

PEPPERMINT: A TASTE OF STIMULATION

Modern peppermint (*Mentha piperita*) is a cultivated hybrid that is thought to be only about three hundred years old. Herbalists in ancient Egypt and China used close mint relatives for many of the same purposes we use peppermint today: as a digestive remedy to treat indigestion, nausea, diarrhea, flatulence, and cramps. Like chamomile, peppermint is popular both as an herb and as an essential oil. Much of the cultivated crop (the United States is a major grower, with the Northwest accounting for the bulk of the crop) is steam-distilled into the very light yellow essential oil. Only a tiny percentage, of course, of the essential oil is used medicinally, as the toothpaste and chewing gum industries require large amounts of Peppermint oil for flavoring purposes.

Fifty percent or more of the essential oil is menthol, an alcohol that has a cooling effect when it is taken into the mouth with air or applied to the skin. Menthol is used in topical creams such as Ben-Gay to help relieve itching and the minor aches and pains of muscles and joints. Menthol's cooling effect on the skin can be so pronounced that you should avoid putting Peppermint oil over more than a small patch of skin at a time. A 1995 double-blind, placebo-controlled study indicated Peppermint oil rubbed into the forehead may be an effective tension-headache treatment capable of relaxing muscles and relieving pain. The oil is also a good insect repellent.

Most people find Peppermint oil to be mildly stimulating to the nervous system and overall circulation when inhaled. It clears the mind, helps to increase alertness, and promotes the ability to focus on mental work. The technical text *Science of Olfaction* includes a report from two researchers who found that the odor of Peppermint can improve the performance of stressful visual tasks.

Though essential oils are not generally taken internally, except with the direct supervision of an experienced aromatherapist, you can take Peppermint in the form of lozenges. Many peppermint candies and lozenges have little if any Peppermint essential oil, but higher quality products exist. For example, Aromatherapy Peppermints, made from only organic cane juice, gum tragacanth, and Peppermint essential oil, are cool and potent (see Resources).

BASIL: THE KING OF PLANTS

This is a large group of annual herbs of the mint family, especially one species (*Ocimum basilicum*) whose aromatic leaves have long been used as a culinary spice in many traditions. The name *basil* is derived from the Greek *basileus,* for king. This royal or "king of plants" had a variety of medicinal uses, not only for the ancient Greeks but in China, India, and parts of Africa. It was recommended in the treatment of colds, bronchitis, digestive complaints, and menstrual problems. Some considered it an aphrodisiac and a circulatory stimulant. Originating in tropical Asia, basil is now widely cultivated throughout the world.

Chemists produce the essential oil by steam-distilling both the leaves and the flowering tops of the plant. The result is a pale yellowish or greenish oil whose fresh, herbal scent has a hint of camphor. Some people associate the fragrance with food dishes that are typically spiced with basil; if you don't like these foods you may not like using the essential oil.

Modern aromatherapists often recommend Basil as a type of inhalable "smart drug" for keeping the mind fresh and energized. Basil is used to increase concentration and strengthen mental function. "It clears the head, relieves intellectual fatigue, and gives the mind strength and clarity," said aromatherapist Marguerite Maury. Some people find that it sharpens the senses, keeps the mind open, and improves memory. Others use it to bolster the nervous system and reduce anxiety, nervousness, and depression.

Basil has the potential to cause adverse effects among some of those who use it.

- -
ROSEMARY: FOR NERVES AND MEMORY
- -

A small evergreen shrub (*Rosmarinus officinalis*) native to the Mediterranean region, rosemary is one of humanity's earliest medicinal plants. The ancient Egyptians and Greeks regarded it as a sacred plant, and it has long been associated with love, death, and remem-

brance. In ancient Greece, rosemary garlands were worn by students to improve memory, and sprigs of rosemary were tossed into graves to ensure remembrance of the dead. Similar associations and practices, such as decorating funerals and weddings with the herb, survived into Shakespeare's England: "There's Rosemary, that's for remembrance: pray, love, remember," Ophelia says in *Hamlet*. Traditional healers from Greece and elsewhere also recognized rosemary as an effective remedy for problems of the liver, circulatory system, and digestion. Perhaps rosemary's most popular use, however, has been to restore a weakened nervous system and revive those who are tired either mentally or physically. It has been used as an herb, in a stimulating tonic wine, and as a scent to alleviate mental fatigue, treat depression, and cure nervous exhaustion.

The flowering tops of the rosemary plant, including its slender, gray-green leaves and tiny, pale blue flowers, are steam-distilled to make the essential oil. The almost colorless oil often has a pleasant minty aroma with undertones of either camphor or eucalyptus. Aromatherapists account for a tiny percentage of the oil's use—most of it is used as a culinary flavoring (such as in meat dishes), an ingredient in perfumes, liniments, and body-care products, and in potpourris and herb pillows. Much of the recent research has focused on apparent antioxidant properties of Rosemary, though a 1987 study found that mice experienced increased physical activity after either inhaling or being given oral doses of the essential oil.

Rosemary's long association with remembrance, and its reputation as a potent nerve tonic, have made the essential oil popular as an enhancer of mental functions and a stimulant for the nervous system. Rosemary invigorates the mind, increases alertness and concentration, and improves memory. It also boosts the spirits and helps to prevent depression. "Rosemary oil can help you cope with stressful conditions and see things from a clearer perspective," says Roberta Wilson, author of *Aromatherapy for Vibrant Health & Beauty.* "It relaxes nerves and restores nerve health, especially after long-term nervous or physical ailments."

Pregnant women should avoid using Rosemary.

PART FIVE

Relaxants

Valerian

◉

NATURE'S VALIUM

Valerian may well be America's break-through herb of the twenty-first century. Because it is relatively safe and effective, and fills a medical niche currently occupied by more toxic substances, it is poised to be the first important mind-altering herb that makes the jump from the limited health food market directly to the mainstream over-the-counter drugstore market. Granted, a half-dozen or so therapeutic herbs, including garlic, the laxative senna, and witch hazel, have already made a similar jump. But the only other widely accepted herb with prominent mind-altering properties, ephedra, is accepted *in spite of* its psychoactive properties—and these very properties may even cause it to be regulated out of circulation (see chapter 4). Valerian is a mild sedative and relaxant that is arguably superior in its benefits to any currently available over-the-counter product of similar purpose. If objective, scientific evidence were the main criterion for determining the best available relaxant and sleep aid, valerian would become as widely accepted in the United States as aspirin. It is quite possible that, within the next two decades, this will happen.

THE PUNGENT ROOT

The genus *Valeriana* includes more than two hundred species of plants growing in temperate areas of both the Northern and Southern hemispheres. Though many of these species have similar properties, the species that is most often used by Western herbalists is *Valeriana officinalis,* which is native to Europe and was transported to the New World by early settlers. A hardy and adaptable plant, it soon escaped colonists' gardens and spread as a wild plant. Naturalized *Valeriana officinalis* now grows in much of the northern United States and southern Canada. In addition, more than a dozen other species of valerian can be found in California and other western states.

Valerian is a perennial that reaches four or five feet in height and generates small white or pink flowers. The psychoactive parts of the plant are the many intertwining roots and rhizome, or underground stem. When the rootstock is harvested, it has only a slight odor. Upon drying, however, valerian takes on a powerful and musty odor. Most people liken the odor to smelly socks, while a few profess to find it pleasantly earthy. Cats like the odor and will play with a valerian-soaked toy as if it were treated with catnip—some cat owners say valerian makes cats too crazy. (Rodents may also like valerian—early retellings of the legend of the Pied Piper credit valerian along with music as the reason he was able to charm the rats into following him out of Hamelin.) Four hundred years ago people used valerian to perfume their clothes, probably an indication not that valerian's odor has worsened since then but that the level of overall hygiene has improved. Gangsters were at one time said to use valerian to make stink bombs as part of their attempts to extort protection money from restaurants.

Despite its strong odor, valerian has a palatable taste when brewed as a tea.

"THE VALIUM OF THE NINETEENTH CENTURY"

Little is known about the earliest uses of valerian. Even the origin of its English name, first used about a thousand years ago, is unclear. The most likely theories are that valerian comes from the Latin *valere,* to be healthy or well; that it derives from *valeo,* to be strong, referring either to its rejuvenating qualities or to the smell of the root; that it is named after a Roman herbalist named Valerius or the Roman emperor Valerianus; or that it refers to the Roman province Valeria, where it may have grown. Greek healers around the time of Christ referred to valerian as *phu,* which has the same derivation as the common expression still used to describe something smelly: phew!

Hippocrates (460–370 B.C.E.) and other early Greek physicians apparently used valerian for a variety of ailments. Some of these ancient uses (particularly as a remedy to soothe digestive ailments) have survived into modern times, while others (a treatment for urinary tract disorders, an epilepsy remedy) have been supplanted. Surprisingly, early references to valerian's appropriateness as a sedative and muscle relaxant are rare, all the way from ancient Greece (though Galen does mention it) to the end of the Middle Ages (the twelfth-century German folk herbalist Hildegard of Bingen is a notable exception). A prominent Italian herbal writer of the early seventeenth century extolled valerian for curing his epilepsy, inspiring renewed investigation and use of the herb. Valerian slowly began to be recognized as the premier herb for calming the body, relaxing muscles, and promoting sleep.

For much of the eighteenth and nineteenth centuries, valerian was indispensable as a treatment for various types of nervous conditions, not only insomnia but also anxiety, nervous headache, panic, exhaustion, and hysteria. Doctors often recommended it to women who suffered from overall nervousness or from two quasi-hypochondriacal conditions that were favorite diagnoses in the nineteenth century but have since gone out of medical favor: neurasthenia (a type of emotionally induced exhaustion of the nervous system) and "the vapors" (melancholy or depressed spirits). The association between women, nervous conditions, and valerian was so strong that valerian has been called the "Valium of the nineteenth century."

Valerian lasted longer than most herbs as an "official drug" among pharmaceutical companies and national pharmacopoeias, which in the past century have switched over almost entirely from natural to synthetic products. Valerian was an official remedy in the *U.S. Pharmacopoeia* from 1820 to 1936 and in the *National Formulary* from 1888 to 1946. As late as World War II it was still sometimes used as a remedy for shell shock or "bombing neurosis." Eli Lilly continued to market valerian tincture until 1985. Valerian remains a "generally recognized as safe" food additive in the United States, where tiny amounts of extracts are used to flavor some processed foods. At one time cooks used valerian as a spice for soups and other dishes.

As an official drug valerian has fared much better in most European countries, where it continues to be listed in the national pharmacopoeias of France, Germany, Italy, and Switzerland and is used to produce over-the-counter sleep remedies. German pharmacies offer more than one hundred valerian-based products, representing sales in the tens of millions of dollars. Furthermore, the influential German Commission E (made up of doctors, pharmacists, toxicologists, and others who as a body regulate the country's use of herbs as medicines) lists valerian as an approved safe-and-effective sleep aid. France and Great Britain also represent bustling valerian markets. Valerian has even attracted the attention of researchers at Nestlé, the giant Swiss-based food company, who have been trying to neutralize the odor and create a calming, sedating drink.

Today, valerian is in the top rank of herbal substances worldwide. While it may not be threatening to overtake Valium anytime soon in the United States, it has many qualities that make it a better remedy for anxiety and sleeplessness.

"STRONG AND SURE OF EFFECT"

Valerian is the ideal herbal remedy for a number of ailments, primarily including nervous conditions related to anxiety, tension, or stress. It works well as a nerve tonic for people who suffer from nervous exhaustion, panic attacks, and emotional disturbances. It also serves as a pain-relieving agent for conditions such as tension-related headaches. Of course, it is an invaluable insomnia remedy, though most herbalists don't consider valerian a classic hypnotic (a substance, such as any of the barbiturates, say, that in sufficient doses quickly causes sleep). Rather, valerian is a "minor tranquilizer" or relaxant that calms anxiety and thereby *allows* or *encourages* sleep, as opposed to directly inducing it. Valerian is "above all a sedative, strong and sure of effect," notes herbalist Michael Moore, author of *Medicinal Plants of the Pacific West*.

Much of the scientific research that has been conducted on valerian in recent decades (an estimated two hundred papers have been published in technical journals worldwide) has focused on the root's complex chemistry. Although a smaller percentage of the research has been in the form of double-blind clinical trials and well-controlled studies, those that have been conducted have tended to confirm that valerian has valuable sedative and muscle-relaxing properties. Some of the most notable studies include the following:

■ In a 1980 controlled clinical trial on forty patients, Italian researchers found valerian to work better than a placebo at relieving minor anxiety and emotional tension.

■ In a 1982 double-blind study on 128 subjects, a group of Nestlé researchers found that valerian extracts significantly improved sleep quality, especially among women who were poor sleepers. Valerian also helped to shorten sleep latency (the time it takes to fall asleep).

■ In studies done in 1984 and 1985 by some of the same researchers, valerian extracts were found to reduce sleep latency and improve the sleep quality of those suffering from mild insomnia. Their findings led these researchers to rate valerian's effectiveness as a sleep aid as similar to small doses of barbiturates or benzodiazepines, with the advantages of greater safety, fewer side effects, and less morning grogginess.

■ In a 1987 study, Russian researchers found that valerian reduced the motor activity of caffeine-drugged mice and rats.

Valerian's success as a mild sedative and minor tranquilizer in studies such as these has led numerous researchers—and even more herbalists—to term it a Valium substitute. The obvious similarity in name (though the drug's developers may have chosen "Valium" to remind consumers of Librium, which it hoped to—and did—surpass in popularity and sales) has caused some confusion among newcomers to herbs. "Valerian is the parent of Valium, isn't it?" queried one person in an on-line forum. To clarify, valerian and Valium are not chemically related. Valium is the trade name for a generic synthetic chemical, diazepam, that is classified as a benzodiazepine. Benzodiazepines are widely prescribed as minor tranquilizers for the relief of anxiety or stress; in larger doses they cause drowsiness and can help relieve insomnia. Valium is a more potent drug than valerian, with more apparent adverse side effects and greater potential for abuse. Neither substance should be used when alertness is crucial, such as while driving, though valerian is not usually so soporific in its effects that it interferes with motor function or induces sleep when the person is trying to remain awake.

IN SEARCH OF ACTIVE COMPOUNDS

Valerian is an interesting example of an ongoing debate within the herbal world concerning the pros and cons of using the whole herb versus certain of the herb's compounds that have been identified, extracted, concentrated, and standardized as its "active ingredients." Defenders of the whole-herb approach note that many herbal compounds often work synergistically, offering a more effective action on the body than any single, isolated chemical. Defenders of standardized extracts contend that there are many advantages to using only those single chemical components that have been conclusively proven to have the desired effects, particularly with regard to consistent manufacturing and dosaging.

Valerian offers some ammunition for proponents of both camps. Like many herbs, it is a complex chemical soup with more than one hundred components identified so far. Prominent in this group are small amounts of alkaloids, essential oil, fatty acids, flavonoids, amino acids, tannins, and choline. The alkaloids first attracted the attention of researchers because alkaloids (from caffeine to morphine) derived from other plants have proved to have strong effects on the mind. During the first half of the twentieth century, researchers discovered and isolated a number of alkaloids in valerian. These alkaloids didn't demonstrate much biological activity, however, and researchers soon shifted their focus to two of the plant's constituents:

■ The essential oil, present in the dried root up to 2 percent. This volatile liquid itself is complex, containing resins, the alcohol borneol, and various hydrocarbon compounds known as terpenes (such as pinene and limo-

lene). The three components of the essential oil that researchers have focused on recently are valerenic acid, valeranone, and valerenal. When the essential oil dries, chemicals within yield valerian's notable odor.

■ A mixture of highly unstable compounds unique to valerian, known as valepotriates, which like the essential oil naturally occur in the root in amounts only up to about 2 percent. Two major valepotriates are valtrate and isovaltrate. (To complicate matters further, chemicals that form in the body when the valepotriates break down may also have therapeutic effects.)

After giving up on the alkaloids, researchers next turned their attention to analyzing and testing the volatile oil and the valepotriates. Chemists began to isolate the valepotriates in 1966 and later developed synthetic derivatives. A number of valerian studies over the next fifteen years found that both the essential oil and the valepotriates, as well as certain isolated components derived from one or the other (such as valerenic acid), are indeed pharmacologically active as sedatives or muscle relaxants. Researchers continued to focus closely on individual components, trying to determine if valerian's prominent relaxant effects could be reduced to a single chemical, and some herbal producers began to standardize valerian products to valepotriates or essential oil content.

There the matter stood until 1981, when the prevailing wisdom about the source of valerian's activity began to shift. In that year researchers found that water extracts, which did not contain valepotriates, as they are non-soluble in water, also showed sedative activity. Seven years later, a more forceful challenge appeared in the form of a convincing animal study published in a German journal. The researchers, J. Krieglstein and D. Grusla, found that rats that were given the whole herb were sedated. Surprisingly, however, lab animals were not affected when they were fed any of a dozen components of either the essential oil or the valepotriates. Varro E. Tyler, Ph.D., author of *The Honest Herbal,* offers the latest best guess for explaining valerian's actions: "Possibly a combination of volatile oil components, valepotriates or their derivatives, and as-yet unidentified water-soluble constituents is responsible." He has noted elsewhere that valerenic acid content "is considered to be the best quality parameter for the drug."

Whatever the active ingredient or ingredients, the direct effect from taking valerian is a depression of some parts of the central nervous system and a relaxation of certain muscles, especially those in the uterus, colon, and bronchial passages.

Exactly how valerian causes these effects is still being determined. The most likely potential mechanism relates to valerian's interaction in the brain with either serotonin or with gamma aminobutyric acid (GABA), both of which are neurotransmitters that play an important role in mood, relaxation, and sleep. The ability to affect GABA levels also happens to be the mode of action for the minor tranquilizers known as benzodiazepines (Valium, Xanax). Recent findings indicate that valerian may work by a slightly different route than the benzodiazepines, which are thought to directly stimulate GABA receptors. Valerian compounds may block or inactivate the enzyme that breaks down GABA, indirectly increasing GABA levels. Compared to the benzodiazepine action, valerian's mechanism may actually allow for a prolonged sedative effect.

Chemists' inability to untangle the threads of valerian's therapeutic compounds and mechanisms of action has caused valerian supplement producers to change their formulations of the herb. Today, many valerian producers use the whole herb or standardize their extracts for tiny percentages of essential oil or valerenic acid. Fewer products are now being standardized for valepotriates, for a number of reasons. One is that, as we've seen, valepotriates may account for some but not all of valerian's effects. Another reason is that valepotriates are so unstable that levels in the finished product are unreliable a few months after production. (In addition to being unstable in the products, valepotriates are not well absorbed in the body.) A final, crucial factor is that a few studies have raised health concerns about certain valepotriates. Experiments done on cell cultures found that high concentrations—beyond naturally occurring levels—of certain valepotriates can cause cell mutations, potentially leading to cancer in organs such as the stomach and liver. Some valerian producers have even removed the valepotriates from their products, citing the possibility of harm from long-term consumption of concentrated valerian extracts with high levels of valepotriates. Subsequent studies, however, have not confirmed the finding of cellular damage.

For example, a 1994 rat study of prolonged administration of valepotriates on mothers and their offspring found no evidence of teratogenic or carcinogenic potential. "No toxicity has ever been demonstrated in intact animals or human beings, so there is no cause for concern," Tyler concludes.

As one of its early names, *all heal,* indicates, valerian has long been recognized as a multipurpose herbal remedy. Among its most popular uses beyond sedation are to:

- Relax muscles, reduce joint tension, and alleviate cramps (you can apply it topically to back spasms or muscle cramps by soaking a pad in the tincture and applying as a compress)
- Soothe the digestive system and relieve some types of indigestion, constipation, irritable bowel, and stomach cramps, especially those that may be due to excess nervous tension
- Relieve pain, especially headaches and other pains due to tension
- Lower high blood pressure, often in combination with other herbs, such as hawthorn (*Crataegus laevigata*)
- Relieve cough, often in combination with other expectorants such as licorice (*Glycyrrhiza glabra*)
- Prevent altitude sickness (a Russian study indicated that valerian may help protect the body from the effects of reduced oxygen supply)
- Help overcome addiction to antidepressants and other drugs (valerian tea is recommended in some drug rehabilitation programs, and people have successfully used it as a mild antidepressant that helps break the smoking habit)

Many women in particular have become fans of valerian. According to herbologist Rosemary Gladstar, author of *Herbal Healing for Women,* "Sometimes called moon root and Undine's herb, valerian has a special affinity with women. Because of its muscle-relaxant properties, it is an excellent treatment for alleviating menstrual tension and stress. Combined with cramp bark [*Viburnum opulus*], it effectively relieves menstrual cramps."

Practitioners of both Ayurveda, the traditional medicine of India, and traditional Chinese medicine also include species of valerian in their practices, primarily for its sedating and digestive-soothing actions and as a remedy for neurasthenia, dizziness, fainting, and similar conditions.

Valerian's calming powers should not be overstated—it's not likely to slow you down to the extent that Valium or any of the prescription tranquilizers do. If you take an especially large dose of valerian—five teaspoons, say—you may notice some of the side effects common to depressants, such as headaches, rubbery legs or heavy muscles, lethargy, or a feeling of mild confusion upon awakening. Occasionally people who are sensitive to valerian may experience heart palpitations.

Another, more unexpected potential side effect is stimulation. Perhaps one in every fifteen or twenty people react to valerian by being energized, with increases in circulation and breathing rate, rather than being calmed. One study found that this stimulant effect was more likely when the person was extremely fatigued; valerian seemed to work best as a sedative on people who are agitated, nervous, or restless. An explanation for this puzzling effect from the Chinese perspective, which considers a person's overall energy state, is that valerian is "heating" and thus most appropriate for people who tend to be cold and nervous; those with a naturally "warm" constitution are more likely to be stimulated by valerian. Another, more scientific explanation that has been proposed for valerian's occasional stimulating effect is that some peoples' bodies don't digest valerian in a way that allows its sedating compounds to be used. If you find that valerian has a stimulating rather than calming effect, try one of the other relaxing substances, such as California poppy (see chapter 14) or melatonin (see chapter 15).

One of valerian's advantages as a calming agent is that it does not multiply the effects of other depressants, particularly alcohol. Taking most prescription sedatives, such as barbiturates, and drinking alcohol at the same time can be a potentially lethal combination. Even so, consuming multiple depressant substances at the same time is not recommended. (It is perfectly safe and effective to adjust the dosage and combine valerian with other calming herbs. For example, instead of taking one teaspoon of valerian extract to promote sleep or alleviate anxiety, you could take ½ teaspoon valerian and ½ teaspoon California poppy.)

Valerian's overall safety when used responsibly is quite remarkable. Huge doses are needed before acute toxicity is reached—a mice study found that the LD50 for one of the valepotriates taken orally was over 4,600 mg/kg. (While mice-to-human extrapolations are admittedly hypothetical, this would amount to an LD50 for a 150-pound human of two-thirds of a pound of this particular valepotriate.) In 1995, a woman tried to commit suicide by taking forty to fifty 470 mg capsules of powdered valerian. The 20 g dose did not kill her, causing instead fatigue, abdominal cramping, chest tightness, lightheadedness, hand tremors, and dilated pupils. Tests of liver function were normal and the symptoms disappeared within twenty-four hours.

Although valerian is not addictive and side effects are rare and not life-threatening, as with any substance problems can arise when valerian is taken in large amounts on a daily basis for weeks or months. In such cases it is more likely that valerian will cause headaches, palpitations, or possibly even depression. Most herbalists suggest using valerian on an occasional basis, or for no longer than a few weeks on a daily basis. According to Moore, while dried root preparations are "fine for occasional, even frequent, use but not for daily regular, daily doses," weaker fresh root preparations have "none of the accumulative effects."

OVER-THE-COUNTER VALERIAN?

Given the relative safety and effectiveness of valerian as a mild sedative, one might wonder why it must be sold in the United States as a "dietary supplement" (as are almost all herbal products) rather than as an over-the-counter (OTC) medicine, like aspirin or Pepto-Bismol. The short answer is that the U.S. Food and Drug Administration usually requires a lengthy and expensive testing procedure to approve new drugs. Also, unlike similar regulatory agencies in other countries, the FDA does not recognize a history of long-term safe use in a foreign market as an alternative approval method. Until producers can prove to the FDA's satisfaction that an herb such as valerian is safe and effective, the substance cannot be promoted as a drug, and health claims made for it are severely restricted.

In June 1994, a coalition of European and North American herbal companies took the first step toward changing valerian's status by filing a citizens' petition with the FDA. The European-American Phytomedicines Coalition (EAPC), which was founded in 1991, hopes to force the FDA to include valerian in the short list of other substances approved as "OTC sleep aids."

"Valerian was chosen because it fit squarely into an existing OTC drug monograph category and because significant substantive evidence of its safety and effectiveness exists in the scientific literature," EAPC co-counsel Robert Pinco told the trade journal *HerbalGram.*

The EAPC notes in its twenty-four-page petition that valerian exhibits a number of attractive qualities as an over-the-counter medicine:

■ As a relatively mild nontoxic substance, it provides a viable alternative to the few conventional drugs available as sleep aids:

There is a paucity of safe and effective insomnia remedies that are available over the counter. Existing OTC remedies, which contain antihistamine, cause sleepiness but like prescription drugs often leave the user with residual drowsiness upon waking. Such drowsiness is a significant drawback for many people who take sleep aids. The scarcity of safe and effective OTC drug products is especially troubling in view of the fact that a significant number of persons experiencing insomnia do not seek a physician's advice. A safe and effective OTC sleep aid that will permit a restful sleep without residual drowsiness is needed. Valerian, with its long history of safe use and its proven efficacy, can meet this need.

■ Peer-reviewed scientific research and double-blind studies, on both animals and humans, confirm that valerian improves sleep quality while having few adverse side effects.

■ Valerian has a long history of safe use, and is currently approved as an effective sleep aid in Germany, France, the United Kingdom, and other developed countries.

"A thorough reading of this petition and its numerous footnotes," comments *Herbal-Gram* editor Mark Blumenthal, "provides a compelling legal and scientific case for the immediate approval of valerian for the petitioned claim. It will be interesting to see how reviewers within the FDA will deal with this petition."

Does this mean your local pharmacy will soon stock a variety of valerian-based products? Don't hold your breath. The FDA's track record on issues relating to approval of herbs and natural products suggests that it will be five years or longer before it rules on the petition. As of late 1997, the FDA still had not responded to a related citizens' petition filed by the EAPC more than five years earlier, in July 1992, "requesting that the agency change its extralegal policy that refuses to recognize foreign marketing histories of well-known botanical drug ingredients." Presumably, if the agency rules in favor of this earlier petition and allows a history of safe foreign use to qualify a substance for OTC use, valerian would be one of the most immediate beneficiaries.

TAKING VALERIAN

Valerian is readily available in many forms in natural foods stores, including as a coarse powder to make tea, in capsules, extracts, and tinctures. Extracts are sometimes standardized for small percentages of valerenic acid or other compounds. Herbal formulas that go by names like Eurocalm, Herbal Calm, and Forty Winks typically combine valerian with other calming herbs such as passionflower (*Passiflora incarnata*), catnip (*Nepeta cataria*), and hops (*Humulus lupulus*). Valerian and skullcap (*Scutellaria lateriflora*) seem to work well together to relieve tension. Products new to the market now combine valerian with melatonin. Some people like to add valerian to their hot bath to make it even more relaxing.

As with other plants, the levels of active compounds in the product may vary considerably, depending upon a variety of factors such as growing conditions and time of harvest, production methods, and freshness. If you're buying the dried root to make tea, check for valerian's characteristic smell—the riper, the better. The dried root often retains its smell and its potency for years. Liquid forms of valerian, however, such as tinctures and concentrated drops, tend to lose some of their potency after four to six months.

How much valerian to take depends a lot on the form of the product and an individual's sensitivity to it. Valerian can be safely taken in relatively generous dosages. "The chief mistake people make in using valerian is that they take too low a dose," remarks Paul Bergner, editor of the Portland, Oregon–based *Medical Herbalism: A Clinical Newsletter for the Herbal Practitioner.* The following are some average dosage suggestions that can be taken up to three times daily. You can safely double these dosages if necessary to achieve the desired effects. On the other hand, if you're new to valerian, you may want to start with slightly lower levels to check for adverse reactions.

- 2 to 3 teaspoons of the dried root per cup of water to make valerian tea (add hot water to the herb and steep; don't boil the infusion, as that would destroy valerian's volatile oils)

- 1 to 2 teaspoons of the tincture or concentrated drops
- 200 to 300 mg of the liquid or solid extract
- 750 to 1,500 mg of the dried root in capsules
- 250 to 500 mg of a dried powdered extract
- 150 to 300 mg of an extract standardized for 1 to 1.5 percent valtrate or 0.8 to 1 percent valerenic acid

Within about an hour of taking any of these doses of valerian, you should start to feel more relaxed and ready to sleep.

California Poppy

◎

OPIUM'S LITTLE SISTER

A striking annual with large and colorful flowers, the opium poppy (*Papaver somniferum*) is thought to be native to somewhere in the eastern Mediterranean. The plant has been molded to humanity's needs for so long that it shares a few traits with house pets: an association with humans that goes back to prehistoric times, adaptation for use by cultures around the world, and cultivation to the point that the plant is so "tame" it may no longer be able to survive in the wild without humanity's help. Among the earliest records of human use is archeological evidence that the Minoans of Crete worshiped a "poppy goddess" circa 4000 B.C.E. The Sumerians and the people of the Late Bronze Age on Cyprus apparently knew of the opium poppy and may have made it into a tea or even smoked it. The evidence suggests that the ancient Egyptians and Greeks were also familiar with the plant's ability to promote sleep.

With the opium poppy's contrasting potentials for medicinal benefit, euphoric exhilaration, and social devastation, it has been both a boon and a bane to humanity for thousands of years. Various cultures have revered opium poppies for their remarkable ability to entrance the mind, cure melancholy, and cause sleep. Today, almost two centuries after the isolation of morphine (named after Morpheus, the Greek god of dreams) by a German pharmacist, that alkaloid and its pharmaceutical relatives remain the most potent useful remedies for the acute pain that accompanies numerous serious medical conditions. On the other hand, addiction to morphine and its semisynthetic relative heroin results in much misery and tragedy, not only in North America but throughout the world.

Not surprisingly, mention *poppy* and many people's immediate associations are words like *opium, morphine, narcotics, addiction*. The poppy family (Papaveraceae) of plants, however, includes an estimated 250 species, only one of which is the opium poppy, the plant that is illegal to grow almost worldwide because of its high concentrations of morphine and other narcotic and addictive alkaloids. Yet, with one minor exception (*P. setigerum*) none of the other poppy species are known to contain more than trace amounts of the phenanthrene alkaloids morphine, codeine, and thebaine. What mind-altering compounds are found in some other poppy species have effects on the body and mind that are milder than those of the opium poppy, and are neither narcotic nor addictive.

The golden-flowering California poppy, for example, is not only legal to grow, it's been the state flower of California for more than a century. In recent years herbal preparations of California poppy have become increasingly popular as a gentle nervous system depressant that is useful for promoting sleep, reducing anxiety, and relaxing muscles.

- -

FIELDS OF GOLD

- -

The California poppy is in the same family as the opium poppy but in a different subfamily, Eschscholtzioideae, which is one of only four in the poppy family. Naturalist Adelbert von Chamisso was the first scientist to collect and study the California poppy on a Russian expedition to what was then the Spanish province of California in 1816. Chamisso named the new genus *Eschscholtzia,* after his close friend Johann Friedrich Eschscholtz, a German-Russian physician and expedition mate. Eschscholtzioideae contains three genera and some eighteen species, fifteen of which are in the genus *Eschscholtzia.* Chief among these species is California poppy (*Eschscholtzia californica*), now in-

creasingly being recognized as a mild but effective calming herb. Other prominent species in the genus are the closely related Mexican gold (*E. californica* ssp. *mexicana*), found mostly in Baja California and northwestern Mexico but occasionally as far east as western Texas, and desert poppy (*E. glyptosperma*), centered around the Mojave Desert and into Arizona and Utah. Dozens of subspecies of California poppy have also been identified. While differences among the various plants of *Eschscholtzia* may be important to botanists and gardeners, the plants are thought to be fairly similar in their compounds and potential mind-altering effects.

California poppy is found throughout California and, sporadically, in Oregon, Nevada, and Arizona. It is also known as the golden poppy—early spring rains can result in an explosion of blossoming, causing some grassy hillside fields to appear almost carpeted with yellow-to-orange flowers. Its seed pods look more like string beans than the familiar ball-shaped capsules of the opium poppy. California poppy can be a perennial or an annual, depending upon the conditions in which it grows. It has been known to blossom more than once between spring and fall.

Until fairly recently California poppy was appreciated chiefly as a disappearing wild-flower and a lovely garden flower rather than as a medicinal plant. Early settlers to the West Coast sent specimens back to Europe, where, according to botanist Christopher Grey-Wilson, author of *Poppies,* a definitive guide to the poppy family, it has been cultivated in gardens since 1790. Others have exported California poppy to parts of Australia and India, where it has become naturalized. West Coast Native Americans included California poppy among their remedies for certain types of pain, such as colic. The flowers as well as the leaves, stems, and seed capsules are harvested and dried, either for use as a tea or to make an alcoholic extract.

CALMING
BUT NOT ADDICTIVE

California poppy has a gentle, calming effect on the body, useful for reducing anxiety and promoting sleep. You can also take it for the dull pain of bruises and other minor injuries. "It ain't opium," notes herbalist Michael Moore, author of *Medicinal Plants of the Pacific West,* "and it will only have a certain degree of analgesic effect, but it always helps, especially when the pain is keeping you awake." He recommends combining California poppy with valerian, which is more "overtly sedative," for added effect. Parents have begun to turn to California poppy for help with children who are so wound up they can't fall asleep at night, and the herb is mild enough that most herbalists consider this a safe course of action.

As mentioned, California poppy does not contain the potent and addictive alkaloids morphine and codeine. Rather, researchers have identified various complex alkaloids, known as isoquinoline alkaloids, in California poppy, such as protopine and sanguinarine. According to Grey-Wilson, "Surprisingly [the isoquinoline alkaloids] have never been thoroughly investigated, which is very strange considering the modern trend toward 'natural

medicines.'" The phenanthrene alkaloids are potent at killing pain and inducing stupor; they're highly addictive. The isoquinoline alkaloids have mild relaxing effects on the central nervous system and on smooth muscles, with much less significant powers of analgesia. The isoquinolines are also neither narcotic nor addictive.

A few people have been known to ingest these alkaloids by smoking the dried plant. Smoking California poppy is said to offer a mild marijuanalike high.

What few studies have been done on California poppy have been conducted mainly in Europe, where California poppy is somewhat more recognized for its medicinal properties than in its native country. The extensive Napralert database (see Resources) includes references to about a dozen studies on California poppy. Human clinical trials are apparently totally lacking, and most of the studies (including all those prior to 1988) were testing for effects irrelevant to its current use as a relaxant. For example, early studies tested California poppy for potential anticancer, antifungal, and liver-protective properties. (Most of the results indicate California poppy is ineffective for these purposes.)

Two studies done on mice have suggested that California poppy is an effective agent for depressing central nervous system activity and relaxing smooth muscles: a 1988 study done by Italian researchers and published in a British journal, and a 1991 study done by French researchers and published in the prominent German botanical journal *Planta Medica.* The latter found that high doses of a water extract induced sleep while lower doses appeared to have an anxiety-reducing action. The mechanism for California poppy's sedative action appears to be through an effect on GABA, a calming neurotransmitter (see chapter 16). A more recent German study found that a mixture of California poppy and another, somewhat poppylike herb, *Corydalis cava,* in the closely related fumitory plant family, inhibited monoamine oxidase, the enzyme found in nerve cells that has been tied to changes in mood.

Though relatively mild, California poppy in large doses can cause headaches, next-day hangovers, and other minor side effects. Like other central nervous system depressants it should not be taken before driving or performing physical tasks that require full coordination and attention, nor should it be combined with other depressants, such as alcohol and prescription sedatives. Pregnant women should avoid it. Another hazard worth mentioning is that recent use of California poppy may cause a urine test to read positive for opiates (as might recent consumption of poppy seeds, for that matter).

TAKING CALIFORNIA POPPY

California poppy is still generally unavailable in capsules; a few companies offer it as a concentrated liquid or tincture. An average dose is 1 to 2 dropperfuls. You can also purchase the dried herb and make an unappetizing tea; infuse one to two teaspoons in a pint of water. Keep in mind that if you live in California and want to harvest California poppy, you must grow your own, as California law protects the plant by prohibiting wildcrafting.

Melatonin

◉

THE BODY'S OWN SLEEP AID

Few supplements have burst onto the health scene with the suddenness of melatonin. Until the early 1990s it was virtually unheard of in health food stores, though researchers had been conducting studies on it since it was identified in the late 1950s and a few travelers had been aware of its noted effects in preventing jet lag. Yet within a few short years melatonin became one of the hottest-selling supplements of all time, so much in demand that for a few months in mid-1995 stores literally couldn't keep it in stock. Melatonin also became the subject of a half-dozen popular books, a few of which appeared briefly on best-seller lists, and the focus of a mostly positive cover story on "Melatonin Mania" in *Newsweek* magazine. Scientific interest also mushroomed. By 1997 the number of published studies on melatonin had grown to an estimated five thousand worldwide. Along with only a few other supplements, such as vitamin E, melatonin gained a rare badge of

medical respect: many of the researchers who studied the substance also began personally to use it. An estimated twenty million Americans have now taken the hormone.

The available evidence indicates that melatonin deserves its sudden success. It is a natural substance that seems to be universally present in plants and animals, from algae to humans. It is central to a number of important physical functions relating to mood and consciousness yet, taken as a supplement, seems remarkably free of any toxicity or adverse effects. As a sleep-inducing agent, it may already deserve to be ranked ahead of any other drug, natural or synthetic, prescription or over-the-counter. Since blood levels of melatonin tend to decrease progressively with advancing age, some researchers are now exploring melatonin's potential to boost immunity, prevent cancer and heart disease, and possibly extend longevity. If melatonin were a proprietary drug instead of a natural substance, it is likely that its success would rival that of another pharmaceutical newcomer—Prozac—with a much more mixed record regarding safety and effectiveness.

Melatonin is a hormone naturally present in the body in fluctuating levels. It is produced by a tiny endocrine organ, the pineal, at the base of the brain. Recent studies have found that the retina also produces small amounts of melatonin, as does the gastrointestinal tract under certain conditions. It is unclear at this point, however, whether intestinally produced melatonin contributes significantly to circulating blood levels, or whether it pretty much stays in the gut to serve as a local free radical scavenger. The pineal produces melatonin from tryptophan, an essential amino acid found in various foods. (Until 1989, when tryptophan supplements were banned due to a contamination incident, they were widely used relaxants; see chapter 16.) The pineal converts tryptophan into 5-hydroxytryptophan (5-HTP; see chapter 16), which is converted into serotonin, the neurotransmitter. With another intermediary step, serotonin is converted into melatonin. Though serotonin and melatonin have a structural resemblance and both have been tied to improvements in mood (melatonin's neurotransmitterlike actions and its multiple effects on the nervous system and the brain have caused some researchers to refer to it as a "neurohormone"), many of

their important functions differ, as we'll see.

Once regarded by doctors as a vestigial or "leftover" organ, the pineal is now recognized as crucial for overall health because of its role in the manufacture and secretion of melatonin. Enzymes in the pineal that promote the conversion of tryptophan into melatonin are sensitive to light and darkness. The process starts at the eyes, which send information about light exposure to a bundle of nerves—the "body clock"—in the brain behind the eyes. Using the neurotransmitter noradrenaline, the body clock relays signals to the pineal to produce melatonin. Melatonin from the pineal is secreted into the blood and carried to various parts of the brain, where it easily passes through the blood-brain barrier. Melatonin is also transported throughout the body, where it seems to have special access to cells in general. Researchers reported in a 1994 study that melatonin may actually operate within the nucleus of the cell, through special melatonin receptors. In the nucleus melatonin can have an intimate impact on cellular functions and even on how cells age.

The pineal's natural rhythm is to secrete only tiny amounts of melatonin during the daytime, and then to begin to increase production at the onset of darkness. The pineal is most active in secreting melatonin in the early hours of the morning, such as between 2 and 3 A.M. By sunrise, melatonin production shuts off again and the hormone's sleep-inducing effects are put on hold for the daylight hours. Melatonin is potent—the pineal probably produces less than 0.1 mg per day. Levels of melatonin in the body are measured in picograms (trillionths of a gram) per milliliter of blood; the notation is pg/ml. A person may have melatonin levels of about 10 pg/ml during the day, rising to a peak somewhere in the range of 50 to 150 pg/ml during the night.

Melatonin levels in the body can also be influenced by various other factors, including certain drugs, diet (foods relatively rich in melatonin include oats, rice, and bananas), and overall health. Numerous studies have established that chronological age is one of the most important determinants. Newborns rely upon breast milk for melatonin for their first three months before they start to produce it themselves. Production increases for the next nine months, so that by age one, an average nighttime peak of 125 pg/ml is typical. Levels stay at this lifetime peak until age six or so, when the usual spurt in growth combined with static melatonin output dilutes the hormone's relative concentration in the body. Most people experience a rapid decline in melatonin levels at puberty, and researchers are investigating whether the hormone is involved in the timing of its onset. The steepest decline has occurred by age thirty (when nighttime peaks may average about 40 pg/ml), but body levels continue to fall throughout adulthood. Beyond age sixty melatonin production is minimal, with nighttime peaks of 10 pg/ml or less—some people may lose entirely their ability to produce the hormone. Melatonin is similar in this last respect to estrogen, dehydroepiandrosterone (DHEA), human growth hormone, and other hormones, which the body tends to produce in declining amounts with advancing years.

Exactly why a person's melatonin output slowly declines with advancing age is not known. A couple of potential culprits have been proposed: an increase in calcium deposits in the pineal, a decrease in the number of actual pineal cells, and a decline in the function of certain of the pineal's noradrenaline-receiving cells. Whatever the reason for the decline, studies on the elderly and others have determined that less melatonin causes a wide range of physical effects.

The most obvious of these effects have to do with sleep. Because of its intimate connection with light and darkness, the body's clock, and sedation, melatonin has come to be known as the rest and recuperation hormone. Researchers have linked melatonin levels with quality of sleep, time required to fall asleep, and time of awakening. Low melatonin levels have been shown to be associated with sleep problems, as in a 1996 study that was done on hard-core insomniacs. These unfortunate people, who had been suffering from insomnia for an average of eighteen years, were determined to have significantly lower melatonin levels than matched control subjects.

Numerous studies have also established that melatonin supplements have the desirable quality of promoting natural sleep. Researchers have tested melatonin's effects on normal, healthy people, on people with chronic insomnia, and on subjects who have been artificially deprived of sleep. The consensus is that melatonin doesn't change normal sleeping patterns or reduce the time spent during the important dream-heavy stage of sleep. Taken orally in small doses at the right time, melatonin can reinforce the body's normal circadian (twenty-four-hour) rhythms. At nighttime, a small dose of supplemental melatonin will help to lower the body's temperature and reduce heart rate, conditions that promote sleepiness. Doctors now use melatonin to treat various sleep disorders, including insomnia and disruptions in the sleep-wake cycle due to either jet lag or changing work shifts. Melatonin can also help alleviate the condition known as delayed sleep phase disorder, characterized by an inability to fall asleep when you want to, although when you wait a few hours you fall asleep only to awaken in the morning feeling drowsy and fatigued. According to a survey of members of the American Sleep Disorder Association, physicians who work in sleep disorder clinics are far more likely to recommend melatonin to their patients than any other sleep aid.

Melatonin has also been shown to have important effects on mood. People often do things that disrupt their normal sleeping patterns—staying up all night to study, flying across five time zones, going to bed early one night and late the next. Frequently, part of the price paid in succeeding days for such behaviors is irritability, depressed mood, and anger. Numerous studies have tied disruptions in melatonin patterns or low nighttime levels to effects on mood. Manic-depressive patients, suicide victims, and schizophrenics have all been shown to have lower levels of melatonin.

Many normal, healthy people now take melatonin at nighttime because they notice that it helps them to feel more calm and relaxed the next day. Some even claim that melatonin is mildly euphoric. Melatonin may have anxiety-lowering properties because of its ability to increase GABA levels (see chapter 16), according to a 1986 study.

Melatonin has not received as much publicity for its potential effects on mood compared to drugs that promote serotonin action, such as Prozac. As Russel J. Reiter, Ph.D., founder and editor of *The Journal of Pineal Research,* author of more than five hundred articles on the topic and coauthor of *Melatonin: Your Body's Natural Wonder Drug,* reports, both melatonin and serotonin may be crucial, though at different times of the day. "A high level of serotonin during the day punctuated by a strong pulse of melatonin at night appears to be nature's formula for vibrant good health. Serotonin keeps you alert and energized during the daytime; melatonin helps you rest and recuperate at night." He says that melatonin may be a "more logical candidate as a treatment for depression." This is because adjusting the body's melatonin levels is easier than affecting its serotonin levels—melatonin more readily crosses the blood-brain barrier than serotonin and is more effective taken orally. "Given the preliminary evidence that melatonin may enhance mood in some people, coupled with its apparent lack of toxicity and negative side effects, it is reasonable to suggest that a few million dollars might be diverted to exploring the antidepressant potential of melatonin."

Melatonin supplements show promise as a

reliable way to stimulate the pineal, regulate sleep cycles, and enhance the moods of those who suffer from seasonal affective disorder (SAD). This condition is not uncommon in climes that get little sunshine during the winter, such as Scandinavia and northern North America. An estimated one in twenty people (four times as many women as men) who live in these sunlight-deprived areas experience notable seasonal depression, while twice as many more people suffer from a more moderate form of SAD known as "winter blues." During the winter months people with SAD tend to be irritable, tired, and lethargic. They gain weight, lose their ability to concentrate, and show no interest in having sex. While scientists are not sure that they know the exact mechanism of SAD, it is possible that the lack of daytime light leads to diminished release of melatonin during the night or to the untimely release of melatonin in the late morning. Researchers who have exposed SAD victims to bright, full-spectrum lights have found they can help these people become happier and more energetic. The SAD-busting lights, however, are expensive, and victims need to be exposed to them for many hours per day.

While much of the research has focused on melatonin's obvious utility as a mild hypnotic and mood-brightening agent, recent studies have extended melatonin's potential benefits into the fields of immunity, cancer prevention, and longevity. Among the most important findings:

■ Researchers have determined that melatonin is a potent antioxidant that can neutralize one of the most harmful of the free radicals, the hydroxyl radical. In fact, melatonin may be the best free radical scavenger known. One dramatic study done by Reiter and colleagues and published in *Mutation Research* in 1995 found that melatonin was five hundred times as powerful in its antioxidant effects compared to the potent synthetic antioxidant DMSO. Melatonin is especially powerful and effective as a free radical scavenger because of its ability to access every cell in the body and to protect the brain in particular.

■ Melatonin strengthens the immune system, especially when you're under stress from ill health, work pressures, or whatever. Various mechanisms have been demonstrated, including that melatonin promotes functioning of the important immune-system organ, the thymus gland; stimulates immune system cells and substances such as T-helpers, phagocytes, natural killers, and interferon; protects the important immune-boosting mineral zinc in the body; and slows the age-related decline of the immune system. As an immune system stimulant melatonin may eventually be used therapeutically to help prevent or treat conditions ranging from the common cold to AIDS.

■ A 1993 study concluded that "aging can be regarded as a process caused by hydroxyl radical pathology and melatonin deficiency." Longevity researchers say that melatonin may be the most important anti-aging compound yet discovered, capable of increasing life expectancy even when its use is started relatively late in life. Some substances and programs, such as the smart drug deprenyl and calorie-restricted diets, are now suspected of accomplishing their life-enhancing effects through melatonin-related mechanisms.

(The strong anti-aging claims for melatonin made by researchers Walter Pierpaoli, M.D., and William Regelson, M.D., authors of *The Melatonin Miracle,* have caused something of a backlash in the media. A story in early 1996 in *Time* magazine on melatonin as the "Lost Fountain of Youth" proclaimed that longevity-related claims for melatonin "are running far ahead of the science." Also, Pierpaoli's proposal that the pineal constitutes the body's "aging clock" is rejected by many melatonin researchers. For example, German researcher Dr. Gerald Huether says, "I don't believe the human body relies on one particular organ or tissue to regulate its aging. The body is incredibly complicated with countless interdependent systems.")

■ Melatonin may slow the growth of some cancers and help to prevent others. In addition to its cancer-preventing effects from antioxidant and immune system actions, melatonin has been shown to kill certain types of cancer cells. Studies have suggested a positive role for melatonin in the prevention or treatment of cancers of the breasts, lungs, prostate, and brain.

■ The latest research suggests melatonin may affect fertility, and women in the near future may be able to take advantage of an apparent contraceptive action from high doses of melatonin. Researchers in the Netherlands are enthusiastic about an ongoing study of B-Oval, a birth control pill composed of 75 mg of melatonin and 0.3 mg of a progesterone hormone.

■ Other conditions that have been shown to benefit from melatonin are high cholesterol levels, osteoporosis, menopausal discomforts, Alzheimer's disease, chronic pain, heart disease, and diabetes.

DIETARY SUPPLEMENT VS. PRESCRIPTION DRUG

The explosion of scientific interest in melatonin has resulted in a wealth of data about the hormone's effects. The consensus among the vast majority of melatonin researchers is that melatonin is remarkably safe and nontoxic. A number of prominent researchers, however, harbor reservations about whether people should be taking supplemental dosages of the hormone on a regular basis. Some of these reservations pertain to melatonin's status as a dietary supplement. Isn't melatonin too potent to be an over-the-counter drug? And aren't dietary supplement producers unreliable as a source for high-quality melatonin products?

Among the most vocal of the "wait for it to be a prescription drug" crowd is Richard Wurtman, M.D., a professor of neuroscience at Massachusetts Institute of Technology and director of the school's Clinical Research Center. He has repeatedly been quoted in news magazines and on network news shows saying that "people should not self-medicate with melatonin." He told *American Health* in late 1994, "I urge everyone to wait until melatonin is available as a drug approved by the Food and Drug Administration. Although this will take several years, it will allow us time to learn more about melatonin's effects on sleep, which dosage is best and any interactions that could arise due to drinking alcohol or taking prescription or over-the-counter medications." He has said that melatonin can cause feelings of dissatisfaction, restlessness, depression, or anxiety, and that taking high doses for a long time might even disturb a person's biological rhythms.

Because Wurtman is a renowned researcher in the melatonin field, his voice carries much authority. Unfortunately for the widespread, largely uncritical exposure he has received for his views, his is not a disinterested point of view. As the *Wall Street Journal* pointed out in August 1994, Wurtman is a major stockholder of Interneuron Pharmaceuticals, Inc., a small Lexington, Massachusetts–based company that he cofounded in 1988. Melatonin is a natural substance and thus can't be patented, but it is possible to create close chemical analogs of melatonin and patent them, and even to patent specific uses of a natural compound such as melatonin. Wurtman has been actively pursuing these possibilities and through MIT has already licensed melatonin patents to Interneuron. Through his involvement in Interneuron, he hopes to market and ultimately profit from melatonin-based drugs. If Interneuron were successful at supplanting the current cheap and readily available melatonin supplements with proprietary melatonin drugs Wurtman developed, he could reap substantial financial benefit.

The other common charge—that much of the melatonin on the market is suspect in some way because the dietary supplement industry is "unregulated"—has a grain of truth to it but vastly overstates the likely problem. Various medical authorities have raised questions about the purity of melatonin supplements as an excuse to recommend that consumers not take the hormone. Within recent years, articles on melatonin in consumer publications such as the *University of California at Berkeley Wellness Letter* and the *Johns Hopkins Medical Letter* have warned against "potential contamination" of supplements and claimed (without evidence) that melatonin products can vary considerably in quality. Stories have even been posted on the Internet claiming that "most of the publicly available melatonin is doped with other much more powerful sleep inducers."

This level of paranoia would be laughable if it weren't so prevalent. In point of fact the dietary supplement industry is hardly "unregulated," and problems with contamination, mislabeling, or adulteration seem no more common than in the mainstream food, cosmetic, and drug industries, as the producers of Tylenol, Perrier, Jack-in-the-Box hamburgers, and various other products that have experienced contamination problems might admit. As Lorri Rosenthal, a member of the board of trustees of the American Herbal Products Association, has pointed out, "The overall percentages of people committing illegal acts on the scale of 'doping' a dietary supplement with a drug are minuscule, and for a reputable U.S. manufacturer to engage in such a practice would be absolutely insane given the magnitude of legal and product liability issues involved." When deceptions have been identified, such as with an obscure Chinese patent medicine (supposedly an herbal sleep remedy) imported from Taiwan that was spiked with Valium, the natural products industry has acted quickly and jointly with the FDA to protect consumers from such fraud.

It is true that the FDA does not have the resources to test dietary supplements. Reputable companies, however, do their own testing of melatonin, have it assayed by an independent lab, or participate in third-party programs that guarantee the purity of melatonin supplements. Nationally established brands typically guarantee the purity and potency (99+ percent pure melatonin) of their melatonin; smaller companies may be more tempted to cut corners. This was demonstrated in early 1996 when CNN tested five brands of melatonin purchased from health food stores in the Atlanta area. The products of four nationally known, well-established supplement companies (KAL, Source Naturals, Alacer, and Natrol) contained 2.5 mg of melatonin, just as their labels stated. A fifth product made by a smaller company had only 1.2 mg of melatonin instead of 2.5 mg. The company recalled the product.

It is also true that, compared to dietary supplements, prescription drugs undergo a somewhat higher degree of regulatory scrutiny and are manufactured using more rigorous standards. For those people who wouldn't mind paying two dollars a tablet for prescription melatonin, and who would prefer to act only on the recommendation of their doctor, perhaps an FDA-approved melatonin drug makes sense.

Something like this scenario did occur recently, in Canada. In the fall of 1995, regulators dramatically altered their approach to melatonin. Health Canada, the federal agency that regulates foods and drugs, changed melatonin's classification from dietary supplement to drug, making it illegal to sell melatonin over the counter until manufacturers had submitted it to an expensive and lengthy approval process. Officials said that regulations forced them to make the change, because melatonin is a hormone and is thus automatically considered a drug. In an "action alert" on melatonin mailed to health food stores, asking store managers to stop selling melatonin, the agency also noted, "We don't have evidence that melatonin is safe, effective, and of high quality." Many Canadians now obtain their melatonin by driving into the United States or buying it through the mail.

In the United States a spokesperson for the FDA commented at the time of the Canadian ban that the agency had not received any complaints about negative side effects from melatonin and had no plans to challenge its status as a dietary supplement.

WHO CAN USE MELATONIN?

Beyond the issues relating to whether melatonin should be a dietary supplement or a prescription drug, there are additional possible reservations about its use that question the substance itself. One is that, as a hormone, melatonin almost by definition has many functions in the body and is still only partially understood. Hormone action is exceedingly complex. Melatonin is no exception. Exactly how it works, and which bodily systems it partially controls, are still being determined. Conservative doctors believe that until more is known about the long-term effects of supplementing with a hormone, daily, unrestricted melatonin use should be discouraged. A few prominent natural health practitioners agree with this assessment. For example, Michael Murray, a naturopathic doctor and the author of *Natural Alternatives to Prozac,* emphasizes that melatonin is a hormone, not a nutrient. "While I am a strong advocate of self-care," he says, "because of potential complications with inappropriate use I feel that melatonin is best utilized when it is prescribed by a licensed health care practitioner."

The second major reservation with regard to taking melatonin has to do with the fact that when you take a melatonin supplement, you supply the body with much more of the hormone than it naturally produces. For example, a 3 mg tablet dissolved in a person's blood supply (roughly 10 pints) causes a melatonin concentration in the range of 600,000 pg/ml. Even adjusting for the fact that oral melatonin supplements are not completely absorbed—perhaps as much as 95 percent is metabolized in the liver and excreted before it can have any effect at all—a 3 mg tablet taken orally can still cause a spike of melatonin concentration of 30,000 pg/ml, many times normal bodily levels. As one researcher has noted, "Does the body need so much melatonin? Maybe adults produce less for some reason."

The question is certainly worthy of further research, though other findings must be taken into consideration. One is that the body is proficient at rapidly metabolizing melatonin. After reaching a peak from ingestion of an oral supplement, total blood levels of melatonin fall by 50 percent as quickly as every half hour to one hour. All of the extra melatonin from taking a supplement is usually metabolized

and eliminated from the body within twelve hours. Another relevant finding is that studies are pointing to the effectiveness of lower and lower doses of melatonin. Many of the early melatonin studies administered huge doses by today's standards. Gradually, the dose that has been shown to be effective has become smaller and smaller. A 1995 study by MIT researchers found that doses of 1.0 mg and 0.3 mg shortened the time it took subjects to fall asleep, with 0.3 mg being as effective as the larger dose.

A third reservation concerns the effect that taking melatonin supplements may have on the body's ability to produce its own melatonin. It could be a problem if the body came to rely on oral supplements and, when the person stopped taking them, he or she could not then resume producing melatonin. This does not, however, appear to be the case. According to Dr. Michael Cohen, director of the Dutch study that is administering the melatonin-based birth control pill, even such high doses of melatonin do not appear to cause the body to stop producing its own supply of the hormone. Cohen says that the body's production of melatonin does not seem to be affected by how much has already been produced, nor did the women who participated in his trials suffer any negative side effects after stopping taking melatonin.

For some people, these reservations carry enough weight to justify taking a wait-and-see attitude with regard to whether daily doses of melatonin are beneficial for boosting the immune system, enhancing longevity, and so forth. For many others, the evidence for melatonin's safety and efficacy is felt to be convincing. They have considered the pros and cons of melatonin and decided to take it on a daily basis, feeling that its risks are minimal compared to the potential benefits.

On the other hand, reservations with regard to melatonin's use on an occasional basis as an insomnia remedy, jet-lag preventive, and anti-anxiety agent seem almost nonexistent at this point, especially when its risks and benefits are compared to conventional prescription drugs used for the same purpose. Prescription barbiturate sedatives, for example, are often addictive and even potentially fatal in large doses. They can cause a long list of side effects, from headaches to liver damage. After a few weeks, they not only lose their effectiveness against insomnia but may begin to cause the condition. The benzodiazepines (Valium, Dalmane) are milder than the barbiturates but can cause dependence, headache, and memory loss. Even the over-the-counter remedies for insomnia, such as those that contain diphenhydramine (Sominex, Sleep-Eze 3), are contraindicated for many people and may cause next-day drowsiness. (Diphenhydramine is basically an antihistamine that causes drowsiness as a side effect.) All of these drugs, as well as another—alcohol—often used to counter insomnia, can interfere with the normal stages of sleep and healthful dreaming patterns.

In contrast, melatonin has an enviable safety profile. Its acute toxicity is virtually nonexistent. An early experiment with animals that attempted to determine what levels of melatonin constitute a lethal dose basically failed. Injecting as much as 800 mg of melatonin per 1 kg of animal body weight was not fatal to the animals. Assuming an equivalency with humans (which may or may not be warranted), this is like giving a 150-pound person 55 g of melatonin. The animal researchers would have tried higher doses of melatonin, but they couldn't force more melatonin into solution. No acute toxicity has been shown in human studies, either. This includes a number of studies that administered whopping doses of melatonin. For example, the Dutch birth-control study has been giving 1,400 women 75 mg of melatonin per day for four years. Other studies have administered, for shorter periods of time, 6,000 mg, 1,000 mg, and 700 mg to test for melatonin's potential usefulness as a cancer remedy or against other serious conditions. Subjects have been monitored for toxic effects on the blood, internal organs, the nervous system, and so forth. Even at these high doses, no toxic effects have ever been shown.

The minor side effects that these and other studies have documented include next-day fatigue or grogginess, mild nausea, diarrhea, bad dreams, headaches, and reduced sex drive. A number of the early studies that suggested high dosages of melatonin cause adverse effects, such as a worsening of mood and slower reaction time, administered melatonin during the day. Administered appropriately, at night, melatonin does not adversely affect mood or cognitive functions the next day, and may actually improve them. Studies on elderly subjects given doses much higher (such as 40 to 50 mg) than normally used to promote sleep found that melatonin did not lead to memory loss, impaired thinking, lack of concentration, or problems with motor control the following day.

Taking melatonin should not cause your skin to become either lighter or darker. That is, melatonin is not thought to affect melanin, the dark pigment that colors skin and hair. Nor does melatonin cause melanoma, the often malignant skin cancer. (In fact, melatonin may actually help treat some cases of melanoma.) Melatonin, melanin, and melanoma share the Greek root *mela* for black. Melatonin was named by researcher Aaron Lerner, M.D., whose discovery of the hormone was announced in a 1958 medical journal report. Lerner coined the name because the hormone was found to lighten the skin of frogs (*tonin* is from *serotonin,* from which melatonin is derived). Lerner wanted to know whether melatonin might lighten human skin and be linked to vitiligo, the condition in which the skin develops light patches (and for which pop singer Michael Jackson was treated). Lerner found that human skin, however, was not affected by the newly identified hormone.

Anecdotal reports exist, on the other hand, of melatonin lightening age or liver spots that often develop in late middle age on people's hands and faces. Age spots are often due to a buildup of the skin pigment lipofuscin, bodily levels of which increase from free radical activity. Melatonin's antioxidant power may help reduce lipofuscin levels and thus prevent or lighten age spots.

Though relatively safe, melatonin is contraindicated for certain people nonetheless. It should not be taken by women who are pregnant or breast-feeding; anyone suffering from kidney disease; and people with autoimmune diseases or immune-system cancers such as lymphoma and leukemia (melatonin's ability to activate the immune system would be countereffective in such conditions). Because it may affect growth or sex hormone levels, melatonin should also be avoided by anyone under the age of eighteen. Though many people are now taking melatonin to alleviate SAD and improve mood, a medical professional should evaluate and monitor any attempt to use melatonin for serious emotional illnesses such as manic-depressive illness and schizophrenia. High doses may act as a contraceptive, so women trying to conceive should avoid high doses.

The question as to how melatonin supplements interact with other drugs, mind-altering or otherwise, is still in the earliest stages of research. Studies have found that certain substances can tend either to increase or reduce the body's natural melatonin levels. Antidepressants seem to have varying effects. The selective serotonin reuptake inhibitor fluoxetine (Prozac) has been shown to reduce nighttime melatonin levels. Some antidepressants of the MAO-inhibitor and tricyclic classes, on the other hand, stimulate melatonin production. Until further research is done, people taking these drugs may want to check with their physician before taking supplemental melatonin. Melatonin should also be avoided by people taking steroid drugs such as cortisone.

Researchers believe that alcohol, tobacco, and caffeine lower melatonin levels. Among the most effective drugs for promoting melatonin production is marijuana. Italian researchers in 1986 discovered that marijuana caused a 4,000 percent increase in melatonin levels two hours after smoking a joint.

TAKING MELATONIN

Melatonin comes in pills and capsules ranging in dosage from 0.2 mg to 20 mg. The most popular products are probably the 0.5, 0.75, 2.5, and 3 mg doses. These are inexpensive (seven dollars or so for a bottle of 100) and readily available not only in natural foods stores but in drugstores and supermarkets.

Melatonin producers are busy innovating. Recently melatonin has begun to appear in combination products, with added vitamin cofactors (such as vitamin B_6, to promote the conversion of tryptophan to serotonin and then melatonin), with relaxant nutrients such as GABA, and even with calming herbs such as kava (see chapter 17) and valerian (see chapter 13). Look for products with names like Sleep Assure and Slumber Tabs. Liquid, sublingual, lozenges, and timed-release products have also come onto the market. Liquid, sublingual, and lozenge products have the advantage over pills and capsules of being more thoroughly and quickly absorbed (they can enter the bloodstream directly from the mouth), while the melatonin in timed-release products is designed to be absorbed slowly. As many as a dozen pharmaceutical firms are also in the process of developing melatonin analogs, close chemical relatives that may have advantages over the natural molecule in terms of factors such as improved bioavailability and longer half-life.

It may take some experimenting to determine what combination of dosage level, product type, and dosage timing work best. Because the timing of melatonin ingestion is so crucial to avoid shifting your biological clock, it is necessary to pay close attention to when you take these different forms of melatonin. In addition, people's reactions to melatonin can vary considerably. Some absorb it readily and feel its relaxant effects within fifteen minutes, while others barely notice a much larger dose. Factors that can influence its effects include how empty your stomach is, how efficiently your liver metabolizes melatonin, how much of the hormone (and its precursor serotonin) you produce naturally, your exposure to light, and so forth. Here are some general guidelines for getting the most from the melatonin you take:

■ Melatonin supplements should support the body's natural biorhythms and normal pattern of melatonin use—low levels during the day, peak release sometime in the midnight to 3 A.M. range. Thus, melatonin supplements are not normally taken during the day, unless you are a night-shift worker who sleeps during the day or are taking it to encourage sleep as a means of preventing jet lag. Taking melatonin during the day may cause you to experience unwanted effects, such as impaired memory, decreased alertness, and possibly even exaggerated symptoms of depression.

■ If you take melatonin every day, avoid side effects and enhance your body's natural biorhythms by taking it at the same time every night (assuming you're not switching among the product types, with their variations in dosage timing).

■ Most people take regular pills or capsules either at bedtime or fifteen to forty-five minutes before bedtime. Pills and capsules cause peak levels of melatonin in the body within one and a half to two hours.

■ Sublingual and liquids will deliver peak levels in an hour or sooner. Taking these too early in the evening could make you sleepy too quickly.

■ Timed-release products may take up to four hours to cause peak levels in the body. If you're used to taking a melatonin capsule at 11:30 at night but instead take a timed-release product at that time, you'd shift your normal circadian rhythm by two hours or more, and probably feel out of sorts in the morning. To keep your body's clock in synch, you'd want to take a timed-release product much earlier in the evening, such as at nine o'clock. According to melatonin researcher Reiter, a slow-release product "may be the best preparation all around because it allows you to take a smaller dose and also mimics the body's own actions. Slow-release tablets may be especially beneficial for those who awaken in the middle of the night and have problems going back to sleep— melatonin will be there when they need it. (Regular tablets can be metabolized so quickly that if taken at bedtime, most of the hormone may be out of circulation by three A.M.)" A recent study published in *The Lancet* found that 2-mg controlled-release pills were especially effective for elderly insomniacs.

■ If it is late at night and you haven't taken melatonin at an appropriate time, it is better to skip it than take it at the wrong time and risk jet-lag-type symptoms the next day. By the same token, if you awaken in the middle of the night, valerian or one of the other natural relaxants would be a better choice than melatonin.

■ Start with a low dose. The most effective dose will vary from one individual to the next. Some people find that as little as 0.1 mg promotes relaxation and elevates mood, while others need to take 9 mg or more. With the most recent data suggesting that doses as low as 0.3 mg are as effective as higher doses, it makes sense to start with a low dose, such as 0.5 mg, and increase it if necessary for greater effect. Older people may benefit from slightly higher doses than younger people.

■ Take smaller average doses for everyday use. In other words, if you intend to take melatonin every day to help boost your immune system, neutralize free radicals, and possibly gain other benefits, the suggested dose range is 1.5 to 3 mg. (Many researchers suggest that only people over the age of forty should consider taking melatonin on a daily basis.) If you take melatonin only occasionally, to promote sleep for example, you can experiment with up to 9 to 12 mg. As mentioned, lower doses may work just as well for some people.

■ The vast majority of melatonin supplements are synthetic melatonin. This melatonin is exactly the same molecule (N-acetyl-5-methoxy-tryptamine) as the natural melatonin found in the body. There is no advantage to so-called natural or animal-derived melatonin supplements, such as melatonin extracted from the pineal glands of cows. In fact, melatonin from animal tissue has a higher likelihood of being contaminated with viruses or other potentially worrisome substances.

■ For best results store melatonin in the refrigerator.

CHAPTER 16

Tryptophan, 5-HTP, and GABA

◉

THE CALMING AMINO ACIDS

Whereas phenylalanine and tyrosine, the amino acids discussed in chapter 6, are stimulating and energizing, taking oral doses of other amino acids can have the opposite effect. These calming, anxiety-reducing, and sleep-promoting supplements include tryptophan, the related amino acid L-5-hydroxytryptophan (5-HTP), and gamma aminobutyric acid (GABA).

Tryptophan is an essential amino acid: we must obtain it from the food we eat. Because tryptophan is found in significant levels in many common foods, humans have been ingesting tryptophan since time immemorial. In the body some tryptophan is converted into 5-HTP and then into the neurotransmitter serotonin, which in turn is converted (especially at night) into the neurohormone melatonin. Serotonin and melatonin are among the most important nerve chemicals. Each has various welcome roles in the body, in optimum amounts and at the right times tending to boost mood, reduce anger and aggression, increase self-confidence, alleviate anxiety, stabilize emotions, and promote normal sleep patterns.

A nonessential amino acid found in high concentrations in the central nervous system, GABA helps to slow down the transmission of messages between nerve cells. Like tryptophan and 5-HTP, it tends to reduce anxiety and promote sleep without causing any of the potentially nasty side effects so common among many of the over-the-counter and prescription relaxants.

TRYPTOPHAN: GONE BUT NOT FORGOTTEN

Tryptophan at one time was widely taken as a natural relaxant, sleep aid, and mood elevator. Although the results of well-controlled trials on tryptophan have been mixed, a number of studies have shown the supplement to be safe and effective at alleviating insomnia without interfering with natural sleep patterns or causing next-day hangovers. Tryptophan may help suppress appetite, lower sensitivity to pain, and reduce alcohol craving. Tryptophan has also been shown to reduce the fatigue, irritability, and sadness associated with forms of depression, in some cases as effectively as conventional antidepressants (such as the tricyclic imipramine) that have much higher levels of toxicity, tolerance, and side effects. Tryptophan-deficient diets and clinically induced states of low blood levels of tryptophan have been tied to depression and even to suicides—a notable 1987 population study linked low tryptophan intakes with increased suicide rates.

Scientists are unsure why the effects from oral doses of tryptophan cannot be more reliably reproduced in human studies. Although serotonin can be made only from tryptophan, questions remain with regard to how reliably oral doses of tryptophan translate into increased serotonin action in the brain and central nervous system. Various complicating factors are still being researched, including:

- the role of enzymes, nutrients such as vitamin B_6, and various cofactors in the process that breaks down tryptophan
- the effect of competing amino acids
- how the brain adapts to large doses of the amino acid
- the effects that tryptophan metabolites may have on the brain
- the impact of other bodily processes (such as infection) on blood levels of tryptophan
- the limitations imposed by the blood-brain barrier in determining how much trypto-

phan and serotonin reach relevant nerve cells

- the fact that most tryptophan is processed by the body for uses unrelated to the nervous system
- the role of gender, as recent findings indicate that men's brains are more efficient than women's at synthesizing serotonin from tryptophan

In spite of tryptophan's mixed scientific record and questions about how, why, and when tryptophan works, its relaxant effects were reliable enough in the late 1980s to have made it into one of the most popular nutritional supplements on the market. Estimates of the number of Americans who were taking tryptophan supplements regularly by 1989 range as high as twelve to fourteen million. Supplements, of course, added to average tryptophan consumption from food, which in industrialized countries is estimated to be 1 to 2 grams per day.

Tryptophan's main drawback as a relaxing supplement today is a whopper: questions about its safety caused the United States and other nations to recall tryptophan supplements from the market in late 1989. In 1990 the FDA banned all further sales in the United States, a ban that remains in effect as of late 1997. These drastic actions were taken because consumption of tryptophan supplements was tied to a rare blood disease called eosinophilia-myalgia syndrome (EMS). More than fifteen hundred cases of EMS and some three dozen deaths were eventually attributed to tryptophan supplements.

Investigations by the federal Centers for Disease Control, the Mayo Clinic, and other medical researchers determined that these deaths and illnesses were caused not by tryptophan itself but by a toxin in the tryptophan produced by a single Japanese company, Showa Denko K.K., that experimented with a new manufacturing process during the first six months of 1989. At the time, Showa Denko was one of a half-dozen Japanese nutrient manufacturers that supplied virtually all of the tryptophan that American supplement companies were encapsulating and selling to consumers. Studies identifying the contaminant (a new, human-made amino acid, ethylidenebis tryptophan or EBT) and the flawed manufacturing process that produced it (reduced filtering and the introduction of a genetically engineered strain of bacteria) were published in leading medical journals in 1990, including the *Journal of the American Medical Association* and the *New England Journal of Medicine*.

Despite this apparent scientific consensus, in the United States the FDA contends that the exact role of tryptophan in the EMS epidemic is still unknown, and that uncontaminated tryptophan may be a factor in causing the condition. In an article in *FDA Consumer* magazine, Lori A. Love, Ph.D., director of the clinical research and review staff in the FDA's Center for Food Safety and Applied Nutrition, said, "Cases of EMS, as well as a related illness, eosinophilic fasciitis, were associated with the use of L-tryptophan even before the 1989 EMS epidemic. And cases of EMS and related illnesses have occurred with the use of a compound (L-5-hydroxytryptophan) that's

similar to L-tryptophan, but not manufactured with the same fermentation process and, therefore, not associated with the same impurities." Because of these concerns, all tryptophan supplements continue to be barred from the over-the-counter market in the United States.

Many nutritional authorities and academic researchers who have followed the tryptophan controversy dispute the FDA's position, saying that the connection between contaminated tryptophan and the EMS epidemic is scientifically solid. Supplement producers in particular contend that uncontaminated tryptophan does not present a danger of causing EMS or any other serious condition and that the suspect supplements have long since disappeared from the market. Not only were cases of EMS rare before 1989 while tryptophan consumption was commonplace, but a study has suggested that (uncontaminated) tryptophan may actually play a beneficial role in the *treatment* of EMS. Critics of the FDA position note that European countries took action against the contaminated supplements but do not currently ban all tryptophan products.

Critics also point out that the federal government's position on tryptophan is inconsistent. While tryptophan supplements are deemed dangerous, the amino acid was never removed from infant formulas and intravenous feeding solutions and remains an important ingredient in these products today. The Department of Agriculture allows tryptophan in animal feed; veterinarians can use it to treat animals. Finally, and perhaps most tellingly, you can now obtain Japanese-produced (though uncontaminated) tryptophan at a number of

U.S. compounding pharmacies if you can get a doctor to write you a prescription. Partly this is because compounding pharmacies are not as tightly regulated by the FDA as are regular pharmacies, although obviously some level of federal complicity is necessary for compounding pharmacies to sell this expensive, prescription-only tryptophan.

More cynical opponents of the continuing FDA ban on tryptophan contend that it is tryptophan's status as an inexpensive and effective sedative that is keeping it off the market, not any public health concerns. From this perspective, it is no surprise that major pharmaceutical companies are not petitioning the FDA to lift its tryptophan ban. Being cheap and natural, amino acids can be sold by almost anyone, but few if any companies will make enormous profits doing so. Why compete with a dozen companies to sell tryptophan at twenty cents a capsule when you can market selective serotonin reuptake inhibitors (SSRIs), such as fluoxetine (Prozac) and sertraline (Zoloft), for two dollars per capsule? In fact, because both tryptophan's and SSRI's effects are traced to increased serotonin action (although the mechanisms are slightly different, as we'll see), the unavailability of one drug tends to promote the success of the other.

According to Dean Wolfe Manders, Ph.D., writing on "The FDA Ban of L-Tryptophan: Politics, Profits, and Prozac" in the journal *Social Policy:*

> *The continuing FDA public ban of L-tryptophan prevents popular access to this most effective serotonin producer. . . . On June 15, 1993, the FDA Dietary Supplement Task Force published a report on the work it had been doing in the area of developing FDA policy around nutritional supplements. On page two, the report admits, "The Task Force considered various issues in its deliberation, including . . . what steps are necessary to ensure that the existence of dietary supplements on the market does not act as a disincentive for drug development." In this case, the FDA has succeeded in carrying out its stated policy goal. With competition from publicly available L-tryptophan removed, the rapidly expanding market in prescription serotonin drugs—now among them L-tryptophan itself—contains no major "disincentives" for the massive accumulation of pharmaceutical industry profits.*

(One wonders if pharmaceutical companies may also be content to keep the suspicion of toxicity on tryptophan because doing so deflects attention from how the disastrous change in a pharmaceutical manufacturing process led to what has been termed "the first actual genetic engineering catastrophe.")

If there is a silver lining to the continuing controversy over tryptophan, it is that two supplements have in recent years managed to avoid being banned, controlled, or proprietized while they have stepped in to fill the vacuum left by tryptophan: Melatonin is now widely recognized as a safe and natural sleep aid, and 5-HTP shows particular promise as a natural antidepressant.

Should tryptophan supplements once again become available, pregnant women should not take them, nor should anyone who is taking MAO-inhibiting drugs, has bronchial asthma, or the autoimmune condition lupus. Taking tryptophan supplements at the same time as taking SSRIs could cause headaches or other symptoms of excess serotonin levels. Tryptophan may also cause side effects such as nausea, headaches, gastric discomfort, or constipation in some people. Large daily doses, such as 6 to 10 g, should be taken only with professional supervision, as it is possible such amounts may reduce rather than increase serotonin availability.

See "Ordering Supplements and Smart Drugs from Foreign Sources" in Resources for information on how to obtain tryptophan by mail order.

Taking Tryptophan

An average dose of supplemental tryptophan is 500 mg. Combine it with 25 to 50 mg of vitamins B_3 and B_6, 250 mg of magnesium, and 500 mg of vitamin C to enhance its effects. To promote sleep, take it on an empty stomach about an hour before your planned bedtime.

Lacking supplemental tryptophan, it is still possible to take advantage of its calming powers through diet. One potential strategy is to eat foods with high levels of tryptophan relative to other amino acids. This is difficult, however, because even many high-protein foods have lower levels of tryptophan than almost every other amino acid. Eggs, poultry, meat, and other protein foods that are rich in tryptophan also contain considerable amounts of other large neutral amino acids (such as phenylalanine and tyrosine) that compete with tryptophan for transport to and uptake in the brain, and are actually delivered to the brain

more efficiently than tryptophan. So it is possible for tryptophan-rich foods actually to *reduce* brain levels of tryptophan, leading to arousal rather than relaxation.

A few foods do have favorable ratios of tryptophan to other amino acids. These include roasted pumpkin seeds, dried sunflower seeds, and soybeans, and to a lesser extent milk, cheddar cheese, peanuts, lentils, and turkey. Still, you must eat relatively large amounts of these foods to approach the levels of tryptophan once widely available in supplements. For example, eating 100 grams, about 3.5 ounces, of pumpkin seeds, or drinking four cups of milk, provides a dose of about 500 mg of tryptophan. To boost mood, eat some of these tryptophan-specific foods while avoiding other sources of protein.

A better way to take advantage of tryptophan's properties is to consume foods rich in carbohydrates, such as potatoes, bread, cereal, or pasta. Carbohydrates promote the secretion of insulin, a hormone that helps amino acids cross from the blood into bodily cells. Insulin has less effect, however, on tryptophan than on the other amino acids that share its transport system into the brain. This leaves relatively more tryptophan in the blood ultimately to cause a gradual rise in serotonin and melatonin levels in the brain.

----

5 - H T P :   B E T T E R   T H A N
       T R Y P T O P H A N ?

Like tryptophan, 5-HTP is a natural amino acid found in high amounts in seeds and other foods. In the body, 5-HTP is formed from tryptophan, with the help of an enzyme and certain cofactors. 5-HTP is the immediate precursor of serotonin in the process that eventually produces melatonin. Because 5-HTP is one step further along this process than tryptophan (and also because tryptophan is banned as a dietary supplement), 5-HTP has begun to garner increased attention as a potential serotonin-enhancing supplement. Of course, this depiction of a nice straight line from amino acid to neurotransmitter—from supplement to effect—is a simplification of a complex, interdependent series of steps and mechanisms that researchers are still in the process of unraveling. Nonetheless, a number of studies have confirmed that oral doses of 5-HTP result in increased brain levels of serotonin as well as beta-endorphins, the body's natural painkillers.

Not-So-Simple Serotonin

Known to scientists as the chemical 5-hydroxytryptamine (5-HT), serotonin is found in various plants (including foods such as bananas and pineapples) and animals. Much attention has been focused recently on its effects on mind and mood, but serotonin also affects various other cardiovascular, respiratory, and gastrointestinal functions. In describing the diverse and complex pharmacologic effects serotonin has on blood pressure, the heart, and smooth muscle, the respected medical text *Goodman and Gilman's The Pharmacological Basis of Therapeutics* uses terms such as "notoriously variable," "uniquely complex," and "complicated by diverse actions." Serotonin may constrict or dilate blood vessels, or stimulate or depress heart output. Serotonin may raise blood pressure and stimulate the gut. Much is still being learned about this compound.

Serotonin can be found in various parts of the body. Like melatonin, a little goes a long way: scientists estimate that at any one time most people have as little as 10 mg of serotonin in their bodies. Approximately 90 percent of this serotonin can be found in cells in the gastrointestinal tract, which both make and use serotonin. Most of the rest is in the blood, while only 1 to 2 percent of all serotonin exists in the central nervous system, including key parts of the brain and spinal cord where it acts as a neurotransmitter.

The serotonin that you ingest in food doesn't much affect bodily levels. Before ingested serotonin can be used by cells, the intestines, liver, and lungs process it and break it down into metabolites that are excreted in the urine. The blood does pick up low levels of serotonin from the intestines, but overall very little serotonin survives intact the journey through the digestive and circulatory systems to the brain. In this regard, serotonin is unlike melatonin, which demonstrates a high degree of bioavailability as a supplement. Even when serotonin reaches the brain, it faces an additional obstacle, the blood-brain barrier, which serotonin (again unlike melatonin) doesn't cross very effectively. These are all reasons why melatonin is a best-selling supplement but serotonin itself is never found in supplement form.

Ingested serotonin is thus a less significant bodily source for the neurotransmitter compared to manufactured serotonin. Cells in the gastrointestinal and nervous systems can manufacture serotonin, and then store it until needed, from tryptophan or 5-HTP derived from food or from dietary supplements. When 5-HTP is taken orally, some of it gets used by the body to make proteins or stays circulating in the blood, but a significant amount also gets transported to the brain, where it readily crosses the blood-brain barrier and is taken up by nerve cells for the production of serotonin.

From Anxiety to Migraine

While it is true that much more research has been conducted on tryptophan than on 5-HTP, scientific interest in the latter is on the upsurge. Early animal studies found that 5-HTP was similar to tryptophan in its ability to promote sleep and relieve sleep disorders. A number of more recent findings suggest that, like tryptophan, 5-HTP may also be effective at improving mood and alleviating anxiety. For example, a 1987 double-blind, placebo-controlled study done on forty-five patients suffering from anxiety disorders found that 5-HTP caused a moderate reduction in symptoms, though it was not as effective as the tricyclic antidepressive drug clomipramine in alleviating certain symptoms associated with depression. A 1985 study on only ten patients with anxiety syndromes found that 5-HTP significantly reduced anxiety as measured by three separate scales.

Researchers have also begun to investigate 5-HTP's potential to help treat panic disorder, narcolepsy, fibromyalgia syndrome, and migraine headache. For example, in 1996 researchers studied twenty children who had frequent migraine headache attacks. The children who took 5-HTP for three months were found to experience fewer and less severe migraines. As the connections between serotonin levels, carbohydrate cravings, and appetite control have become more evident (witness the development of serotonin-affecting diet drugs such as Redux), 5-HTP has also attracted scientific interest as a potential weight-loss agent.

Some recent animal studies also suggest that 5-HTP may enhance spatial memory or help prevent aging-related learning problems.

5-HTP Versus Prozac

Though enhancement of serotonin function is the shared outcome of taking 5-HTP (or tryptophan) and SSRIs, how these two types of substances accomplish that action differs. Prozac and other SSRIs affect the serotonin already present in the brain and central nervous system. SSRIs help to keep the serotonin that has been transported to nerve cell endings active for a longer duration. SSRIs do this by preventing the cells that have released the serotonin into the synapse, the gap between two opposing nerve cell endings, from recapturing or reabsorbing the neurotransmitter. By thus inhibiting reuptake, SSRIs allow serotonin to hang out in the synapse and continue to bind with receptors in the opposing neuron. It is this binding action that serves to pass messages along to further nerve cells, thus eventually translating into feelings of satiation, confidence, relaxation, and other desirable effects on mood and behavior. In other words, while taking SSRIs, blood and brain levels of serotonin may stay low, though what serotonin there is becomes especially active.

One drawback to this approach to increasing serotonin activity may be that inhibiting the reuptake of serotonin can aggravate an existing deficiency. That is, the brain may adjust to having "more active" serotonin by limiting production of new serotonin. This leads to the concept of a "serotonin deficiency syndrome" and the premise that a more effective way to improve serotonin function would be to increase brain levels of serotonin. Unlike SSRIs, 5-HTP doesn't recycle serotonin; it actually increases its synthesis. More can then be released into the synapses, where it imparts its mood-boosting effects.

The possibility that 5-HTP may help address a serotonin deficiency syndrome was supported by a 1991 study done by a team of Swiss and German psychiatric researchers. Using as subjects a group of sixty-three patients between the ages of eighteen and seventy-five with clinical depression, the researchers compared the effects of 5-HTP to the SSRI fluvoxamine. Subjects' responses to the drugs were evaluated according to the Hamilton Rating Scale for Depression, a standard psychiatric test, as well as self-assessments. The researchers determined that 5-HTP was as effective as fluvoxamine in reducing the symptoms of depression (after six weeks both substances averaged better than 50 percent reductions in depression scores). The dietary supplement, however, caused fewer and less severe side effects compared to the prescription drug.

Another distinction between SSRIs and 5-HTP is in their effects on neurotransmitters in addition to serotonin. The advent of SSRIs in

the late 1980s was so readily embraced by psychiatrists in part because, by affecting mainly serotonin, these new drugs were recognized as "cleaner." That is, because SSRIs do not have major effects on other neurotransmitters such as noradrenaline and dopamine, SSRIs are less likely to cause unwanted effects when compared to other classes of antidepressants, such as tricyclics and monoamine oxidase inhibitors (MAOIs). A 1983 study suggests that 5-HTP may not work, as SSRIs do, almost exclusively through serotonin. The researchers found that 5-HTP can stimulate the synthesis of noradrenaline and dopamine, "probably by way of compensation." They noted that it is "conceivable" that these additional effects of 5-HTP contribute to its antidepressant activity. Of course, if these non-serotonic effects were as dramatic as those of the tricyclics and MAO inhibitors, 5-HTP would suffer in comparison to SSRIs. Further studies should clarify 5-HTP's mode of action. Clinical experience so far suggests that 5-HTP is much less toxic and better tolerated than these conventional antidepressants.

5 - H T P a n d M e l a t o n i n

Taking a serotonin-boosting supplement should also have the welcome side effect of increasing the body's melatonin levels, since that is the final stage in the breakdown of tryptophan and 5-HTP. The preliminary evidence regarding 5-HTP's effect on melatonin, including studies on rats, toads, and sheep, suggests 5-HTP increases melatonin levels. Definitive human studies, however, remain to be done. A 1987 study on humans found no appreciable increase in melatonin after administering oral doses of 5-HTP. Only fifteen subjects were tested, however, and ten of these were children, whose naturally high melatonin levels may be less sensitive to change than are adults'. A 1990 study done on twenty patients suffering from panic disorder found that blood levels of melatonin increased significantly after researchers administered 5-HTP.

The Safety Controversy

The most common complaints associated with taking 5-HTP are digestive problems such as nausea and diarrhea. Taking 5-HTP with food may help prevent gastric upset. Daytime grogginess may also be a problem; many people take 5-HTP only at night, with their melatonin supplements. Extremely high doses of 5-HTP (such as 600 to 800 mg) may decrease libido, much as the serotonin-boosting SSRIs are known to do.

Some medical authorities consider 5-HTP to be potentially toxic because of the well-known dangers associated with elevated blood levels of serotonin. The 1997 edition of a large biomedical products catalog cites 5-HTP as a "harmful substance" that "may cause adverse effects if taken up by the body." In the same catalog tryptophan rates no such warning. The controversy relates to whether 5-HTP should be taken only in conjunction with certain other drugs to minimize adverse reactions. These other drugs, known as "peripheral decarboxylase inhibitors" (PDIs), inhibit an enzyme that can convert 5-HTP to serotonin. This enzyme, however, is most active not in the brain but in the intestines and other organs. Theoretically, unless this enzyme is inhibited by PDIs like carbidopa, 5-HTP will cause high levels of serotonin in the blood. High blood levels of serotonin have been associated with some potentially serious health effects, including heart attacks.

Defenders of 5-HTP note, however, that scientific studies have not supported the use of PDIs with 5-HTP. 5-HTP is apparently more effective when used without PDIs, and causes fewer rather than more side effects. Also, no serious health effects such as heart attacks have ever been recorded in 5-HTP studies or clinical use. The authors of a study that looked at 5-HTP's adverse effects noted, "Researchers who reported on the results of various laboratory functions (hematologic, liver, kidney, etc.) found that 5-HTP caused no significant changes. . . . Oral administration of 5-HTP, with or without carbidopa, is associated with few adverse side effects."

Studies have also found that oral doses of 5-HTP don't cause major increases in blood serotonin levels, perhaps because the brain is able to absorb 5-HTP from the blood before the blood does much of its own converting of 5-HTP to serotonin.

Check with your doctor or health care practitioner if you want to take 5-HTP on an ongoing basis to address a potential serotonin deficiency, especially if you are already taking an SSRI or any other antidepressant drug. Even more so than tryptophan, taking 5-HTP supplements at the same time as taking SSRIs may lead to nausea or other adverse effects from excessively high serotonin levels. Users of SSRIs may be able, however, to gradually cut back on their prescription antidepressants by substituting 5-HTP. Such reduction, however, should be done only with the proper medical supervision. Also avoid taking 5-HTP if you are using any other serotonin-affecting compound, such as the diet drug dexfenfluramine (Redux).

Those few people who have the rare condition known as carcinoid syndrome should not take 5-HTP. This disease is characterized by tumors of serotonin-forming cells usually in the gut or lungs and is associated with extremely high levels of serotonin in the blood. Anyone with gastrointestinal diseases such as ulcers or Crohn's disease should also avoid 5-HTP supplements.

Most researchers report that adverse effects from taking 5-HTP are relatively few and benign, though clearly some people don't tolerate it well and should not use it.

A Newcomer to the Supplement Market

Currently, 5-HTP is relatively expensive compared to other nutritional supplements, with the retail price approaching one dollar per capsule for some brands. As expensive as this is, it is still cheaper than most prescription SSRIs. The per-unit price can be expected to fall as supplement manufacturers' production processes begin to respond to market conditions.

The FDA's current ban on the sale of tryptophan does not apply to 5-HTP; the compound apparently exists in a legal gray area, neither banned nor approved for any uses. Some compounding pharmacies sell it by prescription. The first appearance of 5-HTP as a commercial, over-the-counter nutritional supplement came only in 1996. By mid-1997 a half-dozen domestic companies had formulated 5-HTP products and were offering them for sale by mail order (see Resources). Unless the FDA steps in, 5-HTP's popularity will likely continue to increase, causing the large dietary supplement producers to jump on the bandwagon and begin to offer 5-HTP products that will be carried by natural foods stores.

5-HTP is also known as oxitriptan and 5-OHT.

Taking 5-HTP

The effects different dosages of 5-HTP have on any one individual are difficult to predict. Studies that have tested for 5-HTP's effects on insomnia, anxiety, and mild depression typically administer 50 to 300 mg per day. Other studies have tested much higher levels, such as 600 to 1,200 mg per day, as possible treatments for more serious forms of depression and for other conditions. In general, users find 5-HTP to be more potent than tryptophan by a factor of approximately ten. Thus, a 50 mg dose of 5-HTP is approximately equivalent to a 500 mg dose of tryptophan.

5-HTP comes in capsules and powders. An average first-time dose is 25 to 50 mg. Some people may need to take higher levels in divided doses, such as 150 to 200 mg. 5-HTP's antidepressant effects may not be evident until you have taken it daily for two to three weeks.

People who take melatonin supplements at night and want to add 5-HTP to their supplement regimen may also need to reduce their dosage of one or the other supplement to avoid morning grogginess.

Most people take 5-HTP, like melatonin and tryptophan, at bedtime to avoid daytime grogginess. Others, however, have reported taking 5-HTP during the day for its antidepressant effects without experiencing unwanted drowsiness. Taking 5-HTP with 25 to 50 mg of vitamin B_6 may increase the amount that gets converted into serotonin in the brain. As is the case with tryptophan, taking 5-HTP when your stomach is empty of other proteins or with foods high in carbohydrates may somewhat improve its delivery to the brain.

GABA: AMINO ACID AND BRAIN CHEMICAL

Scientists first identified gamma aminobutyric acid as a unique brain chemical in 1950, but only within the past two decades have they realized that in the body GABA functions as a neurotransmitter and a central nervous system depressant. By preventing nerve cells from firing too quickly, GABA acts as a brake on the stimulating and excitatory effects of other neurotransmitters, such as acetylcholine and noradrenaline. Muscles relax, breathing and heart rate slow down, and body temperature drops. Anxiety is reduced, and the whole body starts to feel more at ease.

Valium, Librium, and a number of the other conventional anxiety-reducing and tranquilizing agents are thought to rely in part for their calming effect on their ability to increase the activity of GABA on the central nervous system. In the brain GABA metabolizes to produce the fast-acting sedative substance gamma hydroxybutyrate, or GHB. Like GABA, GHB helps to promote relaxation and induce sleep, though taken orally GHB is much more potent. GABA's effects are more comparable to tryptophan's. Users report that within about an hour of taking GABA, the mind is quieted and sleep is more sound.

Avoid combining GABA with other drugs, especially depressants such as alcohol, and don't drive after taking it. A Chinese study suggested that an increase in brain levels of GABA is "unfavorable" to learning and memory, so don't take GABA before a long study session or an important business meeting, either. Of course, this recommendation could well apply to relaxants in general.

Taking GABA

GABA is sold as a powder, in 750 mg tablets, and in capsules that go by names such as GABA Calm, Gaba-tol, and GABA Plus. An average anxiety-reducing dose is 500 to 750 mg; for insomnia take 750 to 1,500 mg about an hour before bedtime. Some people find that GABA's calming effects are enhanced by combining it with a dose of 25 to 50 mg of the B-complex vitamins niacinamide (B_3) and pyridoxine (B_6), which help the body to synthesize even more GABA and deliver it to the appropriate receptors in the brain.

PART SIX

Inebriants and Aphrodisiacs

cultures' spiritual practices, missionaries sought to ban it as a way to disrupt traditional religion and to pave the way for the likes of Presbyterianism. By the same token, colonial administrators recognized kava-drinking circles as important social and political gatherings. Imperialists knew that such quaint traditions as self-governance and cultural integrity, inimical to the demands of colonial rule, could be disturbed by discouraging kava cultivation and use.

Where colonial pressures and missionary zeal were especially effective, kava use was sometimes abandoned altogether. This was the case in Kosrae (a tiny island in Micronesia) and Tahiti. Kava was also abandoned in Hawaii, which probably originally acquired the plant via Tahiti. Kava was well established in Hawaii by the time Cook arrived in 1778. For a brief time in the early 1800s, Hawaiians even exported kava. Native Hawaiian use of kava peaked by the turn of the twentieth century, and until recently the few plants that could be found on the islands were mostly imported ornamentals in commercial nurseries. In Hawaii as well as Tahiti and other Pacific islands, however, kava is showing signs of making a comeback as native peoples have begun to regain respect for their traditional culture and their unique identity. Hawaiian growers have also begun to embrace kava as a potentially lucrative crop currently in high demand from natural product companies.

Vanuatu remains the kava capital of the world. Though missionary pressures to curtail its use were still in evidence as recently as the late 1940s, today nearly all the adult males of Vanuatu drink kava, and, as is the case in more urban areas throughout the South Pacific, its use has spread to include females. Scores of kava bars, or *nakamals* as natives call them, have opened in recent years in Vanuatu's cities and towns, and in rural areas the average household cultivates more than one hundred kava plants. Vanuatu's reputation for growing the highest quality kava has allowed it to become a major exporter, principally to Germany and a few other European countries that use it pharmaceutically.

K A V A ' S
P S Y C H O A C T I V E
C H E M I S T R Y

Scientific interest in kava's psychoactive properties began soon after it was authoritatively classified by Forster. The first researcher to detail kava's traditional preparation and use, as well as to isolate one of kava's mind-altering compounds, was the French pharmacist G. Cuzent in the late 1850s. Additional nineteenth-century scientific work on kava is credited to the famous German botanist Louis Lewin, whose 1886 publications on kava inspired fellow scientists in Germany and elsewhere to explore kava's fascinating effects on the mind. Lewin's interest in kava spanned decades, from his research into kava's active compounds in the 1880s to his inclusion of kava in 1924 in his classic, interdisciplinary book, *Phantastica: Narcotic and Stimulating Drugs*.

The process of identifying and isolating kava's psychoactive compounds has continued for well over a century now, with much of the pioneering work done in the 1920s.

Kava

◉

THE PACIFIC HERB

Kava is a type of pepper plant whose root is used to make a relaxing, even inebriating, nonalcoholic beverage. At any of the hundreds of kava bars that have sprung up in recent years throughout the South Pacific, native islanders and tourists alike sip this milky, strong-smelling beverage from cups or the traditional coconut shell. For fifty cents or a dollar, you can experience its uniquely sensuous and pleasurable effects. If you're like most people, after a few drinks you'll feel peaceful and friendly and, if the beverage is a potent one, quite possibly a little rubber-legged. Though your body will be so relaxed you may feel as if you've sunk into your chair, your mind will stay sharp, in marked contrast to an alcoholic high. The next day you'll notice another pleasant trait of kava compared to alcohol: kava doesn't cause a hangover.

Termed "the official drink of the Pacific," kava is (with the stimulant betel nut) one of the area's two principal, traditional psychoactive plants. Kava has played a central role in South Sea Island culture and spiritual practice for thousands of years. Though its use tapered off in the past two centuries due to European influence, kava is now being rediscovered in Fiji, Hawaii, and elsewhere, where native peoples are adapting it to modern times. With its potential as an effective anti-anxiety remedy and sleep-inducing aid, as well as a relatively nontoxic and nonaddictive alternative to alcohol, kava has also begun to set sail from the Pacific and infiltrate Australia, mainland Asia, and Europe. In North America kava is one of the hottest new herbs in health food stores, where it is sold both as a beneficial therapeutic substance (primarily as a gentle yet reliable sedative) and as a potential pleasure drug. In mid-1996, restaurateurs even opened what must be North America's first kava bar. The Kava Lounge in Manhattan's trendy TriBeCa area is attracting newcomers to the traditional drink, even though the menu describes it humorously as tasting like "dirty dishwater with a hint of cloves." The taste may be an acquired one, but kava in one form or another now appears poised to become a world-renowned natural mind-alterant.

THE POTENT PEPPER

A large perennial shrub of the diverse pepper family, kava is native to the islands of the tropical South Pacific. It is widely cultivated in Melanesia, which ranges from New Guinea to the Solomon Islands to Fiji and is one of the three main areas of the South Pacific. Kava is less widely cultivated farther east, in Polynesia, which includes Samoa, Tahiti, and Hawaii. Few of the many tiny islands that make up Micronesia, in the West Pacific north of the equator, cultivate kava. Kava is known by diverse names among the widespread native cultures of the South Pacific: as *yaqona* in Fiji; *keu* along the Maclay Coast of Papua New Guinea; *sakau* on Pohnpei; *seka* on Kosrae; and *'awa* in Hawaii.

Kava is not a particularly attractive plant, being a stalky shrub adorned with a paucity of heart-shaped leaves. Plants can grow up to fifteen feet tall but are usually uprooted for their starchy root, stump, and lower stems well before reaching full height. Typically, native South Sea islanders plant kava as one of the lower crops in a multilayered garden, shaded by taller nut or fruit trees. Kava prefers regular rain, high humidity, and summer days of 80° to 90°; it doesn't do well in either swampy or desertlike conditions. Natives harvest the plant when it is at least three to four years old,

at which point the knotty roots attain a weight of about twenty pounds.

What's most interesting about kava the plant (*kava* also refers to the inebriating beverage itself) is that it is as much an invention of humans as a product of nature. Modern kava is a sterile, cultivated species that bears neither fruits nor seeds. It is thought to have originated only within the past three thousand years. Around the time of King David's rule of Israel, native South Sea Islanders first began to domesticate a wild species of kava (*Piper wichmannii*). How these natives first discovered kava's psychoactivity is not known, though some mythical accounts indicate they may have observed rats becoming inebriated by chewing on the lower stems.

Natives began to domesticate kava by cutting off one of the plant's lower stems, setting it aside to sprout, and pulling or digging up the root. If the plant offered desirable psychoactive properties, the natives would return to plant the stem cutting. Over centuries this "natural cloning" process of artificial selection has led to the development of some 120 cultivars—varieties originating and continuing in cultivation and given a name in a modern language—that have been identified throughout fourteen Pacific Island countries. Some of these varieties have no doubt been bred for factors such as yield and hardiness, but the principal trait for which growers have long been selecting kava is its ability to relax the body and calm the mind.

THREE THOUSAND YEARS OF TRADITIONAL USE

Lacking written records, kava researchers have explored various disciplines for clues to kava's early prehistory. For example, by tracing the development of certain words; analyzing the shape and structure of bowls, cups, and other types of pottery associated with kava use; mapping the location of various species or cultivars of kava; and comparing species genetically, researchers now believe that kava use originated in Melanesia and slowly spread outward to other parts of the South Pacific.

After considering the linguistic, botanical, and genetic evidence, the authors of the authoritative *Kava: The Pacific Drug* narrowed the origin of kava cultivation to the northern islands of Vanuatu (formerly New Hebrides), a Melanesian country consisting of a chain of seventy-some islands, at least twenty-one of which cultivate kava. "It is possible that all kava cultivars trace back to a single ancestral plant somewhere in northern Vanuatu that has been repeatedly cloned, developed, and dispersed by stem cuttings over perhaps three millennia," note Vincent Lebot, Mark Merlin, and Lamont Lindstrom. Some eighty-two different kava cultivars have been identified in Vanuatu alone, and native myths also support a Vanuatu origin.

The earliest Europeans to explore the South Pacific, from the initial expeditions of discovery in the sixteenth century to British navigator Captain James Cook's landmark

voyages in the 1760s and 1770s, reported the use of kava. Cook was accompanied on his second trip, from 1772 to 1775, by German writer and scientist Johann G. A. Forster, who in 1786 carefully described kava and classified it as *Piper methysticum* (from the Greek *methy* for wine), or "intoxicating pepper." Crewmen on Cook's and others' voyages often tried kava, with varying results—some sailors likened it to opium, while others said it had little or no effect.

In a number of South Pacific societies kava was a major plant with important medicinal, social, and spiritual applications. As were psychoactive plants in traditional cultures around the world, kava was central to many island societies' religion. Kava allowed those who drank it (usually only men; sometimes only spiritual or political leaders) to commune with the gods or contact deceased relatives. Where kava was abundant, it was usually embraced by elites and commoners alike. As an herb that helped people relax, enjoy each other's company, and expand everyday consciousness, kava played a predominant role in Pacific Island culture.

Kava use went into decline in the late eighteenth and early nineteenth century as it came under fire from European colonialists and from missionaries, who sifted into the South Pacific and began to convert native islanders to Christianity. European sensibilities and notions of hygiene were offended by the traditional method of kava preparation, which required that the root be chewed for ten minutes or so before the pulpy mass was spat out, infused with water, filtered, and then drunk. Because kava was an integral part of many

Chemists have determined that kava's psycho-active ingredients are not alkaloids, the nitro-gen-containing compounds (such as cocaine and caffeine) prominent in many drug plants, but rather certain oxygen-containing, lipidlike resin compounds known as lactones or py-rones. Researchers have identified six major kavalactones and another dozen minor ones. The major ones, which are most abundant and account for much of the mind-altering effect, are:

- Yangonin
- Methysticin
- Dihydromethysticin (DHM)
- Kavain
- Dihydrokavain (DHK)
- Demethoxy-yangonin

It would not be important to know the names of these kavalactones except that their relative concentrations in various kava culti-vars and differences in their rate of absorption in the body determine whether the psychoac-tive effects are potent and desirable. For exam-ple, kava varieties that are richest in DHM have powerful tranquilizing effects but are so strong that they tend to promote nausea. Many kava connoisseurs prefer those kava cultivars, such as certain varieties from Vanu-atu and Fiji, that are richest in methysticin and quickly absorbed kavain.

The lateral roots are the part of the plant with the highest concentrations of kavalac-tones. Kavalactone content is somewhat lower in the main root and continues to decrease progressively into the stump, lower stems, and higher parts of the plant. Scientists have, how-ever, found traces of some kavalactones in the leaves. Although the amounts are tiny and leaves are not abundant on kava plants, this is a promising discovery given that, as a root herb like ginseng, kava plants are destroyed when harvested. (Indeed, at least one herb company has begun to offer capsules of kava derived from the leaves and stems and to promote the product as "an environmentally friendly crop," because the leaves are harvested continually without destroying the plants.) Even the roots of kava are mostly starch and fibers; kavalac-tone content averages only 10 to 15 percent, and rarely rises above 20 percent.

Whether older kava roots are more potent than younger ones is a matter of dispute. In 1989 researchers reported, on the basis of sev-eral trials, that kava roots reach their maxi-mum kavalactone content after about eighteen months, and that older roots are larger but no more potent. This finding is contrary to the experience of many of the native users of kava, who have long considered old roots to be of higher potency than young ones. Roots that are at least seven years old are particu-larly valued and sometimes reserved for spe-cial occasions.

Studies have shown that the kavalactones have a number of important effects on the body's muscles, nerves, and organs. Kava

- Relaxes skeletal muscles, especially those in the arms and legs
- Initially stimulates and then depresses the rate of breathing
- Initially stimulates and then depresses the central nervous system, primarily reducing the activity of the spinal cord rather than the brain

- Promotes sleep
- Relieves pain, whether used orally or topically
- Promotes the production and flow of urine

While all of the major kavalactones help to relax skeletal muscles, some kavalactones have more effect on certain bodily actions than others do. For example, kavain has anti-anxiety effects and seems to be responsible for most of kava's ability to numb tissues in the mouth, while DHK and DHM are more potent general analgesics (almost twice as effective per milligram at reducing pain as is aspirin, though considerably less potent than morphine).

The slightly different actions of the six major kavalactones also help to explain two additional factors: why kava varieties rich in certain kavalactones have varying effects on the mind, and why synthetic kava preparations made up of only one kavalactone are pale imitations of natural kava. The modern pharmaceutical practice of favoring isolated compounds rather than whole herbs as therapeutic agents may have hindered Western medicine's acceptance of kava—researchers in the mid-1960s who determined that large doses (800 to 1,200 mg) of DHM were needed for it to be an effective tranquilizer dismissed further research into kava as apparently unnecessary. This in spite of the fact that a number of studies conducted both before and since have found that the natural blend of kavalactones works synergistically to produce what has been termed kava's "complex and subtle psychoactivity."

Exactly how the kavalactones act on the brain to produce their sweeping mind-altering effects is not yet known. Kavain and other kavalactones pass through the blood-brain barrier and are suspected to alter the action of certain neurotransmitters. It is unclear whether, like Valium and other benzodiazepines, kava's calming effects are due to an influence on GABA, the neurotransmitter that acts as a brake on the central nervous system (see chapter 16). A kava study done in 1992 found no GABA-related interaction, while a 1994 study done on rats' brains found that kavalactones increased the number of binding sites for GABA. The main parts of the brain kava seems to affect are the hippocampus and amygdala, structures in the brain's limbic system (which is concerned especially with emotions and motivation). Whether kava affects other neurotransmitters, such as dopamine, or works through unrelated pathways is still being studied.

Although kava is sometimes classified as a narcotic, this is misleading. Kava is not like the classic narcotics—opium derivatives such as morphine and codeine—which, while reducing pain and promoting stupor, are highly addictive and potentially lethal in high doses. Kava is a narcotic only in the sense of being soothing and lulling. It is more accurately classified as a muscle relaxant, anxiolytic (reduces nervousness and anxiety), soporific or sedative/hypnotic (relaxes and, in larger doses, promotes sleep), and inebriant.

Thousands of years ago, the earliest kava users probably took the most direct route for ingesting kava's active chemicals: chewing lengthily on the root itself, ingesting some if not all of its tough fibers and mind-altering resin. Some kava cultivars can provide quite a kick in this form, but in all likelihood only the most determined and dentally endowed of these early kava fans would have found this practice worth the trouble.

Early traditional peoples no doubt also brewed kava into a tea. They would harvest the roots and lower stems, cut them up, and sun-dry them. A stick and a hollowed log or a bowl-shaped stone served as mortar and pestle to grind the dried kava into a powder. Dissolved in hot water and sweetened, kava tea is appetizing but has minimal effects on the mind. Primitive kava consumers no doubt recognized a fact that scientists confirmed by the late nineteenth century: the most psychoactive compounds in kava don't get released into solution merely by being infused in water.

At some point, Pacific peoples managed to discover a preparation technique that offered some of the potency of root chewing with the convenience of drinking it as a beverage. They found that they could chew on the root but not swallow it. Typically it was children who were tapped for this chore, whether young female virgins (some were known to sacrifice their chastity to avoid this duty) or just chil-dren with strong teeth. After ten minutes or more, the designated chewers would spit the soggy mass into a bowl. When a large handful or so of chewed kava was collected, it would be mixed with coconut milk and drunk. Alternatively, the chewed-up mass would be placed in a large leaf in a way that water or coconut milk could be run over it and a kava liquid would filter through. The kava beverage would then be drunk.

Chewing is indeed an effective method for making kava's psychoactive compounds accessible to the body. The earliest scientific researchers thought that salivary enzymes transformed kava's mind-altering compounds. It's now known that the process is more mechanical than chemical. Chewing emulsifies the root's resin, where the kavalactones are. That is, chewing suspends tiny, kavalactone-rich resin particles in the saliva. After this emulsion is prepared into a beverage, the kavalactones are more easily absorbed into the bloodstream when they reach the stomach. The more finely emulsified or separated in water these particles are, the more likely it is that the kava beverage will be a potent one.

Various forms of the traditional chewing method were widespread in the South Pacific when the first Europeans arrived. They found the practice "revolting" and "unhygienic," and took what steps they could to discourage it, including outlawing it. By the late nineteenth century the chewing method had been abandoned in Fiji and elsewhere. Today only some isolated tribes in Vanuatu and Papua New Guinea are known to still use the traditional chewing method.

Chewing persisted for as long as it did because it was effective. Saliva, however, is not the only liquid capable of emulsifying kava. Water works, though alcohol or lipids such as lecithin or vegetable oil work even better. Nowadays mechanical grinding of either the fresh or dried root mixed with a liquid, along with squeezing of the liquefied mass through some sort of filter, has supplanted chewing. One method is to loosely enclose a half-cup of fine kava powder in a piece of cloth. This "kava ball" is then dunked in two quarts of water and repeatedly squeezed and mashed about. After five or ten minutes, the dunking and mashing creates a milky kava emulsion, enough for about four people to drink.

The use of electric grinders and blenders has further updated these traditional preparation techniques. You can make a version of the traditional kava beverage by starting with a quarter-cup of finely ground kava. Mix the powder with one or two cups of water. You can also add two tablespoons of olive or other vegetable oil, or a similar amount of liquid lecithin. Blend the powder and liquids at high speed in a blender for five minutes or so into a milky froth. Strain this liquid through a filter or fine sieve and drink. The pulp can be reprocessed to make a weaker drink by adding more water, blending, and straining.

As a drink, kava is an acquired taste, at best. Even Pacific natives tolerate rather than embrace the taste—the word *kava* in Polynesian languages also has such meanings as "bitter," "pungent," and "bad-tasting."

More high-tech methods exist for extracting the resin and concentrating it in liquid form. Unless you have some knowledge and practice in basic chemistry, and are comfortable using heat baths and evaporating organic solvents, leave these methods to the professionals. A number of herbal producers offer concentrated liquid extracts of kava (see Resources). As we'll discuss below, kava is also now becoming available in standardized extract capsules.

Cultures in the South Pacific have honed their preparation techniques for thousands of years, and numerous slight variations exist from one island to the next. Some observers say that the results are similar. "From my own experience I suspect that there is little, if any, difference in the effects of kava prepared by the alternative techniques," says Ron Brunton, author of *The Abandoned Narcotic: Kava and Cultural Instability in Melanesia*. "I have drunk kava prepared both by chewing and by grating on many separate occasions in Vanuatu, and with both I have experienced feelings of tranquillity, difficulty in maintaining motor coordinations, and eventual somnolence."

I GET A PEACEFUL, EASY FEELING...

As with any mind-altering substance, kava has different effects on different people. In addition, the strength of kava preparations varies widely, and the atmosphere and the social setting of kava consumption play an important role in determining the user's experience.

For some, kava's effects are too subtle. For others, the relaxation is too pronounced. Also, some people find that they feel no effects at all the first few times they try kava, a "reverse tolerance" trait that kava shares with some other psychoactive substances, such as marijuana.

For most people, the mild high from a moderate kava dose of average potency will last two to three hours, with the initial effects being felt within twenty to thirty minutes. Some people at first feel a pleasant stimulation, while others notice right away that nervousness and anxiety begin to dissipate and muscles start to unwind. As with alcohol, many people feel an initial mild stimulation. Inhibitions dissolve and many people become more talkative, though not in a particularly boisterous way.

After the first half-hour, feelings of peacefulness and deep relaxation become more prominent. Lewin described this harmonious state as one "of happy unconcern, well-being, and contentment, free of physical or psychological excitement." Natural health author Chris Kilham in *Kava: Medicine Hunting in Paradise,* the first popular book on kava, described his first experience with a potent form of kava:

> *I felt the first effects of the kava in about five minutes. The muscles throughout my body became softer, more elastic. My face became relaxed and pliable, as subtle tension seemed to drain out of my facial muscles. I became aware of my breathing, which felt deeper, slightly more full and definitely more pleasurable than usual. Over the course of the next few minutes a sensuous wave of muscular relaxation washed slowly throughout my entire body like India ink spreading on white paper. My visual and auditory acuity also became heightened. . . . My mind was lucid and clear. The overall effect was one of great pleasure and complete mental alertness. It was delightful.*

Like some of the more potent methoxylated amphetamines (particularly MDMA, or ecstasy; see chapter 4), kava is often an effective empathogen—a substance that increases feelings of sociability, friendliness, and empathy with others. One of the kavalactones, methysticin, actually bears some chemical similarity to MDMA. "Kava seems to make you feel closer to other people," one user reports. "You feel like hugging every stranger who walks by; you want to see-hear-feel their world with them." Thus, you may miss some of kava's most dramatic effects if you take it by yourself or experience it only as a sleep-inducing sedative. In traditional societies, kava would rarely be used by the solitary individual.

Taking large doses or especially potent kava kicks in another layer of mind- and body-altering properties that may last a number of hours. (A note on dose: Kava is a weak drug in the sense that you need to take relatively large amounts, such as multiple-gram doses, of the whole herb to feel its most dramatic effects. While kava varieties differ, a rule of thumb is that one serving of the traditional beverage, usually four to six ounces, contains about one gram or so of kavalactone-rich resin, according to Lebot. Kava researchers have estimated the kavalactone content of one serving of the beverage to be approximately 250 to 500 mg of kavalactones. South Sea Islanders sometimes consume three, four, or more such servings in a single night, though a single dose or two of a potent variety of kava can produce the classic symptoms of mild euphoria, heavy limbs, and deep relaxation. Kava is also most potent when consumed on an empty stomach.) Users are more obviously inebriated and the sedative effects are more pronounced. At the same time, there's a surprising level of mental acuity, rather than the dizziness and hazy thinking of alcoholic inebriation. Kava deeply relaxes muscles, almost to the point of numbness. You can still function but not in an energetic or coordinated way—driving is not a good idea. Eventually the arms and legs begin to feel so tired and heavy that they're hard to use, making even walking a chore (physically if not mentally). At this point, you're not eager to do any wild and crazy dancing—quiet contemplation is more appropriate, "an inclination to remain mute in a mood of happy dreaminess," as one observer put it.

Some kava users then feel so deeply relaxed that they lie down and don't move a muscle or they fall into a deep and restful sleep. Vivid dreams are common when using kava. Upon waking most people feel relaxed rather than hungover or disoriented.

"Thinking is certainly affected by the kava experience, but not in the same ways as are found from caffeine, nicotine, alcohol, or marijuana," says kava researcher R. J. Gregory. "I would personally characterize the changes I experienced as going from lineal processing of information to a greater sense of 'being' and contentment with being. Memory seemed to be enhanced, whereas restriction of data inputs was strongly desired, especially with regard to disturbances of light, movements, noise, and so on. Peace and quiet were very important to maintain the inner sense of serenity. My senses seemed to be unusually sharpened, so that even whispers seemed to be loud while loud noises were extremely unpleasant."

Though kava is sometimes described as a hallucinogen (notably in Abram Hoffer and Humphry Osmond's 1967 book, *The Hallucinogens*), this is really an exaggeration of its effects. Kava's mind-altering powers are nowhere near those of the classic entheogens such as LSD and peyote. At most, some kava users report that high doses of potent kava can cause mild visual and auditory distortions, such as objects taking on a soft glow or an overall vagueness. A study done in 1985 described visual effects from drinking a kava beverage, but the findings were based on the experiences of only a single subject, and in any case were minor (a slight change in focus and an increase in pupil diameter). It is true, on the other hand, that the traditional use of kava in ceremonies and rituals resembles the manner in which other cultures use the true entheogens, such as the mind-altering mushrooms.

- -
KAVA VERSUS ALCOHOL
- -

Kava use in the South Pacific in some ways mirrors alcohol use in the West. Both kava and booze are primarily social and recreational drinks, usually consumed in the early evening before dinner and in a relaxing atmosphere. "For South Sea Islanders, drinking kava in groups at night is the equivalent of an American cocktail party, " according to Dr. Andrew Weil and Winifred Rosen, authors of *From Chocolate to Morphine*. Like an ice-breaking round of drinks among friends after work, kava acts initially to mildly stimulate and elevate mood while helping to lower social inhibition and promote conversation and communal feelings.

Though ritual use of kava has declined as South Pacific societies have modernized, kava is also still a tool that can help resolve conflicts, patch up disputes, and welcome friends. Bringing a kava root to a neighbor's serves much the same purpose as offering the gift of a bottle of wine at a dinner party in the West.

Like wine grapes in southern Europe, kava is also becoming an important export crop in the South Pacific. There, however, the similarities end between kava and alcohol. Kava researchers have long noted that kava's general effects on personality, behavior, and overall health are much more benign than alcohol's. In 1927 Lewin said that kava soothes temperaments and makes the drinker silent and drowsy. The kava drinker "never becomes angry, unpleasant, quarrelsome or noisy, as happens with alcohol." South Seas natives who have had experience with both kava and alcohol almost unanimously agree that kava promotes tranquillity and sociability while alcohol makes people become aggressive and even violent. Consuming both substances, as in using an alcoholic beverage as a kava chaser, is done but is, as one native observed, "incompatible with the true kava frame of mind." The owners of New York's Kava Lounge promote the drink with the presumably tongue-in-cheek statement, "The effects of kava differ from alcohol—women prefer their men to drink kava because they come home, want sex and then fall asleep."

For some kava's combination of mental clarity and bodily relaxation is welcomed, while regular drinkers of alcohol may feel kava's effects are too subtle for them. (It is necessary to emphasize that consuming high doses or particularly potent kava can, like drinking alcohol, lead to accidents if appropriate cautions are not taken. In particular, driving is inadvisable.) Finally, kava is less likely than alcohol to cause a hangover or to cause chemical addiction.

Given the relative health advantages of kava over alcohol, it may be surprising that alcohol has gained in popularity in the South Pacific over the past two centuries, while kava use, at least until very recently, has declined. Social and political factors have contributed more to this trend than an unbiased assessment of these drugs' impact on individual and public health. Nineteenth-century missionaries and colonialists often sought specifically to suppress kava drinking, while they tolerated or even promoted the importation of alcohol (as well as another potent and addictive drug, nicotine). Native leaders in Hawaii were encouraged to embrace alcohol as "the water from America," clean and packaged and modern. Hawaii even passed a law in the 1850s that basically made kava a prescription drug, though enforcement was lax. Alcohol rushed into the void.

Ironically, in a number of other Pacific Island countries, health authorities and even some government officials have now actually gone full circle on kava and alcohol: they're calling for the return of traditional kava drinking as a relatively healthful alternative to alcohol consumption. For example, in Vanuatu over the past fifteen years, official sanction has allowed kava use to experience a resurgence while imports of beer and wine have fallen by 60 percent. In Queensland, Australia, Aboriginal leaders familiar with alcohol's propensity for causing debilitation and violence have begun to promote kava as a viable substitute for alcohol, even though kava is not an indigenous plant.

In addition to offering an alternative to alcohol, kava can also be favorably compared to prescription anti-anxiety drugs, such as the exceedingly popular benzodiazepines (Valium, Xanax). A number of studies have demonstrated that kava has notable anti-anxiety effects and that, in contrast to the "minor tranquilizers" often prescribed for anxiety, kava is less likely to cause adverse side effects or promote long-term dependence. Most recently, a double-blind, placebo-controlled study published in *Phytomedicine* in 1996 tested fifty-eight subjects with "anxiety, tension, and excitedness of non-mental origin." The researchers found that a standardized kava extract (subjects were administered 70 mg of kavalactones three times daily for four weeks) reduced anxiety symptoms as measured by various widely used psychological tests. Compared to the placebo subjects, the kava subjects experienced less anxiety after only seven days, while further improvements were noticed after fourteen and twenty-eight days.

Kava is also less likely to impair thinking, though studies conflict on whether the herb can actually benefit cognition and memory. A 1993 study found that the mean cognitive performance (including reaction time and tracking tasks) of a group of volunteers who took kava was generally poorer than the control group, though admittedly the difference was not statistically significant. Other research, such as a 1991 study published in a German journal and a 1993 study published in *Neuropsychobiology,* found that subjects who took a standardized kava extract improved their reaction time and word recognition scores. In the latter study, the kava subjects significantly outperformed subjects who took oxazepam, a benzodiazepine that caused word recognition scores to fall.

BEYOND THE MIND

Kava's primary medical use in the Pacific is related to its social and recreational use: to calm body and mind, reduce anxiety, relax muscles and prevent convulsions, and promote restful sleep. Thus, kava may be prescribed by traditional healers as part of a program to help control epilepsy, muscle spasms, insomnia, and other conditions. Various traditional peoples of the Pacific, however, have also found numerous other medical applications for kava. Perhaps paramount among these is kava's ability to treat urinary tract infections (UTIs) and bladder disorders. A mild diuretic that promotes urine production and flow, kava also has some potential antibacterial and antifungal effects, according to researchers. Contrary to claims, it doesn't cure gonorrhea or other venereal diseases, although it may provide some symptomatic relief or possibly even play some preventive role.

Kava has also been used as an ingredient in topical painkilling lotions. Kava drinkers can confirm that downing a cup of traditional kava brew induces numbness inside the mouth, affecting the gums, tongue, and throat (thus mimicking one of the few truly therapeutic uses of a much more potent drug, cocaine). This property of local anesthesia has been investigated for medicinal uses, and some Pacific peoples treat toothaches, sore throats, insect stings, and other minor pains with kava-based remedies.

While scientific studies or chemical analyses have supported a few of kava's therapeutic uses, some traditional kava remedies have only folklore and myth to back them up. These include claims that kava induces abortion, promotes the flow of breast milk, and relieves gout and rheumatism.

THE DOWN SIDE

Kava is one of the least harmful and safest drugs of its kind. Ronald K. Siegel, Ph.D., author of *Intoxication: Life in Pursuit of Artificial Paradise,* says that among the sedative/hypnotics, kava is the drug easiest to control and the least likely to produce toxicity or dependency. Occasional and even moderate drinking of kava among Pacific peoples seems to have no noticeable adverse effects on long-term health.

Side effects from kava are rare. The German Commission E monograph on kava lists under side effects "none known." Some users do report short-term adverse effects, such as

mild nausea and numbness to the mouth, from taking moderate to heavy doses of kava. More important, potent dosages can reduce your motor control and lead to accidents—including fatal ones if you unwisely attempt to drive or operate heavy equipment.

Adverse long-term health effects may be more prominent, however, with constant heavy consumption of kava. Kava abusers may suffer from diarrhea, photophobia, and double vision. An overall lethargy and apathy may cause loss of interest in sex and decreased appetite, frequently leading to weight loss. Heavy kava users who are susceptible to certain allergens in kavalactones may find that their skin becomes yellow, dried, and scaly. Fortunately, all of these symptoms can be alleviated within about two weeks by eliminating or cutting back on kava consumption.

Whether even heavy daily consumption of kava leads to chemical addiction is unlikely. A 1991 study found that mice do not develop a tolerance to kava, and no studies have firmly established a pattern of kava addiction. Undeniably, however, some Pacific cultures have a minority of kava drinkers whose habitual and debilitating use of kava can be classified as drug abuse. Some of the cultural practices associated with traditional kava consumption, such as rarely drinking alone, may be helping to prevent abuse. Of course, no such cultural safeguards exist in North America, where various (non-beverage) forms of kava have started to appear on health food stores' shelves in recent years. Still, kava must be considered one of the safest and most nontoxic psychoactive substances known to humanity.

Persons suffering from Parkinson's disease

should not consume kava until questions about its effects on dopamine levels are resolved. Pregnant and nursing women should also avoid kava. Taking kava may increase the effects of other relaxant or anxiety-reducing drugs.

Questions were raised about kava's safety in January 1997 when some fifty attendees at a New Year's Eve concert in Los Angeles became ill after consuming vials of a fringe natural-high product called fX that listed kava as its main ingredient. Subsequent laboratory testing, however, determined that the product contained no kava at all but did contain caffeine and a potent sedative chemical (1,4 butanediol).

KAVA COMES TO NORTH AMERICA

Over the past few decades kava has begun to expand beyond its base in the Pacific to become more of a world herb. Pharmaceutical preparations, using both pure kava and kava in combination with other ingredients, have been made from natural kava extracts and from synthetic kavalactones. At one time or another, such drugs have been listed in the official pharmacopoeias of various European countries as well as in the United States, Japan, and Venezuela. Even today you can purchase regulated kava-based products with names like Kaviase (a UTI remedy), Laitan (a relaxant), and Kavaform (a tonic) in France, Germany, Switzerland, and other European countries where kava remains an officially recognized medicine.

Much of the hottest action on kava, however, is taking place in the over-the-counter consumer market for medicinal herbs. According to a recent survey by *Whole Foods* magazine of retail stores that sell herbs and supplements, kava placed in the top ten for the "up-and-coming herbs for 1996." And while fresh kava root, which makes the most potent beverages, generally can't be found outside the South Pacific, herbal companies are now offering a wide variety of kava products.

A limited number of North American herbal companies (see Resources) sell dried kava in various forms: pieces of root, cut and sifted, and as a powder. (Some ethnic food markets in Pacific Rim areas with significant Polynesian communities, such as Hawaii, may also carry dried kava.) As we've seen, using whole kava to make the traditional inebriating beverage is somewhat difficult and time-consuming, and yields an unappetizing brew. An increasing number of herbal companies have begun to market dried and powdered kava in capsules, typically containing 200 to 250 mg of kava. Assuming that the dried herb averages 10 percent kavalactones, two capsules provide only 40 to 50 mg of kavalactones. Like drinking the tea, taking such a limited one-time dose of kavalactones is minimally psychoactive, as is confirmed by most users' experiences with the powdered herb.

North Americans who have experienced kava in the Pacific and then tried to re-create the drink at home have often been disappointed with the quality and potency of dried, imported kava (though their lack of brewing technique may be as important). Unfortunately for consumers, grading of dried kava has taken hold only in Fiji. *Waka* is the most potent and expensive Fijian kava, derived from plants' lateral roots. Less potent and cheaper are *lewena* (rootstock) and *kasa* (lower stems), respectively. Ask your supplier about the freshness and potency of the product before buying. Dried kava powder usually costs only a few dollars an ounce.

Kava is also available in tea bags, but because dissolving kava powder in water does not release the kavalactones, drinking a kava tea results in virtually no psychoactive effect. The water-soluble components of kava, on the other hand, have not been fully studied and may have some positive health effects. In the South Pacific the tea is said to be mildly stimulating and to reduce anxiety and fatigue.

Kava is also available as a liquid herbal concentrate, typically in 1- to 4-ounce dropper bottles. Kavalactone content per milliliter is frequently not stated. Two to three dropperfuls in a single dose is calming for some people, but few experience anything beyond gentle sedative effects. Taking eight to ten dropperfuls may be necessary for more pronounced effects.

Mark Merlin, an associate professor at the University of Hawaii and a coauthor of the 1992 *Kava,* said, "It will be interesting to see if scientific research will discover ways to control the dosage or the lactone content of the substance in a prepared form." Indeed, such an advance has already taken place. Just within the past few years, a number of supplement manufacturers have begun to offer kava in liquid extract formulations standardized at levels such as 150 mg of kavalactones per milliliter, and in standardized extract capsules. Consumers can find kava products in natural foods stores that provide 250 to 400 mg capsules of dried kava standardized for approximately 30 to 55 percent kavalactones, with most yielding an average of 75 mg of kavalactones per capsule. The suggested use is one to three capsules up to three times daily, with meals or at bedtime, for a mildly relaxing, anxiety-relieving effect. To experience kava's more dramatic sedative and inebriating properties, it is necessary to take higher doses. Most users have found that 150 to 250 mg of kavalactones on an empty stomach acts as a gentle soporific. Taking higher doses, such as 500 to 750 mg of kavalactones, still a very safe level, may provide the mild euphoria, heavy limbs, and other effects of a traditionally prepared kava beverage.

Yohimbé

SEX AND SPEED

With the possible exception of ephedra, yohimbé is the most controversial herb widely sold on the market today. Like ephedra, yohimbé is a potent nervous system stimulant that sometimes causes unwanted and even dangerous side effects. It is thus an herb that is shunned by many practicing herbalists and in addition has attracted the ongoing concern of state and federal regulators. Yohimbé, again like ephedra, is also hyped by some herbal producers for powers it does not have—it is neither a hallucinogen nor a muscle-building steroid substitute. Yet many people do have positive experiences with yohimbé. It may be the most effective true aphrodisiac known, and a case can be made that health officials are overstating its dangers. While it's not an herb for everybody, or for everyday use, the best way to determine whether it is a substance you'd like to try is to find out more about it and come to your own conclusions.

OUT OF AFRICA

Yohimbé is a rarity on natural foods store shelves: a traditional herb of Africa. It is derived from the inner bark of a large evergreen tree (*Pausinystalia yohimbé*) in the madder (Rubiaceae) family indigenous to the tropical forests of West Africa. Natives to that part of Africa have used yohimbé for centuries by making a tea from bark shavings. Drinking the tea allowed warriors who were preparing for battle to become more fearless and aggressive. Africans used yohimbé tea selectively to help promote love as well as war. Male members of some tribes would take yohimbé as part of marriage and mating rituals and during special week-long fertility celebrations when sexual relations would be encouraged. Yohimbé gained a reputation for increasing libido as well as improving male performance by enhancing the size and staying power of erections.

Scientific studies on yohimbé conducted since the 1930s have confirmed that the herb has definite effects on aspects of sexual desire and performance. In the past two decades an alkaloid isolated from yohimbé has become generally accepted by the medical establishment as a therapeutic drug to treat some types of male impotence. This alkaloid, yohimbine, has been the subject of at least two-dozen scientific studies, most of which have confirmed its ability to increase blood flow to the penis and cause "erectile stimulation." Today yohimbine is approved by the FDA for treatment of male impotence, whether due to vascular problems, diabetes, or psychogenic causes. Even some veterinarians now turn to yohimbine to treat impotent breeding stallions, for example.

Drug companies have developed various prescription drugs incorporating yohimbine. An early yohimbé-based drug, Afrodex, unfortunately led the way down the path of controversy, having to be pulled from the market in 1973 because of concerns about its toxicity. This product, however, contained not only yohimbine but also methyl testosterone (a form of the male sexual hormone) and small amounts of strychnine (an alkaloid extracted from the seeds of the poison nut plant and once recognized not only as a poison but as a heart stimulant with minor medicinal uses). After studies in the mid-1980s demonstrated yohimbine's effectiveness as a treatment for male impotence, the FDA granted the alkaloid approved-use status for that one condition. A number of pharmaceutical companies currently offer prescription drugs (Yohimex, Yocon, Aphrodyne) with the only active ingredient being the yohimbine compound yohimbine hydrochloride. These drugs are sold in 5.4 mg tablets and in liquid form.

Although yohimbine's sole approved purpose is to treat impotence among males, even the *Physicians' Desk Reference* mentions yohimbine's potential as an aphrodisiac. (Under the entry for Yocon, the *PDR* admits, "It may have activity as an aphrodisiac.") Within the past decade various over-the-counter herbal preparations containing yohimbé have become increasingly popular, primarily as natural aphrodisiacs. Some people also take yohimbé as a stimulant or mood brightener and others use it for its presumed ability to promote weight loss. A growing category of use is in bodybuilding formulas.

THE GOOD YOHIMBÉ...

People who like taking natural yohimbé products point to a variety of pleasurable effects from the herb. If you can figure out the right dose for your body (and find a product containing that dose), within the first hour of taking yohimbé you may experience

- An increase in alertness and stimulation
- Warm shivers or tingling feelings up and down the spine
- Intensified sensory awareness, including increased sensitivity of the skin and the genitals and, during sex, feelings of melding into another's body

- Mild inebriation or euphoria
- Empathogenic actions, such as heightened emotional feelings and openness to others
- A surge in libido, which in men is frequently accompanied by persistent erections (in perhaps one in five men, even in the absence of sexual stimulation)

Some people who have taken doses of yohimbé higher than those usually suggested report that the herb may cause vivid mental images or slight perceptual changes to hearing or vision. Calling such effects "hallucinations," however, seems to be an overstatement of yohimbé's powers. Most people come to yohimbé not for exotic visions but for the stimulation, mild high, and prosexual effects. Sexual activity after taking yohimbé can be truly revelatory, according to some reports. One user says that yohimbé "completely changes the meaning of orgasm—for men, anyway."

Men who take yohimbé sometimes report that it causes them to get prodigious erections of unprecedented size, hardness, and duration. Orgasms are said to be more powerful and numerous, without the penis becoming limp between orgasms. Ejaculations are amazing in quantity of semen and forcefulness of ejection. These results have led actors in the porn movie industry to become some of yohimbé's most ardent fans.

When yohimbé works as hoped, its effects wear off after four to six hours with no ill after-effects or hangover. The user feels both relaxed and invigorated.

...AND THE BAD

Most of yohimbé's positive traits have negative flip sides. For example, what some people experience as mild stimulation others experience as unwelcome anxiety and uncomfortable restlessness. Instead of warm spinal shivers, some users report the kind of shakes, chills, and jitters associated with an overdose of caffeine. Yohimbé's stimulation of the nervous system can last into the night, interfering with sleep, and even keep some users awake through the night.

Also, one man's amazing, spontaneous erection is another man's annoyance or embarrassing situation. Even in the best of circumstances, after—what?—an hour or so, an erection can become more bothersome and painful than exciting and useful. Because in many circumstances (one thinks of locker rooms, riding a bicycle, being at work) an erection can be an extremely uninvited guest, it is best to plan accordingly if you intend to take yohimbé.

Finally, in addition to yohimbé's most common minor side effects (dizziness, anxiety, insomnia, headache), which may happen to some people even when relatively low dosages are taken, higher doses of yohimbé may lead to more serious symptoms such as rapid heartbeat and a dramatic rise in blood pressure. The number and frequency of negative reactions from taking yohimbine prompted one prominent yohimbé researcher, Julian Davidson, to note that while it does help men get an erection, "They don't know what do with it because they feel so lousy."

Indeed, when the shakes, anxiety, and other adverse side effects all happen at once, you have the proverbial herb-from-hell experience. Consider the report one user recently posted in cyberspace, in which he said that after taking yohimbé he started to speed as if he'd taken a megadose of coffee. The overall effect was "not pleasant at all." He relates that he got an erection so persistent that he tried to masturbate it away but his heart was beating so fast he thought, "I am going to have a heart attack." He finally reached a prolonged orgasm but "I did not give a flying shit because my heart was beating so hard that the room was turning black." He fell on the floor and waited for his heart to slow down, which it eventually did. He went to bed but couldn't sleep the whole night, partly because "I had a constant feeling that I was going to throw up."

Surprisingly, this intrepid consciousness explorer says that he would think about repeating the experiment, though by using a lower dose of yohimbé. (He drank several cups of yohimbé tea; as we'll see, it is very difficult to gauge yohimbine content in such cases.)

Less commonly, people have the opposite reaction to yohimbé: they feel no increase in sexuality or mind-altering effects at all. Yohimbé is a potent herb, but those who come to it expecting hallucinations instead of a relatively subtle stimulation may be disappointed.

H·O·W Y·O·H·I·M·B·I·N·E WORKS

Virtually all of the scientific studies into yohimbé's effects have focused on the alkaloid yohimbine rather than the whole herb. What researchers have found is that yohimbine works by blocking certain types of neurotransmitter-receptors in nerve cells. Yohimbine affects primarily a part of the adrenaline-related or "adrenergic" nervous system, which helps control aspects of various bodily functions, including motor activity and sexuality. Yohimbine is thought to have a relatively minor effect on adrenaline, the hormone that stimulates the heart and temporarily increases muscular strength. The alkaloid has a major impact, however, on blood levels of noradrenaline, a neurotransmitter secreted by certain nerve endings and by the adrenal gland. Noradrenaline levels affect blood pressure, sex drive, bodily metabolism, alertness, and other aspects of bodily function.

Less well established are yohimbine's possible effects on blood levels of other neurotransmitters, particularly serotonin, acetylcholine, and dopamine. Serotonin is concentrated in certain regions of the brain, where it is thought to affect mood and consciousness. Acetylcholine is the neurotransmitter that operates between the endings of nerves and muscles; it also plays a role in the control of various organs and the physiology of male erection. Dopamine helps to control muscular movement and plays a role in sex drive.

The various biochemical adjustments caused by ingesting yohimbine can help to explain some of both its positive and negative effects on the body. Yohimbine stimulates the central nervous system, increases resting heart rate, and slightly raises body temperature. It dilates small arteries in the skin and increases blood flow to peripheral parts of the body. In men this surge of arterial blood to the penis is accompanied by slight compression of veins there, thus preventing blood from flowing out of the organ. Yohimbine's possible inhibiting effect on serotonin may override some of serotonin's noted sex-deadening side effects. (An inability to reach orgasm and lack of sex drive are common complaints among some users of Prozac and other antidepressants of the serotonin-reuptake inhibitor class, drugs that boost serotonin action.) Yohimbine's aphrodisiac effects may also be partially attributed to the chemical's effects on the hypothalamus, the region in the brain that controls, among other functions, sexual motivation. Yohimbine is also thought to activate a part of the lower spinal cord with clusters of nerve connections to the sexual organs.

Scientific studies have not confirmed that yohimbine can increase testosterone levels, which early researchers had assumed was the primary reason for yohimbine's ability to boost male sexual desire. These negative research findings, however, have been largely ignored by various supplement manufacturers who continue to promote yohimbé as an anabolic, or muscle-building, herb. If yohimbé has any muscle-building effect, according to John Morgenthaler, coauthor of *Better Sex Through Chemistry,* it is indirect and probably due to the feeling of increased physical energy. "Many people like to use it," he says, "before a workout because of the increased intensity it makes possible. And, if you work out more intensely you will get a greater release of growth hormone and testosterone."

Too much yohimbine can result in the same kind of nervousness, sweating, elevated heart rate, and shaking associated with the body's fight-or-flight reaction to circumstances that cause a sudden boost in circulating adrenaline. Lower levels, however, have been shown to cause fewer adverse reactions and to be moderately effective after two or three weeks in promoting erections in impotent males. Clinical studies have shown that approximately four out of ten impotent men benefit from taking yohimbine hydrochloride. Many of these men are glad to have found yohimbine, as conventional treatments are otherwise limited to more invasive measures such as penile implants. Yohimbine's effectiveness seems to be unrelated to whether the cause of the impotence is structural malfunctions in the body, mental conflicts, or other pharmaceutical drugs.

Yohimbine's actions on the body are complex and still not thoroughly understood by scientists. Yohimbé, because it also has other chemical components, by extension is even more complex.

- -

BEYOND MALE IMPOTENCE

- -

Scientific acceptance of yohimbine as an aphrodisiac began to build in 1984 after a noted study conducted by researchers at the department of physiology at Stanford University was published in *Science.* Until then, yohimbine was recognized by some mainly as a drug capable of causing erections. Merely having an erection, however, is not the same thing as exhibiting the desire to use it. Even a statistical increase in the number of copulations by itself could be seen in terms of a generalized activation of behavior rather than a more selective activation of sex-related behavior. The term *aphrodisiac* means different things to different people, but the ideal substance would not only stimulate the genitals but also increase sexual desire and enhance the pleasure of sex.

The Stanford University scientists tested yohimbine's effects on laboratory rats. They found that yohimbine increased arousal in male rats that had been identified as "sexually experienced." Surprisingly, it also induced randy behavior in low-libido rats—those that had not previously displayed sexual activity. When the researchers concluded that the "data suggest that yohimbine may be a true aphrodisiac," both public and scientific interest in yohimbé and yohimbine took off.

Follow-up studies done by the Stanford group as well as other studies done in the United States and abroad have demonstrated that yohimbine's effects are not due merely to "behavioral stimulation." For example, a 1992 study done on motor behaviors of male rats concluded that yohimbine's ability to facilitate copulation is apparently not mediated by "nonspecific activation" of behavior. Scientists have also conducted studies in which rats' sex drive was found to be increased by yohimbine even after the rats' penises were anesthetized, demonstrating an increase in sex drive rather than mere use of handy erections. Studies have found that yohimbine causes male animals to mount females more readily and ejaculate more quickly. Yohimbine has also been shown to increase the amount of ejaculate and shorten the period between copulations.

A notable 1992 study was done on eigh-teen captive male Nile crocodiles. Eight of the crocodiles were given 30 mg capsules of yohimbine twice a day for one week. Although the treated animals did not copulate more frequently, their reproductive period was significantly prolonged, from eight to eleven weeks. The researchers also found a marked increase in the percentage of fertile eggs laid by females who were in the yohimbine-treated group (39 percent of the eggs resulting from sex with the yohimbine-treated males were fertile, compared to 30 percent in the control group). The researchers speculated that the fertility increase might be due to more successful copulations.

A double-blind, placebo-controlled human study published in the *Archives of Sexual Behavior* in 1996 confirmed that yohimbine can benefit men who suffer from erection-related problems. Thirty-one male subjects who took 15 mg of yohimbine daily for seven weeks experienced significant increases in the hardness and rigidity of their erections.

Anecdotal evidence for yohimbine's reputation as a prosexual herb also continues to grow. Many users' experiences have been posted on cyberspace bulletin boards. For every account of "no reaction" or ill effects, there are plenty more from men (and a few women) who have found yohimbé or yohimbine has dramatically improved a moribund sex life.

Researchers have documented a number of possible applications for yohimbine as a stimulant. More than a dozen studies in the past ten years have determined that yohimbine is useful for arousing animals (including horses, elk, sheep, gray wolves, cats, and dogs) and shortening their recovery after they have been sedated or anesthetized. A few studies have also explored yohimbine's potential in the treatment of narcolepsy (uncontrollable sleepiness), congestive heart failure, and weight loss. Two studies using dogs indicated yohimbine can enhance thermogenesis (fat burning) during fasting, though a 1991 study on 47 men found that a six-month program involving high doses of yohimbine (up to 43 mg per day) had no effect on such factors as body weight, body fat, and fat distribution.

- -
WHOLE HERB OR ALKALOID EXTRACT?
- -

As is the case with ephedra, yohimbé represents an interesting example of an herb with relative advantages and disadvantages to taking the whole herb or an extracted compound, in this case the alkaloid yohimbine. Though yohimbé also contains other compounds and up to about 6 percent of total alkaloids (such as yohimbiline and ajmaline), yohimbine doubtless accounts for much of the herb's actions on the body. Several other potent medicinal plants, including Indian snakeroot, also known as rauwolfia (*Rauvolfia serpentina*), the source of the potent alkaloid reserpine used in drugs to lower blood pressure, also contain yohimbine and bear some chemical resemblance to yohimbé. (The presence of long-lasting reserpine and other compounds in Indian snakeroot prevents the whole herb from being a useful yohimbé substitute.)

While yohimbine probably accounts for most of the mind-altering effects of the herb, it is possible that it does not account for *all* of the

effects. Unfortunately, it is difficult to draw objective distinctions between yohimbé and yohimbine. Both the whole herb and the alkaloid have diverse and complex actions on the body. Though some of yohimbine's actions on specific neurotransmitters have been identified, researchers have not yet fully explored its various effects. Even less is known about yohimbé's full range of actions.

Looking at yohimbé's composition indicates that the whole herb probably does have effects that go beyond those caused by yohimbine. In fact, "The whole plant is potentially so evil and insidious," says herbalist Michael Moore, director of the Southwest School of Botanical Medicine in Albuquerque, New Mexico, "*because* its complex chemistry contains both adrenergics [substances that affect the adrenergic nervous system] and cholinergics [substances that affect the action of acetylcholine]. . . . It contains both yohimbine alkaloid groups (stimulating and hypertensive) and several potent reserpinoid (*Rauvolfia*) alkaloids (tranquilizing and hypotensive) . . . a warlock's brew."

Some herbal authorities contend that the complex mix of compounds found in the whole herb is a reason to avoid it. "Consistent use will, because of its wildly opposite effects, find and widen metabolic chinks in almost anybody," claims Moore.

Moore also notes that the whole plant is a monoamine oxidase (MAO) inhibitor whereas yohimbine is not. (Indeed, no mention of MAO inhibition is made in the *PDR* coverage of yohimbine products; reserpine does merit the warning against use with MAO inhibitors.) Monoamine oxidase is an enzyme found in nerve cells. In the brain, it oxidizes various neurotransmitters that have mood-boosting effects, inactivating them. The end result is that a substance that inhibits MAO, like yohimbé, allows these neurotransmitters to work longer in the brain and thereby brighten mood.

The reason that drugs whose antidepressant effect is due to MAO inhibition are not more popular has to do with the potentially dangerous side effects they can cause. When MAO inhibitors in the body react with the chemical tyramine, the person may experience a dramatic increase in blood pressure or possibly even a stroke. Because tyramine is found in many common foods and drinks (cheese, chocolate, red wine, coffee), nutrients (the amino acids tryptophan and tyrosine), and drugs (decongestants, diet aids), the typical precaution for taking an MAO-inhibiting substance such as yohimbé is extensive.

The most obvious advantage to using the whole herb is that it is widely available without a prescription. Though not all health food stores carry yohimbé products, many do, or will order it for you. It is also easily purchased from many mail-order sources (see Resources). Yohimbine, on the other hand, requires a prescription, and few doctors will write one for you just because you want increased sexual pleasure or stimulation. And if you're a woman, forget it, since the only officially sanctioned use is for male impotence.

On the other hand, an obvious and significant advantage to using yohimbine is control of dose. The standard recommendation for prescription yohimbine is to take one of the 5.4 mg tablets three times daily. The liquid

forms of the prescription drugs also offer explicit information on yohimbine content per dosage. In contrast, the vast majority of herbal producers don't offer any information about yohimbine content on their labels. Thus, you have little idea how much yohimbine is in Product X's 500 mg capsules, Product Y's 1,500 mg capsules, or Product Z's concentrated drops. A 1991 analysis of ten yohimbé products found a three-fold variation, with yohimbine levels ranging from 4.5 mg per dose to 14.4 mg. (Most of the products averaged in excess of the 5.4 mg found in prescription yohimbine drugs.)

In recent years some products have begun to offer yohimbine content per dose. For example, Life Enhancement Products of Petaluma, California, has developed a liquid Yohimbé Tonic that is standardized for yohimbine content so that half a dropperful (20 drops) will always provide a 2.5 mg dose of yohimbine. Standardized extract capsules have also begun to appear on the market; a 400 mg capsule of one is standardized for 8 mg yohimbine. Providing such information is an immense benefit to the consumer, because controlling dosage levels is crucial for reducing the risk of negative experiences.

YOHIMBÉ AND WOMEN

Women's sex drive is still, it seems, a taboo area of medical research. While numerous studies back up the claims for yohimbine's effects on men, very little research has been conducted on yohimbine's effects on women.

Two studies, both done on female rats, indicate yohimbine may enhance female sexual response. Researchers in the first study, published in 1977, gave the test animals a drug that artificially suppressed their sexual receptivity while in heat; yohimbé reversed this sex-deadening effect. Another study, published in 1985, fed yohimbine to female rats during a part of their cycle when they were normally nonreceptive to sex. The drug stimulated sexual activity.

Unfortunately, these provocative results seem not to have inspired much research into how yohimbine might benefit women suffering from lack of libido or from anorgasmia (inability to reach orgasm). Both of these are increasingly common complaints among post-menopausal women and among women taking serotonin-boosting antidepressants such as Prozac as well as various other drugs. (The authors of one study, published in the *Journal of Clinical Psychiatry* in 1992, did state, "Yohimbine may be an effective treatment for the sexual side effects caused by serotonin reuptake blockers.")

Lacking sufficient controlled studies, much of what can be said about yohimbé and women is based upon conjecture (a number of substances that affect sex-linked physical processes, such as increases in certain neurotransmitters and circulatory changes in the area of the genitals, seem to work similarly for men and women) and limited anecdotal experience (women who have taken yohimbé often report similar experiences to men's, including pleasurable skin sensations, a feeling of pressure in the groin area, increased sexual activity,

and stimulation). Some women have also reported the equivalent of male erections: clitoral engorgement. Nor are women immune to yohimbé's occasional adverse effects.

IS YOHIMBÉ FOR YOU?

Yohimbé is clearly among the most potent mind-altering herbs found in health food stores today. Though many people have pleasurable experiences taking it, others find that one or more of the side effects overwhelm any potential fun. A look at the five types of caveats that accompany the literature on the prescription yohimbine products indicates the range of potential problems from both yohimbé and yohimbine.

■ **Contraindications.** Only two are specifically mentioned: patients with kidney disease and anyone with a sensitivity to yohimbine. One product manufacturer adds, "In view of the limited and inadequate information at hand, no precise tabulation can be offered of additional contraindications."

■ **Warnings.** Those who should not use yohimbine include children, pregnant women, and the elderly; people with psychiatric conditions; anyone with a history of problems related to the heart or kidneys; and persons who have gastric or duodenal ulcers. Yohimbine manufacturers also state that yohimbine is generally not for use by women.

■ **Drug interactions.** Yohimbine should not be taken with mood-modifying drugs and antidepressants.

■ **Adverse reactions.** Yohimbine produces "a complex pattern of responses" that may include elevated blood pressure and heart rate, decreased flow of urine, increased motor activity, irritability, tremor, nervousness, headache, skin flushing, and dizziness.

■ **Overdosage.** Daily doses of 20 to 30 mg may increase heart rate and blood pressure or cause the nose to run and hair to stand on end. More severe symptoms may include paresthesias (abnormal sensations such as numbness, tingling, and heightened sensitivity), incoordination, tremulousness, and a dissociative state.

Other individuals who are not good candidates for experimenting with yohimbé include anyone prone to panic attacks, schizophrenia, or manic-depressive illness, and persons with diabetes or hypoglycemia. Some authorities also warn that yohimbine can cause a rapid *decrease* in blood pressure, thus disqualifying anyone with hypotension. Anyone who has experienced an allergic reaction to rauwolfia or its alkaloids, including reserpine, should not take yohimbé.

Many herbalists agree with Moore and feel that both yohimbé and yohimbine are so potent and have such potential for abuse that they should be used only under supervision of an herbalist or physician. Naturopath Michael Murray, coauthor of *Encyclopedia of Natural Medicine,* says, "I have used yohimbine in my practice and have found that, because of side effects, it is very difficult to work with." Germany's Commission E does not recommend therapeutic use of yohimbé, citing, "insuffi-cient proof of activity" as well as a poor trade-off of risks to benefits.

Still, many people do take yohimbé on their own and derive pleasure if not health benefit from it. Those who are best-suited to experiment with yohimbé are persons relatively sound in mind and body and adventurous or curious enough to risk the adverse effects. Yohimbé is also only for those who like stimulants. If caffeine and ephedra don't appeal to you, you're unlikely to appreciate yohimbé's effects. One user notes that yohimbé gives him "little body shakes" and that he likes these feelings: "They don't interfere with sleep, and they seem very natural." As with ephedra, if you are tired, nutritionally depleted, or weak, you are less likely to find yohimbé's effects welcome or pleasurable.

REGULATORS ON THE PROWL

State and federal health authorities and regulators take a dim view of yohimbé, being a relatively potent herb taken more frequently for its psychoactive and prosexual effects than for its alkaloid's accepted medical use against male impotence. When the FDA had its unofficial list of "unsafe herbs" from 1977 to 1986, yohimbé was included. It is likely that if the agency had more enforcement resources it would attempt to ban all over-the-counter sales of yohimbé-containing products. Lacking a tryptophan-type disaster, however, the agency makes do with periodic warnings about the herb and unallowable claims made for it.

For example, in 1990 the FDA ruled that no herbs or dietary supplements could claim they offer powers of aphrodisia, including that they increase sexual desire, improve sexual performance, or build sexual virility and sexual potency. Yohimbé was specifically recognized as "not effective." In 1992 yohimbé was included with GHB and three other substances in an "Automatic Detention" alert for "foreign-manufactured unapproved drugs promoted as alternatives to certain anabolic steroids." The alert noted that "these products appear to be new drugs which are being commercially distributed without an approved New Drug Application." Government agents were instructed to "automatically detain all shipments of finished dosage forms (both commercial and personal)." More recently the FDA has said, "Serious adverse effects including kidney failure, seizures, and death have been reported to FDA with products containing yohimbé and are currently under investigation."

The regulatory interest has had limited effect on herbal producers. The American Herbal Products Association, a trade group of herbal manufacturers, does not endorse yohimbé use but has not joined in the efforts to ban its sale. Product manufacturers who want to suggest yohimbé's aphrodisiac powers have taken to using "fuzzwords" or suggestive product names, such as Hot Stuff and Man Power. Health food stores and supplement catalogs that specialize in bodybuilding products are chock full of yohimbé products with names like Yohimbé Power Max and Super Yohimbé. One company even offers a Yohimbé Bar Chocolate. Label claims ("widely used by bodybuilders and weight lifters"; "can stimulate your body to produce higher levels of testosterone"; "helps increase endogenous hormone levels, which can transform into a stronger, more muscular body") make it clear that, FDA or no FDA, these products are still being promoted for their unproven ability to stimulate muscle growth.

FDA scrutiny of yohimbé has caused jitters in some parts of the retail natural food industry. One of the largest natural foods chains, Fresh Fields, has discontinued selling any products it considers unsafe or unproved. Included with yohimbé in this group are two other herbs with mildly mind-altering properties, ephedra (see chapter 4) and kola nut (see chapter 5). Some natural foods stores don't stock yohimbé but are willing to special order it for customers.

- -
HOW MUCH IS ENOUGH?
- -

The usual adult dose for prescription yohimbine products is one 5.4 mg capsule three times daily, for a total of 16.2 mg per day. Most of the studies that have been done on yohimbine as a treatment for male impotence have administered this standard dosage or more, up to approximately 40 to 45 mg of yohimbine per day (in divided doses). Researchers generally describe the adverse side effects from consuming these levels of yohimbine as limited. For example, a double-blind study published in the *Journal of Urology* in 1989 in which researchers administered daily doses of up to 42 mg of yohimbine to a Veterans Administration population of impotent men resulted in side effects described by the researchers as "only few and benign." (Approximately one-third of the eighty-two men in this study achieved either "restoration of full and sustained erections" or a partial response to the drug.) Even much higher single doses of yohimbine may have relatively little effect on some people. A 1993 report in the *Journal of Emergency Medicine*, entitled "Benign Course After Massive Ingestion of Yohimbine," described the case of a sixty-two-year-old man who took a single dose of 200 mg of yohimbine and experienced mainly rapid heartbeat, raised blood pressure, and "anxiety of brief duration."

While it is possible that higher single doses of yohimbine would more reliably provide the kind of stimulant and prosexual effects people are seeking from it, such usage should be approached with caution as it is difficult to draw direct parallels between the experiences of patients using prescription yohimbine drugs and consumers of herbal yohimbé products. As noted, the whole herb may differ substantially in its actions from yohimbine; herbal product manufacturers typically fail to inform users of yohimbine content, and yohimbine levels may vary widely from one product to another. Also, some people are more sensitive to yohimbé than others. Yohimbé users have reported noticing either the stimulating and prosexual effects or side effects, such as stomach cramps and dizziness, from taking as few as ten drops of concentrated liquid, which probably amounted to only a few milligrams of yohimbine. Others have taken single doses of 100 drops of the concentrated liquid, per-

haps 15 mg or more of yohimbine, and felt next to nothing.

Of course, in addition to the wide range in product potency, other factors such as body size and differences in the ability to absorb and process yohimbine may be crucial. A 1990 human study found that oral doses of yohimbine are rapidly absorbed and eliminated, but that the bioavailability exhibits a wide variation from one person to the next— among the seven young healthy male subjects it ranged from 7 to 87 percent and averaged 33 percent. The researchers said that it is unclear whether these variations are due to how the gastrointestinal tract absorbs yohimbine or how the liver filters yohimbine in its first pass through the organ.

Even psychological or neurochemical factors may be relevant. A 1992 study done on eight macaque monkeys, four of which were "normally reared" and four of which had experienced early maternal and social deprivation, found that yohimbine caused different patterns of response among the two groups. Another study, done in Italy in 1991, found that psychological stress potentiates yohimbine's effects.

Furthermore, a number of studies have reported results that indicate yohimbine's effects may become reversed rather than enhanced at high dosages. Thus high doses won't increase stimulation but rather may have an enervating effect on some individuals. High doses have also been shown to decrease the amount of ejaculate rather than increase it.

The bottom line is that if you want to be conservative and avoid adverse reactions, begin by experimenting with low levels of yohimbé, not more than 500 mg of an encapsulated powder. If the yohimbine content is stated, start by taking only 2 to 3 mg of yohimbine to see how it affects you. Many people will notice only subtle stimulation, or no effects at all, from such a small dose. Even at the dosage of the prescription drugs, 5.4 mg of yohimbine, mind-altering effects are likely to be mild. As the *Physicians' Desk Reference* admits, "Yohimbine exerts a stimulating action on mood and may increase anxiety. Such actions are not adequately studied, although they appear to require high doses." For most people, a single yohimbine dose of 6 to 8 mg will probably be sufficient for stimulation and aphrodisiac effects.

TAKING YOHIMBÉ

Yohimbé is sold in the form of dried bark, encapsulated powder, and liquids. Capsules range in size from 500 to 1,500 mg. Yohimbé is also found as an ingredient in various combination products, usually promoted either as aphrodisiacs or bodybuilding products. These combination formulas use other herbs (smilax, ginseng, damiana) as well as nutrients (vitamin E, zinc, OKG, creatine).

Because yohimbé is a relatively exotic herb and there are no easy methods for measuring potency of samples in the field, it is important to find products made by companies with experience and explicitly stated quality-control guidelines. For example, Gaia Herbs, a Massachusetts-based producer of liquid plant extracts, including yohimbé and five other African herbs, offers the following guidelines: "We work in close association with an herbalist in Africa who instructs native wildcrafters to harvest these important plants according to our specifications. We guarantee these plants are freshly harvested and carefully shade-dried. They are then air-freighted to our laboratory for production into extracts. We keep plant specimens of each lot to authenticate correct genus and species."

If taking yohimbé appeals to you and your health allows it, keep in mind a few common-sense guidelines to increase the odds that your experience will be pleasurable. On the day that you intend to take yohimbé, avoid taking any other drugs, including alcohol and caffeine. Also avoid consuming tyramine-containing substances. Don't take yohimbé late at night unless you're not planning on getting much sleep. Also, reserve yohimbé for special occasions rather than everyday use. Perhaps most important, start with a low dose. As we've seen, this is more easily said than done, given the fact that few yohimbé products offer information on yohimbine content.

The following dosage suggestions usually provide low enough levels of yohimbine that side effects are avoided:

■ 15 to 20 drops of the tincture or concentrated drops. Add them to water or juice to dilute the taste and swallow.

■ 250 to 500 mg of dried herb in capsules.

■ One cup of tea. Obviously, the potency of the dried herb, how much you use, and how long you brew it will determine the tea's strength. Since the potency of the dried herb will be unknown, start by limiting the amount used and brewing time. For example, add three to four teaspoons of bark shavings to one pint of water, boil for about five minutes, and then lower the heat and simmer for ten to fifteen minutes. After straining and cooling, the yohimbé tea will taste bitter, not as unpleasant as traditional kava beverage but still nothing you'd drink for the taste. Add honey or sweetener and sip slowly.

If your first batch is too weak, next time try using five to six teaspoons of dried herb, and increasing the simmer time to twenty to thirty minutes. You can also dissolve 500 to 1,000 mg of vitamin C in the finished tea, which may boost the potency by increasing the assimilation of yohimbine. By the same token, taking 500 mg of vitamin C when you consume yohimbé capsules or liquids may increase their potency.

PART SEVEN

Conclusion

Better Safe
Than Sorry

◉

GUIDELINES FOR USING MIND-ALTERANTS

The almost three-dozen natural mind-alterants described in detail in parts two through six vary widely in their chemistry, uses, and effects. As a rule they are dramatically less toxic than alcohol and tobacco, which have higher rates of addiction and more serious long-term health effects. These substances are also, in many cases, as safe as caffeine and most of the over-the-counter drugs taken for their psychoactive properties. Nevertheless, mind-altering substances are drugs, and in some circumstances they have the potential to disrupt one's life in a number of adverse ways.

What circumstances? That will vary from one individual to another. How you personally use the substance will determine whether it provides you with the pleasures and benefits you seek or whether it becomes just another burden of modern life. *"Any drug can be used successfully, no matter how bad its reputation, and any drug can be abused, no matter how accepted it is.* There are no good or bad drugs; there are

only good and bad relationships with drugs," as Dr. Andrew Weil and Winifred Rosen note in *From Chocolate to Morphine* (italics in original).

Two of the most important factors in determining the nature of your relationship with a drug are how often and in what dosage you take it, and how and where you use it. The same criteria that we might apply to drinking alcohol and using caffeine can fruitfully be applied to the natural mind-alterants. (Nicotine's extreme addictiveness makes it almost impossible to have a good relationship with it.) Do you take the drug every day? At all times of the day? How often in amounts beyond moderation? By yourself or with friends? Only with meals? The answer to only one of these questions is probably insufficient to judge your relationship to any drug. Perhaps you drink every day, ordinarily an indication that the relationship between person and drug is possibly harmful. But if you limit yourself to one drink, and it is taken with family at the dinner meal, you probably qualify as a controlled user in a good relationship with your drug.

Still, frequency and dosage are major considerations. With some exceptions (melatonin, choline, some of the smart drugs, green tea, the mild herbal mood boosters such as ginkgo), the substances considered here are best reserved for occasional rather than everyday use. In part, this is because few scientific studies have been conducted on the long-term health effects of daily use (though kava, ginseng, and others do have established safety records from a history of traditional use). Also, most of these substances belong to the same categories of pleasurable drugs—stimulants, depressants, euphoriants—as do alcohol, tobacco, and caffeine, and current experience indicates that for various reasons, compulsive everyday use of such substances has become commonplace in modern society.

SET AND SETTING

The "how and where" aspects of drug use have been termed "set and setting" by Norman E. Zinberg, M.D., a psychiatrist who for more than three decades has been a leading authority on substance use and abuse. He defines *set* as "the attitude of the person at the time of use, including his personality structure" and *setting* as "the influence of the physical and social setting within which the use occurs." In *Drug, Set, and Setting,* he describes the results of two studies, one lasting five years, that he performed in the 1970s. He recruited some 250 subjects who were exhaustively interviewed on their use of any of three potent illicit drugs: marijuana, psychedelics, and opiates. Subjects were questioned on how they were introduced to the substances, under what conditions they used them, how drugs made them feel, how drugs influenced their lives, how they managed to control their use, and so forth. The subjects were then classified as either "controlled" (moderate, occasional) or "compulsive" users (those who engage in repeated periods of daily use, often in multiple doses). Zinberg found that not the drug itself but set and setting are the factors that, through the development of patterns of behavior and values and rules of conduct, determined whether the person used drugs with control or with compulsion.

Cross-cultural studies of psychoactive drug use have confirmed the importance of set-and-setting factors in controlling the experience. In *Hallucinogens: Cross-Cultural Perspectives,* Marlene Dobkin de Rios described her extensive analysis of various traditional cultures' use of potent hallucinogens, including the mushroom fly agaric (*Amanita muscaria*) and nightshade family plants such as jimson weed (*Datura stramonium*). She notes that anthropological studies consistently report that the effects of the drug itself must be seen in the context of a whole host of variables, including the user's particular

- body weight, physical condition, and diet
- motivation, personality, mood, and past experiences
- relationship to a group or a guide, or participation in ritual performance
- expectation of the experience, belief systems, and values.

Even the presence of particular music or odors can affect the drug experience. Because of these many attendant factors, Dobkin de Rios found that even potent hallucinogens were not generally harmful either to individuals or to the group in traditional societies. When used outside a spiritual or learning context, however, such as for escape in many modern societies, problems such as cultural disorganization, alienation, and abuse are not uncommon.

Prior to the work of researchers like Zinberg and Dobkin de Rios, most people had considered the drugs themselves—their composition, potency, and effects—the primary determinant of usage. And for the three types of illicit drugs he studied, Zinberg noted that "controlled use" was hardly recognized as a possibility, and to a great extent any use was defined as "abuse." As he quotes one medical authority, "For the sake of clarity and at the risk of simplification, misuse [abuse] will be viewed as nonmedical use of psychoactive drugs." This same bias against the notion of controlled use of these illicit drugs remains in evidence today, and is in some respects even stronger. Many conventional physicians and government regulators also carry over this bias against a few of the natural mind-alterants, particularly ephedra and yohimbé. That is, any over-the-counter use of these is considered "nonmedical" and dangerous and therefore should be banned.

Though the popular mind-altering herbs and nutritional substances are much less potent than pot, acid, and heroin, similar lessons can be learned from controlled users of these more controversial drugs. Extrapolating from set-and-setting studies of various drugs, we might say that among the general rules for controlled use of most inebriants are avoiding regular solitary use; planning in advance and reserving special times, events, or circumstances (weekends, finishing a project at work) for using them; knowing your limits; and not using inebriants during work, school, or study. Rules for stimulants, including caffeine and ephedra, may be slightly different—avoid using them more than two days in a row; don't get to the point where you need to take them every time a particular task presents itself (the student who comes to depend on stimulants to study); don't get caught in a cycle of taking stimulants in the morning to overcome the effects of last night's depressants, which you needed to take to counter the previous morning's stimulants.

Mind-altering substances, whether natural or synthetic, legal or illegal, medical or recreational, can be tools for achieving pleasure, creativity, sociability, relaxation. But if the substance becomes the *only* tool that brings the desired benefits, it is time to reexamine your life and determine how you can regain your innate capacity for experiencing these states.

- -

FURTHER TIPS FOR CONTROLLED USE

- -

See the individual chapters in parts two through six for safety and use guidelines specific to the substances described. Potency, effects, and rules for use vary markedly from one substance to another. Blanket statements meant to encompass all of these substances by nature must be broad. In addition to the considerations about frequency, set, and setting just mentioned, here are some additional general guidelines to keep in mind that will allow you to maintain a positive relationship with whatever you decide to take:

■ Whenever you try a new substance, start with low doses to see how it affects you, increasing your intake slowly each successive time you try the substance to find out what works best without causing adverse side effects.

■ Avoid combining and mixing mind-altering substances, and taking numerous types on any one day. Substances with similar effects taken simultaneously can magnify potency. Taking stimulants such as ephedra and yohimbé at the same time could dangerously imbalance your body's energy system, while taking valerian and kava could overdepress vital organs. The combined effects could also be totally unpredictable. Also, keep in mind that many medical drugs have psychoactive effects, as their main effect (tranquilizers) and as side effects (drowsiness or stimulation caused by any number of pharmaceutical drugs). Be aware of the possibility of compounded or unpredictable effects from taking OTC mind-alterants and prescription drugs within a few hours of one another.

■ Don't use mind-altering drugs as excuses for not taking the everyday steps necessary to maintain wellness, including eating a healthful diet, getting enough rest and sleep, maintaining a positive outlook, sustaining a social network, and staying physically active. For example, relaxants can occasionally help you to calm down or go to sleep, but they

shouldn't take the place of daily habits that over the long term encourage restful sleep as a matter of course.

■ Learn to recognize the early warning signs that your relationship to a substance is becoming one of compulsion and psychological dependence, defined as craving and emotional distress when the drug is withheld. (None of these substances cause true physical dependence, defined as an adaptation by the body to the drug such that withdrawal symptoms occur when the substance is withheld.) Watch for the feeling that you need to take a substance for help in doing some everyday task, whether it is getting up in the morning, being at work, or keeping the house clean; or the practice of adapting any occurrence into a reason for taking a drug ("to victory . . . to defeat"); or the insistence on continuing to use the substance even in the face of adverse effects clearly tied to its use.

■ Be open to reliable new information on these substances. New studies are constantly being done, new products developed, new findings revealed. If information offers a new perspective, consider its effect on your own use, recognizing that the information may not be value-free but rather may carry along with it a host of often unstated assumptions, biases, and philosophies. By the same token, if you choose to use some of the more controversial substances discussed here, such as ephedra or yohimbé, keep abreast of the changing regulations coming from agencies such as the FDA and the DEA. Recognize that they can and sometimes do make decisions based upon assumptions quite in variance with those held by scientific researchers, health authorities, and producers and users of the substance in question.

■ If you're new to a substance and wary of its effects, seek the advice of an experienced user or health practitioner. This book has provided the most important information, but there is no substitute for talking directly to knowledgeable sources about dosages, effects, and health concerns. Also, on-line chat groups can be invaluable for their lists of frequently-asked-questions (FAQs) and their files of users' reports. As Zinberg notes:

> *Without doubt the most important source of precepts and practices for control is the peer using group. Virtually all of our subjects had been assisted by other noncompulsive users in constructing appropriate rituals and sanctions out of the folklore and practices circulating in their drug-using subculture. The peer group provided instruction in and reinforced proper use; and despite the popular image of peer pressure as a corrupting force pushing weak individuals toward drug misuse, our interviews showed that many segments of the drug subculture have taken a firm stand against drug abuse.*

■ Some of the natural highs should be taken only in certain types of places, for safety and other considerations. Kava's ability in high doses to cause inebriation is especially relevant in this regard. Take steps to insure that your experiences with mind-alterants won't be harmful as a result of an inappropriate setting.

■ Don't use mind-alterants as routine and automatic accompaniments to life's normal pleasures, whether you derive such pleasures from listening to music, engaging in conversation, enjoying nature, painting a picture, playing tennis, or having sex. These are all activities that deserve to have their unadorned pleasures recognized, at least most of the time.

■ As much as possible, avoid mind-altering substances altogether during child conceiving (this goes for men and women), during pregnancy, and while breast-feeding. Even melatonin has not been tested on pregnant women and represents an unknown risk. Almost all substances that a mother consumes are passed on to the fetus or are incorporated into her breast milk. With only a few exceptions (for example, if the pregnant woman and thus her fetus are addicted to opiates, discontinuing the drug could put the fetus's life at risk), women who are pregnant or trying to become pregnant should take only drugs that are medically necessary.

■ People with serious mental illnesses such as schizophrenia, manic-depressive illness, and forms of psychosis should check with their doctor before using mind-altering substances, which may have adverse effects on neurotransmitter levels or bodily functions that could worsen the mental condition. Melatonin and a few of the smart drugs may actually benefit some forms of mental illness, but it is best to check first with a doctor or knowledgeable health practitioner.

■ Some of the mind-altering herbs and supplements should also be avoided by those with serious illnesses such as cancer, severe high blood pressure, cardiovascular disease, and liver conditions. For example, the amino acid tyrosine is contraindicated for melanoma; ephedra can raise blood pressure; and melatonin should be avoided by people with auto-immune conditions since it stimulates the immune system and could exaggerate an auto-immune response. Again, check with your doctor if you're unsure.

■ Certain activities that require one's full mental and physical faculties obviously should not be attempted after taking the more potent mind-alterants. Of special concern are the relaxant properties of central nervous system depressants. Just as responsible people don't drink and drive, those who experiment with natural depressants, including kava, should take into account their potential to cause drowsiness and loss of motor control.

■ Mind alterants should normally be used when you're relatively healthy in body and mind. If you're weak or debilitated, concentrate on taking herbs and nutritional substances that balance the system and boost immunity (such as the herb echinacea, vitamin C, and shiitake mushrooms) rather than substances that cause stimulation, sedation, or elation. Melatonin, green tea, ginkgo, and possibly ginseng may be the exceptions among the mind-alterants discussed here, in that evidence indicates they boost immunity and have other positive health effects.

■ Don't purchase products from unknown sources, especially not "off the street." There is a growing underground market for natural-high stimulants and ecstasy knockoffs, many containing ephedra, yohimbé, or amino acids such as phenylalanine, and being sold at rock concerts, all-night raves, on college campuses, and the like. Unless a product is professionally packaged (with name and location of manufacturer) and legally labeled, you have no idea what's really in it, and in all likelihood neither does the person selling it to you.

■ Avoid poorly labeled, overhyped products sold in head shops, too. In the early 1990s at least four people died when they orally ingested a fringe product that was a purported aphrodisiac meant to be applied topically. Health officials determined that the product contained a traditional Chinese cardiac medication with high levels of compounds that caused heart failure. If you can't be sure of what you're taking, don't take it.

■ Favor the products of companies that offer full information on ingredients, growing and manufacturing processes, and especially levels of active ingredients. Ideally, before you take a substance, find out how many milligrams per dose it contains of recognized compounds such as caffeine, ephedrine, yohimbine, kavalactones, phenylalanine, melatonin, and so forth. Some companies are more forthcoming about this information than others.

Weil and Rosen offer a useful shorthand formula for avoiding problems with mind-altering substances: "Take dilute forms of natural drugs by mouth on occasion . . . for positive reasons according to rules you set for yourself." This remains the best approach for reaping the benefits that natural mind-alterants have to offer while reducing to a minimum the adverse effects sometimes associated with their use.

Resources

CHAPTER-BY-CHAPTER RESOURCES

In the following resource sections for each chapter, the mail-order sources listings are, by necessity, representative rather than comprehensive. Company names and product type are listed; see the section on "Mail-Order Sources of Herbs, Nutritional Supplements, Essential Oils, and Smart Drugs" that follows "Chapter-by-Chapter Resources" for the companies' full addresses. (In the interests of full disclosure, I have no financial interest in any company mentioned, nor have I ever acted as a consultant or provided any other service to a natural product company.) Note that many of the substances are widely available in natural food and health food stores.

Many of the chapter-by-chapter listings also include representative Internet sources for further information. No attempt has been made to offer a comprehensive list of Internet sites. Doing a World Wide Web search using words such as *valerian* and *melatonin* will result in hundreds or even thousands of hits. The listed sites offer large amounts of information, unique personal reports about users' experiences with the substance, or multiple connections to other relevant WWW sites.

Citations for scientific studies mentioned in the text, as well as for important journal articles that may not be directly mentioned, are listed under the sections on "relevant research."

CHAPTER 1:
TYPES OF MIND-ALTERANTS

Print Sources for Further Information

The Age of Entheogens & The Angels' Dictionary by Jonathan Ott (Kennewick, Washington: Natural Products Company, 1995)

From Chocolate to Morphine: Everything You Need to Know About Mind-Altering Drugs by Andrew Weil, M.D., and Winifred Rosen (New York: Houghton Mifflin, 1983; rev. ed. 1993)

Pharmacotheon: Entheogenic Drugs, Their Plant Sources and History by Jonathan Ott (Kennewick, Washington: Natural Products Company, 1993)

Relevant Research

Ruck, C.A.P., et al., "Entheogens," *Journal of Psychedelic Drugs* (1979), 11(1/2):145–46

CHAPTER 2: GREEN TEA

Mail-Order Sources

Allies
seeds

Botanical Preservation Corps
bulk sencha

CFIDS and Fibromyalgia Health Resource
standardized extract (encapsulated powder); decaffeinated standardized extract

Frontier Cooperative Herbs
bulk gunpowder, sencha, jasmine

Gaia Herbs
liquid extract

Olympia
standardized extract (encapsulated powder)

Vitamin Research Products
standardized extract (encapsulated powder)

Supplement discounters (see the section on "Mail-Order Supplement Discounters" below)
Most natural foods stores carry green tea in the tea and coffee section, plus a variety of encapsulated, standardized extract green tea products in the supplement section.

Print Sources for Further Information

All About Tea by William H. Ukers, Vols. I and II (New York: The Tea and Coffee Trade Journal Company, 1935)

All the Tea in China by Kit Chow and Ione Kramer (San Francisco: China Books and Periodicals, 1990)

The Book of Tea by Alain Stella, Nadine Beauthéac, Gilles Brochard, and Catherine Donzel, translated by Deke Dusinberre (Paris: Flammarion, 1992)

The Chinese Art of Tea by John Blofeld (Boston: Shambhala Books: 1985)

The Tea Book by Sara Perry (San Francisco: Chronicle Books, 1993)

Relevant Research

Anon., "Proceedings and abstracts presented at the First International Symposium on the Physiological and Pharmacological Effects of *Camellia sinensis* (Tea)," *Preventative Medicine* (1992), 21:329–553

Dulloo, A.G., et al., "Tealine and thermogenesis: Interaction between polyphenols, caffeine and sympathetic activity," *International Journal of Obesity* (1996), 20(S4):71

Gutman, R.L., and B.-H. Ryu, "Rediscovering tea: An exploration of the scientific literature," *HerbalGram* (1996), 37:33–48

Hertog, M.G.L., et al., "Dietary antioxidant flavonoids and risk of coronary heart disease: The Zutphen Elderly Study," *The Lancet* (1993), 342:1007–11

Imai, K., and K. Nakachi, "Cross-sectional study of effects of drinking green tea on cardiovascular and liver diseases," *British Medical Journal* (1995), 310:693–96

Katiyar, S.K., and H. Mukhtar, "Tea in chemoprevention of cancer: Epidemiologic and experimental studies," *International Journal of Oncology* (1996), 8:221–38

Pozniak, P.C., "The carcinogenicity of caffeine and coffee: A review," *Journal of the American Dietetic Association* (1985), 85:1127–33

Serafini, M., et al., "In vivo antioxidant effect of green and black tea in man," *European Journal of Clinical Nutrition* (1996), 50:28–32

CHAPTER 3: THE GINSENGS

Mail-Order Sources

Allies
Siberian ginseng/eleuthero seeds

CFIDS and Fibromyalgia Health Resource
Asian ginseng capsules; Siberian ginseng/eleuthero capsules

Frontier Cooperative Herbs
Asian and American ginseng whole root, powder; Siberian ginseng/eleuthero root cut and sifted, powder

Gaia Herbs
American ginseng wildcrafted liquid extract, woods-grown liquid extract; Siberian ginseng/eleuthero root wildcrafted liquid extract, tonic elixir

Health Center for Better Living
Asian ginseng cut and sifted, powder, tea bags, capsules

Herb Pharm
Korean ginseng liquid extract; American ginseng wildcrafted liquid extract; Siberian ginseng/eleuthero root wildcrafted liquid extract, alcohol-free liquid extract

Penn Herb Company
Asian ginseng whole root, powder; American ginseng powder; Siberian ginseng/eleuthero powder

Smart Basics
Asian ginseng standardized capsules; American ginseng standardized capsules; Siberian ginseng/eleuthero standardized capsules

Supplement discounters (see the section on "Mail-Order Supplement Discounters")
Virtually all of the major herbal companies carry Asian, American, and Siberian ginseng products

Print Sources for Further Information on Ginseng and Other Tonic Herbs

Adaptogens: Nature's Key to Well-Being by Mikael Wahlström (Göteborg, Sweden: Skandinavisk Bok, 1987)

Ginseng: A Concise Handbook by James A. Duke (Algonac, Michigan: Reference Publications, 1989)

The Ginseng Book: Nature's Ancient Healer by Stephen Fulder, Ph.D. (Garden City Park, N.Y.: Avery Publishing Group, 1996)

Ginseng: How to Find, Grow, and Use America's Forest Gold by Kim Derek Pritts (Mechanicsburg, Pennsylvania: Stackpole Books, 1995)

The Ginsengs: A User's Guide by Christopher Hobbs (Santa Cruz, Calif.: Botanica Press, 1996)

Herbal Tonic Therapies by Daniel Mowrey, Ph.D. (New Canaan, Ct.: Keats Publishing, 1993)

The Tao of Medicine: Ginseng, Oriental Remedies, and the Pharmacology of Harmony by Stephen Fulder (New York: Destiny Books, 1982)

Relevant Research

Asian ginseng:

Bhattacharya, S.K., and S.K. Mitra, "Anxiolytic activity of *Panax ginseng* roots: An experimental study," *Journal of Ethnopharmacology* (1991), 34(1):87–92

Petkov, V.D., and A.H. Mosharrof, "Effects of standardized ginseng extract on learning, memory, and physical capabilities," *American Journal of Chinese Medicine* (1987), 15(1/2):19–29

Rhee, Y.H., et al., "*Panax ginseng* extract modulates sleep in unrestrained rats," *Psychopharmacology* (1990), 101(4):486–88

Siegel, R.K., "Ginseng abuse syndrome," *Journal of the American Medical Association* (1979), 241:1614–15

Watanabe, H., et al., "Effect of *Panax ginseng* on age-related changes in the spontaneous motor activity and dopaminergic nervous system in the rat," *Japanese Journal of Pharmacology* (1991), 55(1):51–56

Yoshimura, H., et al., "Psychotropic effects of ginseng saponins on agonistic behavior between resident and intruder mice," *European Journal of Pharmacology* (1988), 146(2/3):291–97

American ginseng:

Li, J.J., "Pharmacognostical studies on the medicinal parts of *Panax quinquefolius* L.," *Chung Kuo Chung Yao Tsa Chih* (1993), 18(2):73–76

Martinez, B., and E.J. Staba, "The physiological effects of Aralia, Panax, and Eleutheroccocus on exercised rats," *Japanese Journal of Pharmacology* (1984), 35(2):79–85

Zheng, Y.L., et al., "A comparison between Chinese *Panax quinquefolius* and imported *Panax quinquefolius*: Analysis of composition of essential oil in Panax quinquefolius," *Yao Hsueh Hsueh Pao* (1989), 24(2):118–21

Siberian ginseng/eleuthero:

Ben-Hur, E., and S. Fulder, "Effect of *Panax ginseng* saponins and *Eleutherococcus senticosus* on survival of cultured mammalian cells after ionizing radiation," *American Journal of Chinese Medicine* (1981), 9(1):48–56

Bespalov, V.G., et al., "The inhibiting effect of phytoadaptogenic preparations from bioginseng, *Eleutherococcus senticosus,* and *Rhaponticum carthamoides* on the development of nervous system tumors in rats induced by N-nitrosoethylurea," *Voprosy Onkologii* (1992), 38(9):1073–80

Bohn, B., et al., "Flow cytometric studies with *Eleutherococcus senticosus* extract as an immunomodulatory agent," *Arzneimittel-Forschung* (1987), 37(10):1193–96

Dowling, E.A., et al., "Effect of *Eleutherococcus senticosus* on submaximal and maximal exercise performance," *Medicine and Science in Sports and Exercise* (1996), 28(4):482–89

Farnsworth, N.R., et al., "Siberian ginseng (*Eleutherococcus senticosus*): Current status as an adaptogen," *Economic and Medicinal Plant Research* (1985), 1:155–215

Fujikawa, T., et al., "Protective effects of *Acanthopanax senticosus* Harms from Hokkaido and its components on gastric ulcer in restrained cold water stressed rats," *Biological and Pharmaceutical Bulletin* (1996), 19(9):1227–30

CHAPTER 4: EPHEDRA/MA HUANG

Mail-Order Sources

Gaia Herbs
liquid extract

Herb Pharm
liquid extract

Frontier Cooperative Herbs
cut and sifted, powder

Legendary Ethnobotanical Resources
cut and sifted, powder

Penn Herb Co.
cut, powder

Supplement Discounters (see the section on "Mail-Order Supplement Discounters" below)
Solaray: capsules

Relevant Research

Astrup, A., et al., "The effect of ephedrine/caffeine mixture on energy expenditure and body composition in obese women," *Metabolism* (1992), 41(7):686–88

Betz, J.M., et al., "Chiral gas chromatographic determination of ephedrine-type alkaloids in dietary supplements containing ma huang," *Journal of AOAC International* (1997), 80(2):303–15

Blumenthal, M., and P. King, "Ma huang: Ancient herb, modern medicine, regulatory dilemma: A review of the botany, chemistry, medicinal uses, safety concerns, and legal status of ephedra and its alkaloids," *HerbalGram* (1995), 34:22–57

Breum, L., et al., "Comparison of an ephedrine/caffeine combination and dexfenfluramine in the treatment of obesity: A double-blind multi-center trial in general practice," *International Journal of Obesity* (1994), 18:99–103

Dulloo, A.G., et al., "The thermogenic properties of ephedrine/methylxanthine mixtures: Animal studies," *American Journal of Clinical Nutrition* (1986), 43:388–94

Horton, T.J., et al., "Postprandial thermogenesis with ephedrine, caffeine and aspirin in lean, predisposed obese and obese women," *International Journal of Obesity* (1996), 20:91–97

Kalix, P., "The pharmacology of psychoactive alkaloids from *Ephedra* and *Catha*," *Journal of Ethnopharmacology* (1991), 32:201–08

CHAPTER 5: GUARANA, MATÉ, AND KOLA NUT

Mail-Order Sources

Allies
guarana plants; guarana-related yoco plants; maté-related guayusa treelets; yerba maté seeds, live plants

Botanical Preservation Corps
guarana powder, extract, and honey; kola nut powder; maté leaf; "Herbal Stimulant Sampler" with kola nut powder, maté leaf, cacao seed powder, and green tea

The Basement Shaman
guarana whole nuts; kola whole nuts

Frontier Cooperative Herbs
guarana ground, whole; kola cut and sifted, powder; maté leaf cut and sifted, roasted cut and sifted

Gaia Herbs
maté root liquid plant extract

HerbPharm
kola nut liquid extract

JLF
kola powder, nut pieces

Legendary Ethnobotanical Resources
guarana whole, ground; kola nut cut and sifted, powder; yerba maté cut and sifted, roasted cut and sifted

Penn Herb Company
guarana cut, powdered; maté leaves cut, powdered

Smart Basics
guarana standardized extract capsules; kola nut standardized extract capsules

Supplement Discounters (see the section on "Mail-Order Supplement Discounters")
Nature's Answer/Bio-Botanica: guarana liquid extract; kola nut liquid extract

Print Sources for Further Information

Caffeine:

America's Favorite Drug: Coffee and Your Health by Bonnie Edwards, R.N. (Berkeley, California: Odonian Press, 1992)

Caffeine: The Most Popular Stimulant by Richard J. Gilbert, Ph.D. (New York: Chelsea House Publishers, 1986)

Guarana, maté, and kola:

Guarana: The Energy Seeds and Herbs of the Amazon Rainforest by Michael Van Straten (Marvel Cave Park, Mo.: C.W. Daniel, 1994)

Plant Intoxicants: A Classic Text on the Use of Mind-Altering Plants by Baron Ernst von Bibra, translated by Hedwig Schleiffer (Rochester, Vt.: Healing Arts Press, 1995; originally published: Nuremburg, Germany: Wilhelm Schmid, 1855)

Internet Sources for Further Information

Guarana reports:

www.hyperreal.com/drugs/natural/guarana.rpts

Relevant Research

Guarana:

Bempong, D.K., and P.J. Houghton, "Dissolution and absorption of caffeine from guarana," *Journal of Pharmacy and Pharmacology* (1992), 44(9):769–71

Erickson, H.T., et al., "Guarana (*Paullinia cupana*) as a commercial crop in Brazilian Amazonia," *Economic Botany* (1984), 38(3):273–86

Henman, A.R., "Guarana (*Paullinia cupana* var. *sorbilis*): Ecological and social perspectives on an economic plant of the Central Amazon Basin," *Journal of Ethnopharmacology* (1982), 6(3):311–38

Salvadori, M.C., et al., "Determination of xanthines by high-performance liquid chromatography and thin-layer chromatography in horse urine after ingestion of guarana powder," *Analyst* (1994), 119(12):2701–03

Schultes, R.E., "A caffeine drink prepared from bark," *Economic Botany* (1987), 41(4):526–27

Maté:

Patiño, V.M., "Guayusa, a neglected stimulant from eastern Andean foothills," *Economic Botany* (1968), 22:310–16

Vasques, A., and P. Moyna, "Studies on maté drinking," *Journal of Ethnopharmacology* (1986), 18(3):267–72

Victora, C.G., et al., "Patterns of maté drinking in Brazilian city," *Cancer Research* (1990), 50(22):7112–15

Kola nut:

Agatha, M., et al., "Some preliminary observations on the effects of kola nut on the cardiovascular system," *Nigerian Medical Journal* (1978), 8(6):501–05

Ajarem, J.S., "Effects of fresh kola-nut extract (*Cola nitida*) on the locomotor activities of male mice," *Acta Physiologica et Pharmacologica Bulgarica* (1990), 16(4):10–15

CHAPTER 6: PHENYLALANINE AND TYROSINE

Mail-Order Sources

CFIDS and Fibromyalgia Health Resource
L-phenylalanine 500 mg tablets; tyrosine 500 mg capsules

Olympia
L-phenylalanine 500 mg capsules; tyrosine 500 mg capsules; N-acetyl L-tyrosine 300 mg capsules

Smart Basics
tyrosine 500 mg capsules

Sunburst Biorganics
DL-phenylalanine 500 mg tablets; L-phenylalanine 500 mg tablets; tyrosine 500 mg capsules

Vitamin Research Products
L-phenylalanine 400 mg capsules; DL-phenylalanine 500 mg capsules; tyrosine 500 mg capsules

Supplement Discounters (see the section on "Mail-Order Supplement Discounters")
Twinlab: L-phenylalanine 500 mg capsules, tablets; tyrosine 500 mg capsules, tablets; Source Naturals: L-phenylalanine powder, 500 mg tablets; DL-phenylalanine 375 mg and 750 mg tablets; tyrosine powder, 500 mg tablets

Print Sources for Further Information

Thorsons Guide to Amino Acids by Leon Chaitow, N.D., D.O. (London: Thorsons, 1991)

Relevant Research

Beckman, H., et al., "DL-phenylalanine versus imipramine: A double-blind controlled study," *Archiv fur Psychiatrie und Nervenkrankheiten* (1979), 227:49

Beckman, H., "Phenylalanine in affective disorders," *Advances in Biological Psychiatry* (1983), 10:137–47

Ehrenpreis, S., et al., "Naloxone reversible analgesia in mice produced by D-phenylalanine and hydrocinnamic acid, inhibitors of carboxypeptidase A," *Advances in Pain Research and Therapy* (1979), 3:479–87

Gelenberg, A. J., et al., "Tyrosine for the treatment of depression," *American Journal of Psychiatry* (1980), 137:622–23

Gibson, C., and A.J. Gelenberg, "Tyrosine for depression," *Advances in Biological Psychiatry* (1983), 10:148–59

Sabelli, H.C., et al., "Clinical studies on the phenylethylamine hypothesis of affective disorder: Urine and blood phenylacetic acid and phenylalanine dietary supplements," *Journal of Clinical Psychiatry* (1986), 47(2):66–70

Mail-Order Sources

Allies
seeds

CFIDS and Fibromyalgia Health Resource
capsules

Frontier Cooperative Herbs
cut and sifted

Gaia Herbs
liquid extract

Health Center for Better Living
cut and sifted, capsules

Herb Pharm
liquid extract

LifeLink
standardized extract capsules

Olympia
standardized extract capsules

Peggy's Health Center
standardized extract capsules

Penn Herb Company
cut, powdered

Smart Basics
standardized extract capsules

Vitamin Research Products
standardized extract capsules

Supplement Discounters (see the section on "Mail-Order Supplement Discounters")
Nature's Herbs: capsules, liquid extract; Nature's Way: capsules; Futurebiotics: capsules; Solgar: capsules

Print Sources for Further Information

Hypericum and Depression by Harold H. Bloomfield, M.D., and Peter McWilliams (Los Angeles: Prelude Press, 1996)

Internet Sources for Further Information

Definitive St. John's wort links:

www.geocities.com/~ottthoma/depression/sjw.html

Hypericum:

www.hypericum.com

Relevant Research

Hansgen, K.D., et al., "Multicenter double-blind study examining the antidepressant effectiveness of the hypericum extract LI 160," *Journal of Geriatric Psychiatry and Neurology* (1994), 7 Suppl 1:S15–18

Harrer, G., and H. Sommer, "Treatment of mild/moderate depressions with hypericum," *Phytomedicine* (1994), 1:3–8

Hobbs, Christopher, "St. John's wort," *HerbalGram* (1989), 18/19:24–33

Holzl, J., et al., "Investigations about antidepressive and mood changing effects of *Hypericum perforatum*," *Planta Medica* (1989), 55:643

Hubner, W.D., "Hypericum treatment of mild depressions with somatic symptoms," *Journal of Geriatric Psychiatry and Neurology* (1994), 7 Suppl 1:S12–14

Linde, K. et al., "St. John's wort for depression: An overview and meta-analysis of randomised clinical trials," *British Medical Journal* (1996), 313:253–58

Muldner, V.H., and M. Zoller, "Antidepressive effect of a hypericum extract standardized to an active hypericin complex," *Arzneimittel-Forschung* (1984), 34(8):918–20

Reuter, H.D., "Psychotropic herbal drugs: Results of recent pharmacological clinical studies with *Hypericum perforatum*," presentation at the Second International Conference on Phytothcrapcutics, National Herbalists Association of Australia, March 1995, Sidney

Suzuki, O., et al., "Inhibition of monoamine oxidase by hypericin," *Planta Medica* (1984), 50:272–74

CHAPTER 8: ROSE, JASMINE, AND NEROLI

Mail-Order Sources:

See "Mail-Order Sources of Herbs, Nutritional Supplements, Essential Oils, and Smart Drugs."

Print Sources for Further Information on Essential Oils

See Bibliography for books on aromatherapy and essential oils.

Relevant Research

Stevenson, C, "Orange blossom evaluation," *International Journal of Aromatherapy* (1992), 4(3):22–24

CHAPTER 9: VASOPRESSIN, DEPRENYL, PIRACETAM, AND HYDERGINE

Mail-Order Sources:

See "Ordering Supplements and Smart Drugs from Foreign Sources."

Print Sources for Further Information

See Bibliography for books on smart drugs.

For further information on the remarkable properties of ergot:

LSD, My Problem Child: Reflections on Sacred Drugs, Mysticism, and Science by Albert Hofmann (Los Angeles: Jeremy P. Tarcher, 1983)

Poisons of the Past: Molds, Epidemics, and History by Mary Kilbourne Matossian (New Haven, Conn.: Yale University Press, 1989)

The Road to Eleusis: Unveiling the Secret of the Mysteries by R. Gordon Wasson, Albert Hofmann, and Carl A.P. Ruck (New York: Harcourt Brace Jovanovich, 1978)

Internet Sources for Further Information

Experiences with Hydergine:

www.damicon.fi/sd/hydergine.exp.html

Experiences with Vasopressin:

www.damicon.fi/sd/vasopressin.exp.html

Relevant Research

Vasopressin:

Laczi, F., et al., "Effects of lysine-vasopressin and l-deamino-8-D-arginine-vasopressin on memory in healthy individuals and diabetes insipidus patients," *Psychoneuroendocrinology* (1982), 7(2):185–92

Nebes, R.D., et al., "The effect of vasopressin on memory in the healthy elderly," *Psychiatry Research* (1984), 11:49–59

Deprenyl:

Brandeis, R., et al., "Improvement of cognitive function by MAO-B inhibitor L-deprenyl in aged rats," *Pharmacology, Biochemistry & Behavior* (1991), 39(2):297–304

Knoll, J., et al., "Striatal dopamine, sexual activity and lifespan: Longevity of rats treated with (-)deprenyl," *Life Sciences* (1989), 45(6):525–31

Knoll, J. "(-)Deprenyl-medication: A strategy to modulate the age-related decline of the striatal dopaminergic system," *Journal of the American Geriatric Society* (1992), 40(8):839–47

Sabelli, H.C., "Rapid treatment of depression with selegiline-phenylalanine combination," *Journal of Clinical Psychiatry* (1991), 53(3):137

Piracetam:

Ammassari-Teule, M., et al., "Avoidance facilitation in adult mice by prenatal administration of the nootropic drug Oxiracetam," *Pharmacological Research Communications* (1986), 18(12):1169–76

Ammassari-Teule, M., et al., "Enhancement of radial maze performances in CD1 mice after prenatal exposure to Oxiracetam: Possible role of sustained investigative responses developed during ontogeny," *Physiology and Behavior* (1988), 42(3):281–85

Chleide, E., et al., "Enhanced resistance effect of piracetam upon hypoxia-induced impaired retention of fixed-interval responding in rats," *Pharmacology, Biochemistry and Behavior* (1991), 40(1):1–6

Dimond, S.J., and E.Y.M. Bowers, "Increase in the power of human memory in normal man through the use of drugs," *Psychopharmacology* (1976), 49:307–09

Huber, W., et al., "Piracetam as an adjuvant to language therapy for aphasia: A randomized double-blind placebo-controlled pilot study," *Archives of Physical Medicine and Rehabilitation* (1997), 78(3):245–50

Saletu, B., et al., "Double-blind, placebo-controlled, pharmacokinetic and -dynamic studies with 2 new formulations of piracetam (infusion and syrup) under hypoxia in man," *International Journal of Clinical Pharmacology Therapy* (1995), 33(5):249–62

Schaffler, K., and W. Klausnitzer, "Randomized placebo-controlled double-blind cross-over study on antihypoxidotic effects of piracetam using psychophysiological measures in healthy volunteers," *Arzneimittel-Forschung* (1988), 38(2):288–91

Stoll, L., et al., "Age-related deficits of central muscarinic cholinergic receptor function in the mouse. Partial restoration by chronic piracetam treatment," *Neurobiology of Aging* (1991), 13:39–44

Wilsher, C.R., et al., "Piracetam and dyslexia: Effects on reading tests," *Journal of Clinical Psychopharmacology* (1987), 7(4):230–37

Hydergine:

Amenta, D., et al., "Effects of long-term Hydergine administration on lipofuscin accumulation in senescent rat brain," *Gerontology* (1988), 34(5–6):250–56

Hindmarch, I., et al., "The effects of an ergot alkaloid derivative (Hydergine) on aspects of psychomotor performance, arousal, and cognitive processing ability," *The Journal of Clinical Pharmacology* (1979), 19(11–12):726–32

Huber, F., et al., "Effects of long-term ergoloid mesylates ('Hydergine') administration in healthy pensioners: 5-year results," *Current Medical Research and Opinion* (1986), 10(4)

CHAPTER 10: CHOLINE, DMAE, AND PYROGLUTAMATE

Mail-Order Sources

CFIDS and Fibromyalgia Health Resource
lecithin softgels, DMAE capsules

Life Enhancement Products
DMAE capsules

LifeLink
DMAE tablets

Olympia
lecithin gels; DMAE tablets; L-pyroglutamic acid tablets

Smart Basics
phosphatidylcholine softgels; DMAE capsules; arginine pyroglutamate capsules

Sunburst Biorganics
lecithin granules, capsules; phosphatidylcholine capsules

Vitamin Research Products
lecithin granules; phosphatidyl choline capsules; choline capsules, powder, liquid; DMAE capsules, powder; pyroglutamate capsules, powder

Supplement Discounters (see the section on "Mail-Order Supplement Discounters")
Twinlab: choline capsules, powder; DMAE capsules; Source Naturals, KAL, Country Life: pyroglutamate combination formulas

Print Sources for Further Information

Mind Food & Smart Pills by Ross Pelton, R.Ph., Ph.D., with Taffy Clarke Pelton (New York: Main Street Books/Doubleday, 1989)

Relevant Research

Choline:

Meck, W.H., et al., "Pre- and postnatal choline supplementation produces long-term facilitation of spatial memory," *Developmental Psychobiology* (1988), 21(4):339–53

Petkov, V.D., et al., "Effects of cytidine diphosphate choline on rats with memory deficits," *Arzneimittel-Forschung* (1993), 43(8):822–28

Safford, F., et al., "Testing the effects of dietary lecithin on memory in the elderly: An example of social work/medical research collaboration," *Research on Social Work Practice* (1994), 4(3):349

Zeisel, S.H., et al., "Choline: An essential nutrient for humans," *FASEB Journal* (1991), 5:2093–98

Zeisel, S.H., et al., "Choline and hepatocarcinogenesis in the rat," *Advances in Experimental Medicine and Biology* (1995), 375:65–74

DMAE:

Haubrich, D.R., et al., "Deanol affects choline metabolism in peripheral tissues of mice," *Journal of Neurochemistry* (1981), 37(2):476–82

Hochschild, R., "Effect of dimethylaminoethyl p-chlorophenoxyacetate on the life span of male Swiss Webster albino mice," *Experimental Gerontology* (1973), 8:177–83

Osvaldo, R., "2-Dimethylaminoethanol (Deanol): A brief review of its clinical efficacy and postulated mechanism of action," *Current Therapeutic Research* (1974), 16(11):1238–42

Pfeiffer, C.C., et al., "Stimulant effect of 2-dimethyl-1-aminoethanol: Possible precursor of brain acetylcholine," *Science* (1957), 126:610–11

Pyroglutamate:

Antonelli, T., et al., "Pyroglutamic acid administration modifies the electrocorticogram and increases the release of acetylcholine and GABA from the guinea-pig cerebral cortex," *Pharmacological Research Communications* (1984), 16(2):189–98

Drago, F., et al., "Pyroglutamic acid improves learning and memory capacities in old rats," *Functional Neurology* (1988), 3(2):137–43

Grioli, S., et al., "Pyroglutamic acid improves the age-associated memory impairment," *Fundamental and Clinical Pharmacology* (1990), 4(2):169–73

Sinforiani, E., et al., "Sulla reversibilita dei disordini cognitivi negli alcolisti cronici in fase di dissauefazion," *Minerva Psichiatrica* (1985), 26:339–42

Spignoli, G., et al., "Effect of pyroglutamic acid stereoisomers on ECS and scopolamine-induced memory disruption and brain acetylcholine levels in the rat," *Pharmacological Research Communications* (1987), 19(12):901–12

Mail-Order Sources

Allies
seeds

Botanical Preservation Corps
leaves, extract

CFIDS and Fibromyalgia Health Resource
dried extract capsules

Gaia Herbs
liquid extract

Herb Pharm
liquid extract

Life Enhancement Products
dried standardized extract capsules

Olympia
dried standardized extract capsules

Smart Basics
dried standardized extract capsules

Vitamin Research Products
dried standardized extract capsules

Supplement Discounters (see the section on "Mail-Order Supplement Discounters")
Numerous producers offer high-quality standardized extracts, including Nature's Way, Source Naturals, Nature's Herbs, KAL, Natrol, Futurebiotics, and others.

Print Sources for Further Information

Ginkgo biloba Extract (EGb 761): Pharmacological Activities and Clinical Applications by F.V. DeFeudis (Paris: Elsevier Scientific Editions, 1991)

Ginkgo: Elixir of Youth by Christopher Hobbs (Santa Cruz, Calif.: Botanica Press, 1991)

Ginkgo: Ginkgo biloba by Steven Foster (Austin, Tx.: American Botanical Council, 1991)

Rökan (Ginkgo biloba): Recent Results in Pharmacology and Clinic edited by E.W. Fünfgeld (Berlin: Springer-Verlag, 1988)

Relevant Research

Fünfgeld, E.W., "A natural and broad spectrum nootropic substance for treatment of SDAT—The *Ginkgo biloba* extract," *Progress in Clinical and Biological Research* (1989), 317:1247–60

Gessner, B., et al., "Study of the long-term action of a *Ginkgo biloba* extract on vigilance and mental performance as determined by means of quantitative pharmaco-EEG and psychometric measurements," *Arzneimittel-Forschung* (1985), 35(9):1459–65

Hindmarch, I., "Activity of *Ginkgo biloba* extract on short-term memory," *Presse Medicale* (1986), 15(31):1592–94

Hofferberth, B., "The efficacy of EGb 761 in patients with senile dementia of the Alzheimer type: A double-blind, placebo-controlled study on different levels of investigation," *Psychopharmacology* (1994), 9:215–22

Kleijnen, J., and P. Knipschild, "Ginkgo biloba," *The Lancet* (1992), 340(7):1136–39

Paick, J., and J. Lee, "An experimental study of the effect of *Ginkgo biloba* extract on the human and rabbit corpus cavernosum tissue," *Journal of Urology* (1996), 156:1876–1880

Semlitsch, H.V., et al., "Cognitive psychophysiology in nootropic drug research: Effects of *Ginkgo biloba* on event-related potentials (P300) in age-associated memory impairment," *Pharmacopsychiatry* (1995), 28:134–142

Subhan, Z., and I. Hindmarch, "The psychopharmacological effects of *Ginkgo biloba* extract in normal healthy volunteers," *International Journal of Clinical Pharmacology Research* (1984), 4:89–93

Warburton, D.M., "Clinical psychopharmacology of *Ginkgo biloba* extract," *Presse Medicale* (1986), 15(31):1595–604

White, H.L., et al., "Extracts of *Ginkgo biloba* leaves inhibit monoamine oxidase," *Life Sciences* (1996), 58:1315–21

CHAPTER 12: PEPPERMINT, BASIL, AND ROSEMARY

Mail-Order Sources

See "Mail-Order Sources of Herbs, Nutritional Supplements, Essential Oils, and Smart Drugs."

Print Sources for Further Information

See Bibliography for books on aromatherapy and essential oils.

Relevant Research

Ehrlichman, H., and L. Bastone, "Olfaction and emotion," in *Science of Olfaction* (New York: Springer-Verlag, 1992; ed. by M.J. Serby and K.L. Chobor), 410–17

Göbel, H., et al., "Essential plant oils and headache mechanisms," *Phytomedicine* (1995), 2(2):93–102

Hirsch, A., and L.H. Johnston, "The effect of floral odor on learning," *Chemical Senses* (1994), 19(5):77–78

Kovar, K.A., et al., "Blood levels of 1,8-cineole and locomotor activity of mice after inhalation and oral administration of rosemary oil," *Planta Medica* (1987), 53(4):315–18

Nasel, C., et al., "Functional imaging of effects of fragrances on the human brain after prolonged inhalation," *Chemical Senses* (1994), 19(4):359–64

CHAPTER 13: VALERIAN

Mail-Order Sources

Allies
seeds

CFIDS and Fibromyalgia Health Resource
capsules

Gaia Herbs
liquid extract

Herb Pharm
liquid extract

Legendary Ethnobotanical Resources
cut and sifted, powder, capsules

Smart Basics
capsules

Supplement Discounters (see the section on "Mail-Order Supplement Discounters")
Valerian is among the most widely distributed herbal products; virtually every herbal company offers one or more valerian-based remedies.

Print Sources for Further Information

Citizen Petition to Amend FDA's Monograph on Nighttime Sleep-Aid Drug Products for Over-the-Counter ("OTC") Human Use to Include Valerian by the European-American Phytomedicines Coalition (available for $10 plus postage and handling from American Botanical Council; see address, page 249)

Valerian: The Relaxing and Sleep Herb by Christopher Hobbs (Capitola, Calif.: Botanica Press, 1993)

Valerian: Valeriana officinalis by Steven Foster, Botanical Series No. 312 (Austin, Texas: American Botanical Council, 1990)

Internet Sources for Further Information

Experiences with Valerian:

www.hyperreal.org/drugs/natural/valerian.info

Relevant Research

Cavadas, C., et al., "In vitro study on the interaction of *Valeriana officinalis* L. extracts and their amino acids on GABAA receptor in rat brain," *Arzneimittel-Forschung* (1995), 45(7):753–55

Delsignore, R., et al., "Placebo controlled clinical trial with valerian," *Settimana Medica* (1980), 68(9):437–47

Houghton, P., "The biological activity of valerian and related plants," *Journal of Ethnopharmacology* (1988), 22(2):121–42

Krieglstein, J., and D. Grusla, "Central depressant constituents in valerian," *Deutsche Apotheker Zeitung* (1988), 128:2041–46

Leathwood, P.D., et al., "Aqueous extract of valerian

root (*Valeriana officinalis*) improves sleep quality in man" *Pharmacology, Biochemistry & Behavior* (1982), 17(1):65–71

Leathwood, P.D., and F. Chauffard, "Aqueous extract of valerian reduces latency to fall asleep in man," *Planta Medica* (1985), Apr(2):144–48

Lindahl, O., and L. Lindwall, "Double-blind study of a valerian preparation," *Pharmacology, Biochemistry & Behavior* (1989), 32(4):1065–66

Tufik, S., et al., "Effects of prolonged administration of valepotriates in rats on the mothers and their offspring," *Journal of Ethnopharmacology* (1994), 41:39–44

CHAPTER 14: CALIFORNIA POPPY

Mail-Order Sources

Allies
seeds

Botanical Preservation Corps
bulk

Herb Pharm
liquid extract

Gaia Herbs
liquid extract

Legendary Ethnobotanical Resources
liquid extract

Frontier Cooperative Herbs
cut and sifted

Print Sources for Further Information

Poppies: The Poppy Family in the Wild and in Cultivation by Christopher Grey-Wilson (Portland, Oregon: Timber Press, 1993)

Internet Sources for Further Information

The genus Eschscholzia—California poppies and their relatives:

www.is.csupomona.edu/~jcclark/poppy/

Relevant Research

Rolland, A., et al., "Behavioural effects of the American traditional plant *Eschscholtzia californica:* Sedative and anxiolytic properties," *Planta Medica* (1991), 57(3):212–16

Schafer, H.L., et al., "Sedative action of extract combinations of *Eschscholtzia californica* and *Corydalis cava*," *Arzneimittel-Forschung* (1995), 45(2):124–26

Vincieri, F.F., et al., "An approach to the biological study of *Eschscholtzia californica* Cham.," *Pharmacological Research Communications* (1988), 20(5):41–44

CHAPTER 15: MELATONIN

Mail-Order Sources

CFIDS and Fibromyalgia Health Resource
tablets, sublingual

Life Enhancement Products
sublingual

LifeLink
sublingual

Olympia
capsules, sublingual

Peggy's Health Center
capsules, sublingual

Smart Basics
capsules

Vitamin Research Products
capsules

Supplement Discounters (see the section on "Mail-Order Supplement Discounters")
Virtually all of the established dietary supplement companies now offer melatonin products, including Source Naturals, Alacer, Natrol, KAL, and Schiff.

Print Sources for Further Information

The Melatonin Miracle by Walter Pierpaoli, M.D., Ph.D., and William Regelson, M.D., with Carol Colman (New York: Simon & Schuster, 1995)

Melatonin: Nature's Sleeping Pill by Ray Sahelian, M.D. (Marina Del Rey, Calif.: Be Happier Press, 1995)

Melatonin: Your Body's Natural Wonder Drug by Russel J. Reiter, Ph.D., and Jo Robinson (New York: Bantam Books, 1995)

Stay Young the Melatonin Way: The Natural Way to Beat Fatigue and Combat Aging by Stephen J. Bock and Michael Boyette (New York: Penguin Books, 1995)

Internet Sources for Further Information

PharmInfoNet (Pharmaceutical Information Network) sci.med.pharmacy Selected Archives: Melatonin Threads:

pharminfo.com/drugdb/mela_arc.html

Worldwide Labs' Melatonin Central:

www.melatonin.com

The Melatonin Page:

www.tenzing.com/m.html

Yahoo: Melatonin:

www.yahoo.com/Health/Medicine/Sleep_Medicine/Melatonin

Relevant Research

Attenburrow, M.E.J., et al., "Case-control of evening melatonin concentration in primary insomnia," *British Medical Journal* (1996), 312:1263–65

Becker-Andre, M., et al., "Pineal gland hormone melatonin binds and activates an orphan of the nuclear receptor superfamily," *Journal of Biological Chemistry* (1994), 269(46):28531–34

Neville, K., and N. McNaughton, "Anxiolytic-like action of melatonin on acquisition but not performance of DRL," *Pharmacology, Biochemistry & Behavior* (1986), 24:1497–1502

Poeggeler, B., et al., "Melatonin, hydroxyl radical-mediated oxidative damage, and aging: A hypothesis," *Journal of Pineal Research* (1993), 14:151–68

Vijayalaxmi, B.Z., et al., "Melatonin protects human blood lymphocytes from radiation induced chromosome damage," *Mutation Research* (1995), 346(1):23–31

Zhdanova, I.V., et al., "Sleep-inducing effects of low doses of melatonin ingested in the evening," *Clinical Pharmacology and Therapeutics* (1995), 57:552–58

CHAPTER 16: TRYPTOPHAN, 5-HTP, AND GABA

Mail-Order Sources

CFIDS and Fibromyalgia Health Resource
GABA tablets

Life Enhancement Products
5-HTP capsules, 5-HTP formula ("5-HTP SeroTonic," a combination of 5-HTP, St. John's wort, and four nutrients)

LifeLink
5-HTP capsules

Olympia
5-HTP capsules, "5-HTP SeroTonic"; GABA capsules, sublingual tablets

Peggy's Health Center
5-HTP capsules

Smart Basics
5-HTP capsules

Vitamin Research Products
5-HTP capsules

The FDA has prohibited the sale of tryptophan supplements in the United States since 1990. Tryptophan can be obtained with a prescription from some compounding pharmacies (as can 5-HTP). Tryptophan can also be purchased from overseas mail-order sources (see "Ordering Supplements and Smart Drugs from Foreign Sources," page 248).

Print Sources for Further Information

Thorsons Guide to Amino Acids by Leon Chaitow, N.D., D.O. (London: Thorsons, 1991)

Relevant Research

Tryptophan:

Huether, G., et al., "Effect of tryptophan administration on circulating melatonin levels in chicks and rats: Evidence for stimulation of melatonin synthesis and release in the gastrointestinal tract," *Life Sciences* (1992), 51:945–53

Kitahara, M., "Dietary tryptophan ratio and suicide in the United Kingdom, Ireland, the United States, Canada, Australia, and New Zealand," *Omega Journal of Death and Dying* (1987), 18:71–76

Schneider-Helmet, D., et al., "Evaluation of L-tryptophan for treatment of insomnia: A review," *Psychopharmacology* (1986), 89(1):1–7

Slutsker, L., et al., "Eosinophilia-myalgia syndrome associated with exposure to tryptophan from a single manufacturer," *Journal of the American Medical Association* (1990), 264:213–17

5-HTP:

Byerley, W.F., et al., "5-Hydroxytryptophan: A review of its antidepressant efficacy and adverse effects," *Journal of Clinical Psychopharmacology* (1987), 7(3):127–37

Kahn, R.S., et al., "Effect of a serotonin precursor and uptake inhibitor in anxiety disorders: A double-blind comparison of 5-hydroxytryptophan, clomipramine and placebo," *International Clinical Psychopharmacology* (1987), 2(1):33–45

Kahn, R.S., et al., "L-5-hydroxytryptophan in the treatment of anxiety disorders," *Journal of Affective Disorders* (1985), 8:197–200

Pöldinger, W., et al., "A functional-dimensional approach to depression: Serotonin deficiency as a target syndrome in a comparison of 5-hydroxytryptophan and fluvoxamine," *Psychopathology* (1991), 24(2):53–81

Ursin, R. "The effect of 5-hydroxytryptophan and L-tryptophan on wakefulness and sleep patterns in the cat," *Brain Research* (1976), 106:106–15

Van Praag, H.M., "Studies in the mechanism of action of serotonin precursors in depression," *Psychopharmacology Bulletin* (1984), 20:599–602

Van Praag, H.M., and H.G. Westenberg, "The treatment of depressions with L-5-hydroxytryptophan: Theoretical backgrounds and practical application," *Advances in Biological Psychiatry* (1983), 10:94–128

GABA:

Zhang, S.S., et al., "Effects of cerebral GABA level on learning and memory," *Acta Pharmacologica Sinica* (1989), 10(1):10–12

CHAPTER 17: KAVA

Mail-Order Sources

Allies
plants

Botanical Preservation Corps
roots, liquid drops, massage oil, powder, resin extract

The Basement Shaman
chopped dried roots

CFIDS and Fibromyalgia Health Resource
tablets

Frontier Cooperative Herbs
roots, cut and sifted, powder

Gaia Herbs
liquid extract, alcohol-free herbal glycerite

Health Center for Better Living
cut and sifted, powder, tea bags, capsules (powder)

Herb Pharm
liquid extract

JLF
roots, root resin extract

Kava Kaua'i
powder (Waka grade, Fiji), liquid concentrated extract, honey and kava-powder blends

Legendary Ethnobotanical Resources
cut and sifted, powder

Life Services Supplements
standardized extract capsules

Olympia
standardized extract capsules

Smart Basics
standardized extract capsules

Vitamin Research Products
standardized extract capsules

Supplement Discounters (see the section on "Mail-Order Supplement Discounters")

Most herbal companies are in the process of developing kava products. Some that already have products on the market include the following: Rainbow Light: liquid concentrate; Nature's Way: capsules; Jade Chinese Herbals: liquid extract; Solgar: capsules

Print Sources for Further Information

The Abandoned Narcotic: Kava and Cultural Instability in Melanesia by Ron Brunton (New York: Cambridge University Press, 1989)

Ethnopharmacologic Search for Psychoactive Drugs (Symposium Proceedings), edited by Daniel H. Efron et al. (Washington, D.C.: U.S. Government Printing Office, 1967; New York: Raven Press, 1979)

Kava: The Pacific Drug by Vincent Lebot, Mark Merlin, and Lamont Lindstrom (New Haven, Ct.: Yale University Press, 1992)

Kava: Medicine Hunting in Paradise by Chris Kilham (Rochester, Vt.: Park Street Press, 1996)

Internet Sources for Further Information

Lee Kagan's Kava Page:

www.prairienet.org/~kagan/kavabib.html

Kava users' experiences:

www.hyperreal.com/drugs/natural/kava.rpts

Relevant Research

Cawte, J., "Psychoactive substances of the South Seas: Betel, kava and pituri," *Australian and New Zealand Journal of Psychiatry* (1985), 19(1):83–87

Davies, L.P., et al., "Kava pyrones and resin: Studies on GABAa, GABAb and benzodiazepine binding sites in rodent brain," *Pharmacology and Toxicology* (1992), 71(2):120–26

Duffield, P.H., and D. Jamieson, "Development of tolerance to kava in mice," *Clinical Experiments in Pharmacology and Physiology* (1991), 18(8):571–78

Garner, L.F., and J.D. Klinger, "Some visual effects caused by the beverage kava," *Journal of Ethnopharmacology* (1985), 13(3):307–11

Gatty, R., "Kava: Polynesian beverage shrub," *Economic Botany* (1956), 10:241–49

Jussofie, A., et al., "Kavapyrone-enriched extract from *Piper methysticum* as modulator of the GABA binding site in different regions of rat brain," *Psychopharmacology* (1994), 116(4):469–74

Kinzler, E., et al., "Effect of a special kava extract in patients with anxiety, tension, and excitation states of non-psychotic genesis," *Arzneimittel-Forschung* (1991), 41:584–88

Lehmann, E., et al., "Efficacy of a special kava extract (*Piper methysticum*) in patients with states of anxiety, tension, and excitedness of non-mental origin: A double-blind placebo-controlled study of four weeks' treatment," *Phytomedicine* (1996), 3:113–19

Mathews, J.B., et al., "Effects of the heavy usage of kava on physical health: Summary of a pilot survey in an Aboriginal community," *Medical Journal of Australia* (1988), 148:548–55

Munte, T.F., et al., "Effects of oxazepam and an extract of kava roots (*Piper methysticum*) on event-related potentials in a word recognition task," *Neuropsychobiology* (1993), 27(1):46–53

Prescott, J., et al., "Acute effects of kava on measures of cognitive performance, physiological function, and mood," *Drug and Alcohol Review* (1993), 12(1):49–58

Singh, Y.N., "Kava: An overview," *Journal of Ethnopharmacology* (1992), 37(1):13–45

Singh, Y.N., and M. Blumenthal, "Kava: An overview," *HerbalGram* (1997), 39:33–55

CHAPTER 18: YOHIMBÉ

Mail-Order Sources

Botanical Preservation Corps
bark, liquid extract

CFIDS and Fibromyalgia Health Resource
capsules

Gaia Herbs
liquid extract

Herb Pharm
liquid extract

JLF
bark

Legendary Ethnobotanical Resources
whole herb

Life Enhancement Products
liquid extract

Life Services Supplements
standardized liquid extract

Olympia
liquid extract

Supplement Discounters (see the section on "Mail-Order Supplement Discounters")
Universal: capsules

Print Sources for Further Information

Better Sex Through Chemistry by John Morganthaler and Dan Joy (Petaluma, Calif.: Smart Publications, 1994)

Internet Sources for Further Information

yohimbé.reports:

www.damicon.fi/drugs/stimulants/yohimbe.rpts

Relevant Research

Bowes, M.P., et al., "Effects of yohimbine and idazoxan on motor behaviors in male rats," *Pharmacology, Biochemistry & Behavior* (1992), 41(4):707–13

Clark, J.T., et al., "Enhancement of sexual motivation in male rats by yohimbine," *Science* (1984), 225(4664):847–49

Clark, J.T., et al., "Testosterone is not required for the enhancement of sexual motivation by yohimbine," *Physiology and Behavior* (1985), 35(4):517–21

Coplan, J.D., et al., "Behavioral effects of oral yohimbine in differentially reared nonhuman primates," *Neuropsychopharmacology* (1992), 6(1):31–37

Costa, R., and A. Marino, "Further experimental and clinical data on yohimbine with special reference to its anxiogenic action: An experimental contribution," *Clinica Terapeutica* (1991), 136(1):3–9

Davis, G.A., and R. Kohl, "The influence of alpha receptors on lordosis in the female rat," *Pharmacology, Biochemistry & Behavior* (1977), 6(1):47–53

Friesen, K., et al., "Benign course after massive ingestion of yohimbine," *Journal of Emergency Medicine* (1993), 11(3):287–88

Guthrie, S.K., et al., "Yohimbine bioavailability in humans," *European Journal of Clinical Pharmacology* (1990), 39(4):409–11

Hollander, E., and A. McCarley, "Yohimbine treatment of sexual side effects induced by serotonin reuptake blockers," *Journal of Clinical Psychiatry* (1992), 53(6): 207–09

Mann, K., et al., "Effects of yohimbine on sexual experiences and nocturnal penile tumescence and rigidity in erectile dysfunction," *Archives of Sexual Behavior* (1996), 25:1–16

Morpurgo, B., et al., "Effect of yohimbine on the reproductive behavior of the male Nile crocodile (*Crocodylus niloticus*)," *Pharmacology, Biochemistry & Behavior* (1992), 43(2):449–52

Sax, L., "Yohimbine does not affect fat distribution in men," *International Journal of Obesity* (1991), 15(9):561–65

Susset, J.G., et al., "Effect of yohimbine hydrochloride on erectile impotence: A double-blind study," *Journal of Urology* (1989), 141(6):1360–63

CHAPTER 19: BETTER
SAFE THAN SORRY

Print Sources for Further Information

Drug, Set, and Setting: The Basis for Controlled Intoxicant Use by Norman E. Zinberg, M.D. (New Haven, Ct.: Yale University Press, 1984)

From Chocolate to Morphine: Everything You Need to Know About Mind-Altering Drugs by Andrew Weil, M.D., and Winifred Rosen (New York: Houghton Mifflin, rev. ed. 1993)

Hallucinogens: Cross-Cultural Perspectives by Marlene Dobkin de Rios (Albuquerque, N.M.: University of New Mexico Press, 1984)

Psychoactive Drugs and Harm Reduction: From Faith to Science edited by Nick Heather et al. (London: Whurr Publishers, 1993)

MAIL-ORDER SOURCES OF HERBS, NUTRITIONAL SUPPLEMENTS, ESSENTIAL OILS, AND SMART DRUGS

The following are mail-order suppliers of herbs in various forms (whole, capsules, liquid extracts, etc.).

Allies
P.O. Box 2422
Sebastopol, CA 95473
(no phone)

The Basement Shaman
P.O. Box 1255
Elgin, IL 60121
(847) 695-2447

Botanical Preservation Corps
P.O. Box 1368
Sebastopol, CA 95473
(no phone)

The Eclectic Institute
14385 S.E. Lusted Rd.
Sandy, OR 97055
(503) 668-4120
(800) 332-4372

Frontier Cooperative Herbs
3021 78th St.
P.O. Box 299
Norway, IA 52318
(800) 669-3275
www.natnet.com/frontier/

Gaia Herbs
12 Lancaster County Rd.
Harvard, MA 01451
(508) 772-5400
(800) 831-7780

Health Center for Better Living
6189 Taylor Rd.
Naples, FL 33942
(813) 566-2611
www.gate.net/~van/
   herbalcatalog.html

Herb Pharm
P.O. Box 116
Williams, OR 97544
(541) 846-6262
(800) 348-4372

JLF
P.O. Box 184
Elizabethtown, IN 47232
(812) 379-2508 (answering
machine)

Kava Kaua'i
6817 Kahuna Rd.
Kapaa, Kauai HI 96746
(808) 821-1039
www.kauaisource.com
kava@kauaisource.com

**Legendary Ethnobotanical
Resources**
16245 S.W. 304 St.
Homestead, FL 33033
(305) 242-0877
www.shadow.net/~heruka

Mountain Rose Herbs
P.O. Box 2000
Redway, CA 95560
(707) 923-7867
(800) 879-3337

Nature's Way
10 Mountain Springs Parkway
P.O. Box 4000
Springville, UT 84663
(800) 962-8873

Rainbow Light
207 McPherson St.
Santa Cruz, CA 95060
(408) 429-9089
(800) 227-0555

Terra Firma Botanicals
P.O. Box 5680
Eugene, OR 97405
(541) 485-7726
(800) 837-3476
(541) 485-8600 (fax)
terrafirm@continet.com

The following are mail-order suppliers of a variety of nutritional supplements as well as various nutrient-based smart products, amino acids, and in some cases a few herbs:

CFIDS and Fibromyalgia Health Resource
1187 Coast Village Rd.,
　Suite 1-280
Santa Barbara, CA 93108
(800) 366-6056
(800) 965-0042 (fax)
health@silcom.com

Home Health
1160 Millers Ln.
Virginia Beach, VA 23451
(800) 284-9123

J M Pharmacal
251-B East Hacienda Ave.
Campbell, CA 95008
(408) 374-5920
(800) 538-4545

Life Enhancement Products
P.O. Box 751390
Petaluma, CA 94975
(800) 543-3873
(707) 762-6144
(707) 769-8016 (fax)
www.life-enhancement.com

LifeLink
P.O. Box 1299
Grover Beach, CA 93483
(805) 473-1389
(888) 433-5266 (toll-free)
(805) 473-2803 (fax)
www.lifelinknet.com

Life Services Supplements
3535 Highway 66
Neptune, NJ 07753
(800) 542-3230
(908) 922-0009
(908) 922-5329 (fax)
lifeservic@aol.com

NutriCology/Allergy Research Group
P.O. Box 489
400 Preda St.
San Leandro, CA 94577
(510) 639-4572
(800) 782-4274

NutriGuard Research
P.O. Box 865
Encinitas, CA 92023
(800) 433-2402
(619) 942-3223

Nutrition Plus
4747 E. Elliot Rd., #29
Phoenix, AZ 85044
(800) 241-9236
(970) 872-8664
(970) 872-3862 (fax)

Olympia
1765 Garnet Ave., #66
San Diego, CA 92109
(619) 275-6477
(619) 276-2831 (fax)
www.smart-drugs.com
olympia@smart-drugs.com

Peggy's Health Center
151 First St.
Los Altos, CA 94022
(800) 862-9191
(415) 948-9191
(415) 941-9512 (fax)
www.peggyshealth.com
pegshealth@aol.com

Smart Basics
1626 Union St.
San Francisco, CA 94123
(800) 878-6520
(415) 749-3990
(415) 351-1348 (fax)
www.smartbasic.com
smartnet@sirius.com

Vitamin Research Products
3579 Highway 50 East
Carson City, NV 89701
(800) 877-2447
(702) 884-1300
(800) 877-3292 (fax)
(702) 884-1331 (fax)
www.vrp.com
vrp@delphi.com

Wholesale Nutrition
P.O. Box 3345
Saratoga, CA 95070
(800) 325-2664
(800) 858-6520

The following are mail-order suppliers of aromatherapy products. In addition to offering essential oils and blends, most of these companies also sell diffusers, aromatherapy equipment and accessories, body-care products, and in some cases books and posters, videos, home-study courses, and seminars.

Aromatherapy Seminars
117 N. Robertson Blvd.
Los Angeles, CA 90048
(800) 677-2368
(310) 276-1191
(310) 276-1156 (fax)

Aroma Véra
5901 Rodeo Rd.
Los Angeles, CA 90016
(800) 669-9514
(310) 280-0407
(310) 280-0395 (fax)
www.aromavera.com

Aura Cacia
P.O. Box 399
Weaverville, CA 96093
(916) 623-3301
(800) 437-3301

Essential Aromatics
205 North Signal St.
Ojai, CA 93023
(800) 211-1313
(805) 640-1300
(805) 640-1413 (fax)

Mountain Rose Herbs
P.O. Box 2000
Redway, CA 95560
(707) 923-7867
(800) 879-3337

Quality of Life Associates
9 Demars St.
Maynard, MA 01754
(508) 897-8343
(800) 688-8343
(508) 897-3631 (fax)

Rocky Mountain Pure
P.O. Box 541
Morrison, CO 80465
(303) 777-9474

Simplers Botanical Co.
Box 39
Forestville, CA 95436
(707) 887-2012

MAIL-ORDER SUPPLEMENT DISCOUNTERS

The following companies produce catalogs in which they offer discounted prices on the full product lines of nutritional supplements, herbs, essential oils, and other natural substances from a wide variety of producers:

Nutrition Express
P.O. Box 4076
Torrance, CA 90510
(800) 338-7979
(310) 370-6365
(310) 784-8522 (fax)

Sunburst Biorganics
832 Merrick Rd.
Baldwin, NY 11510
(800) 645-8448
(516) 623-8478
(516) 623-2413 (fax)

Vitamin Discount Connection
35 N. 8th St.
P.O. Box 1431
Indiana, PA 15701
(800) 848-2990
(412) 349-2367
(412) 349-3711 (fax)

The Vitamin Shoppe
4700 Westside Ave.
North Bergen, NJ 07047
(800) 223-1216
(800) 497-1122 (catalog request)
(201) 866-7711
(800) 852-7153 (fax)

Vitamin Specialties
8200 Ogontz Ave.
Wyncote, PA 19095
(800) 365-8482
(215) 885-1310 (fax)

The Vitamin Trader
6501 Fourth St. NW
Albuquerque, NM 87107
(800) 334-9310
(505) 344-6060
(800) 334-9320 (fax)

Wellness Health & Pharmacy
2800 South 18th St.
Birmingham, AL 35209
(800) 227-2627
(800) 369-0302 (fax)

Willner Chemists
330 Lexington Ave.
New York, NY 10016
(800) 633-1106
(212) 685-0448
(212) 545-0951 (fax)

ORDERING SUPPLEMENTS AND SMART
DRUGS FROM FOREIGN SOURCES

Tryptophan and the four smart drugs discussed in chapter 9 (vasopressin, deprenyl, piracetam, and Hydergine) are currently unavailable as over-the-counter supplements in the United States. These substances can legally be purchased, however, from a dozen or so overseas mail-order sources. FDA guidelines can be interpreted as allowing Americans to order limited quantities (up to a three-month supply for personal use) of "experimental" drugs not sold in the United States. These FDA guidelines, however, are not uniformly enforced. The FDA occasionally puts foreign import companies on "import-alert status," meaning that their shipments may be seized by customs and returned to the shipper. As *Smart Drug News* noted recently, "Their detentions are quite troublesome to those unlucky enough to become subjected to their bureaucratic whims, but most packages are getting through. InHome [a foreign importer], for example, has been on import alert for five years, but their successful delivery rate is now in the high nineties!"

Any list of foreign importers that could be provided here would soon be dated. Cognitive Enhancement Research Institute (CERI) of Menlo Park, California, maintains an up-to-date "Resources Listing (Sources and Practitioners)," a directory of mail-order sources for prosexual, life-extension, and smart drugs, and nutrients. The listing includes import-alert status and whether any unresolved customer complaints are pending. Readers are encouraged to contact CERI for the most current information. The list is free to subscribers to CERI's *Smart Drug News* (published ten times annually; $44 per year); it's also provided on CERI's home page on the Internet (www.ceri.com). Changes to the listing are first published in the newsletter and then posted on the Web page. *Smart Drug News* is a valuable resource for breaking news, product analyses, book reviews, and other types of information not only on tryptophan and the smart drugs but also DMAE, phenylalanine, pyroglutamate, and other substances.

The CERI "Resources Listing" also provides an up-to-date list of

- Compounding pharmacies in the United States that can fill physician prescriptions for substances such as tryptophan. (Compounding pharmacies were partially exempted from FDA regulation when the Food Drug & Cosmetic Act passed in 1938, allowing them to offer various products off-limits to the pharmaceutical industry.)
- AIDS drug buyers' clubs

- Approximately seventy-five physicians and other practitioners nationwide who are knowledgeable about smart drugs

Finally, CERI's Web page contains the document "FDA Policy on Mail Importations." This is the full text of the July 20, 1988, memo from the director of the Office of Regional Operations to Regional Food and Drug Detectors on the subject "Pilot Guidance for Release of Mail Importations." Based on these guidelines and the experiences of those who have imported drugs from foreign sources, CERI has developed a set of "Import Policy Recommendations" (also available on their Web page). Among their chief recommendations are to send a letter to the importing company to be returned with your shipment that provides your name, address, and phone number; affirms that the drug is for personal use and constitutes less than a three-month supply; and acknowledges that you were responsible for requesting the drug and the importing company did not promote the drug to you. If you have a doctor and a "life-threatening or debilitating condition," provide the specifics. If you are basically healthy, CERI suggests either providing no details on the reason for ordering the substance or stating that you suffer from "age-related mental decline (a debilitating illness) or from aging (a life-threatening illness). . . . Everybody over thirty suffers from those conditions."

Foreign companies generally ship material to the United States through the U.S. Postal Service. You can request that they use a private carrier such as United Parcel Service or Federal Express, although this does not protect your order from being examined or seized. In fact, regular mail originating overseas is subject to more protection from government intervention (basically, a reasonable cause must exist to suspect that the package violates regulations in some way) than are packages coming into the country on private carriers, as these packages are technically considered "cargo" and are subject to the additional burden of random U.S. Customs inspections.

Some foreign companies will not ship substances to purchasers who live in states that have passed laws controlling or outlawing the substance.

Contact CERI at:

Cognitive Enhancement Research Institute
P.O. Box 4029
Menlo Park, CA 94026
(415) 321-2374
(415) 323-3864 (fax)
www.ceri.com
orders@ceri.win.net

- -

ASSOCIATIONS, TRADE JOURNALS, AND DATABASES

Herbs

American Botanical Council (ABC)
P.O. Box 201660
Austin TX 78720
(800) 373-7105
(512) 331-8868
(512) 331-1924 (fax)
www.herbalgram.org

Herb Research Foundation
1007 Pearl St., Suite 200
Boulder, CO 80302
(303) 449-2265
(303) 449-7849 (fax)
www.herbs.org

HerbalGram is a quarterly publication of the American Botanical Council and the Herb Research Foundation. Educational and business offices are at the ABC. The ABC also sells a wide range of technical herb-related texts, including the most comprehensive English translation of the *German Commission E Monographs* (covering 327 monographs on 190 herbs and herbal formulas; cost is $189).

Napralert, an acronym for natural products alert, is an on-line commercial database maintained at the University of Illinois at Chicago of world literature on the chemical constituents and pharmacology of plant, microbial, and animal (primarily marine) extracts. It contains more than 125,000 scientific articles and books on various aspects of natural products, primarily post-1975 but also going as far back as 1650. For further information about access and costs, contact:

Napralert
Program for Collaborative Research in the
    Pharmaceutical Sciences
College of Pharmacy
University of Illinois at Chicago
833 S. Wood St.
Chicago, IL 60612

Nutrients and Smart Drugs

Nutritional supplement companies that produce informative newsletters include Vitamin Research Products, Life Enhancement Products, Smart Basics, and Life Services Supplements. See addresses in the section on "Mail-Order Sources of Herbs, Nutritional Supplements, Essential Oils, and Smart Drugs." Also see the "Ordering Supplements and Smart Drugs from Foreign Sources" for the CERI and *Smart Drug News.*

The newly organized federal Office of Dietary Supplements is creating a Computer Access to Research on Dietary Supplements (CARDS) dababase that is scheduled to be available by late 1997. For further information contact:

Office of Dietary Supplements
National Institutes of Health
7550 Wisconsin Ave.
Federal Building, Rm. 610
Bethesda, MD 20892
(301) 435-2920

The Life Extension Foundation publishes *Life Extension Magazine,* provides a toll-free hotline to answer members' questions, and offers members discounted prices on various nutrients and formulas. For further information contact:

Life Extension Foundation
P.O. Box 229120
Hollywood, FL 33022
(888) 715-5433
www.lef.org

The Longevity Research Center publishes *Longevity Research Update,* a quarterly newsletter (annual subscription is $16), and books authored by Dr. Ray Sahelian on melatonin, kava, and other supplements. For further information contact:

Longevity Research Center
P.O. Box 12619
Marina Del Rey, CA 90295
(310) 821-2409

Essential Oils and Aromatherapy

Aromatherapy Quarterly
for North American subscriptions
P.O. Box 421
Inverness, CA 94937
(415) 663-9519
(415) 663-9128 (fax)
in the U.K.: 01144181 392 1691

Aromatherapy Seminars
1830 S. Robertson Blvd., #203
Los Angeles, CA 90035
(310) 838-6122
(800) 677-2368

National Association for Holistic Aromatherapy
Scentsitivity Newsletter
P.O. Box 17622
Boulder, CO 80308
(800) 566-6735
(303) 258-3791

The International Journal of Aromatherapy
(U.S. Edition)
c/o American Alliance of Aromatherapy
P.O. Box 309
Depoe Bay, OR 97341
(800) 809-9850

Bibliography

Herbs

The Healing Herbs by Michael Castleman (Emmaus, Pa.: Rodale Press, 1991)

The Healing Power of Herbs by Michael T. Murray, N.D. (Rocklin, Calif.: Prima Publishing, 1991)

Herbal Emissaries: Bringing Chinese Herbs to the West by Steven Foster and Yue Chongxi (Rochester, Vt.: Healing Arts Press, 1992)

An Herbal Guide to Stress Relief by David Hoffman (Rochester, Vt.: Healing Arts Press, 1986)

Herbal Healing for Women: Simple Home Remedies for Women of All Ages by Rosemary Gladstar (New York: Fireside, 1993)

Herbal Renaissance by Steven Foster (Layton, Utah: Gibbs Smith, 1993)

Herbs of Choice: The Therapeutic Use of Phytomedicinals by Varro E. Tyler, Ph.D., Sc.D. (Binghamton, N.Y.: Haworth Press, 1994)

The Herbs of Life by Lesley Tierra, L.Ac. (Freedom, Calif.: The Crossing Press, 1992)

The Honest Herbal by Varro E. Tyler, Ph.D. (Binghamton, N.Y.: Haworth Press, 3d ed., 1993)

The Information Sourcebook of Herbal Medicine edited by David Hoffman (Freedom, Calif.: The Crossing Press, 1994)

Medicinal Mushrooms by Christopher Hobbs, L.Ac. (Santa Cruz, Calif.: Botanica Press, 2d ed., 1995)

Medicinal Plants of the Mountain West by Michael Moore (Santa Fe, N.M.: Red Crane Books, 1993)

Medicinal Plants of the Pacific West by Michael Moore (Santa Fe, N.M.: Red Crane Books, 1993)

Natural Alternatives to Over-the-Counter and Prescription Drugs by Michael T. Murray, N.D. (New York: William Morrow, 1994)

The New Age Herbalist edited by Richard Mabey (New York: Macmillan, 1988)

The New Holistic Herbal by David Hoffman (Rockport, Mass.: Element, 1992)

Out of the Earth: The Essential Book of Herbal Medicine by Simon Y. Mills (New York: Viking Arkana, 1991)

Mind-Altering Plants and Substances

Ecstasy: The MDMA Story by B. Eisner (Berkeley, Calif.: Ronin Publishing, 1989)

Hallucinogenic Plants by Richard Evans Schultes (New York: Golden Press, 1976)

Flowering Plants: Magic in Bloom by P. Mick Richardson, Ph.D. (New York: Chelsea House Publishers, 1986)

LSD, My Problem Child: Reflections on Sacred Drugs, Mysticism, and Science by Albert Hofmann (Los Angeles: Jeremy P. Tarcher/Perigee Books, 1983)

Moksha: Writings on Psychedelics and the Visionary Experience by Aldous Huxley, edited by Michael Horowitz and Cynthia Palmer (Los Angeles, Calif.: Jeremy P. Tarcher, 1982)

Narcotic Plants by William Emboden (New York: Macmillan, 1979)

Pharmacotheon: Entheogenic Drugs, Their Plant Sources and History by Jonathan Ott (Kennewick, Wash.: Natural Products Company, 1993)

Pharmako/Poeia: Plant Powers, Poisons, and Herbcraft by Dale Pendell (San Francisco: Mercury House, 1995)

Plant Intoxicants: A Classic Text on the Use of Mind-Altering Plants by Baron Ernst von Bibra, translated by Hedwig Schleiffer (Rochester, Vt.: Healing Arts Press, 1995; originally published Nuremberg, Germany: Wilhelm Schmid, 1855)

Plants of the Gods: Their Sacred, Healing, and Hallucinogenic Powers by Richard Evans Schultes and Albert Hofmann (Rochester, Vt.: Healing Arts Press, 1992; originally published New York: McGraw Hill, 1979)

Psychedelic Drugs Reconsidered by Lester Grinspoon and James B. Bakalar (New York: Basic Books, 1979)

Psychedelics Encyclopedia by Peter Stafford (Berkeley, Calif.: Ronin Publishing, 1978; 3d ed., 1992)

True Hallucinations by Terence McKenna (San Francisco: HarperSanFrancisco, 1993)

APHRODISIACS

Better Sex Through Chemistry by John Morganthaler and Dan Joy (Petaluma, Calif.: Smart Publications, 1994)

Love Potions: A Guide to Aphrodisiacs and Sexual Pleasures by Cynthia Mervis Watson, M.D., with Angela Hynes (New York: Jeremy P. Tarcher/Perigee, 1993)

The Magical and Ritual Use of Aphrodisiacs by Richard Alan Miller (Rochester, Vt.: Destiny Books, 1993)

Male Sexual Vitality by Michael T. Murray, N.D. (Rocklin, Calif.: Prima Publishing, 1994)

MEDICAL TEXTS

The American Medical Association Encyclopedia of Medicine edited by Charles B. Clayman, M.D. (New York: Random House, 1989)

Current Emergency Diagnosis and Treatment edited by Charles E. Saunders and Mary T. Ho (Norwalk, Ct.: Appleton & Lang, 4th ed., 1992)

Drug Evaluations prepared by the Department of Drugs, American Medical Association (Chicago: American Medical Association, 6th ed., 1986)

Drugs and the Brain by Soloman Snyder, M.D. (New York: Scientific American Books, 1986)

Goodman and Gilman's The Pharmacological Basis of Therapeutics edited by Alfred Goodman Gilman, Louis S. Goodman, and Alfred Gilman (New York: Macmillan Publishing Co., 6th ed., 1980)

Medical Botany: Plants Affecting Man's Health by Walter H. Lewis and Memory P. F. Elvin-Lewis (New York: John Wiley & Sons, 1977)

Pharmacognosy by Varro E. Tyler, Lynn R. Brady, and James E. Robbers (Philadelphia: Lea & Febiger, 1936; 9th ed., 1988)

Physicians' Desk Reference (Montvale, N.J.: Medical Economics Data, 47th ed., 1993)

A Primer of Drug Action by Robert M. Julien (San Francisco: W. H. Freeman and Company, 3d ed., 1981)

Receptors by Richard M. Restak, M.D. (New York: Bantam Books, 1994)

DRUG USE GUIDES

From Chocolate to Morphine: Everything You Need to Know About Mind-Altering Drugs by Andrew Weil, M.D., and Winifred Rosen (New York: Houghton Mifflin, 1983; rev. ed., 1993)

Guide to Psychoactive Drugs by Richard Seymour and David E. Smith, M.D. (New York: Harrington Park Press, 1987)

Legal Highs: A Concise Encyclopedia of Legal Herbs and Chemicals with Psychoactive Properties by Adam Gottlieb (Manhattan Beach, Calif.: Twentieth Century Alchemist, 1992)

Licit and Illicit Drugs by Edward M. Brecher and the Editors of Consumer Reports (Boston: Little, Brown and Company, 1972)

SOCIAL AND CULTURAL HISTORIES OF MIND-ALTERANTS

The Age of Entheogens and the Angels' Dictionary by Jonathan Ott (Kennewick, Wash.: Natural Products Company, 1995)

Buzz: The Science and Lore of Alcohol and Caffeine by Stephen Braun (New York: Oxford University Press, 1996)

Essential Substances: A Cultural History of Intoxicants in Society by Richard Rudgley (New York: Kodansha America, 1994)

The Forbidden Game: A Social History of Drugs by Brian Inglis (New York: Charles Scribner's Sons, 1975)

Hallucinogens: Cross-Cultural Perspectives by Marlene Dobkin de Rios (Albuquerque, N.M.: University of New Mexico Press, 1984)

Intoxication: Life in Pursuit of Artificial Paradise by Ronald K. Siegel, Ph.D. (New York: E. P. Dutton, 1989)

Murder, Magic, and Medicine by John Mann (New York: Oxford University Press, 1992)

Perspectives on the History of Psychoactive Substance Use edited by Gregory A. Austin, Ph.D. (Rockville, Md.: National Institute on Drug Abuse, 1978)

Storming Heaven: LSD and the American Dream by Jay Stevens (New York: The Atlantic Monthly Press, 1987)

Ups and Downs: Drugging and Duping by Julius Rice, M.D. (New York: Macmillan, 1972)

NUTRIENTS AND SMART DRUGS

Brain Boosters: Foods and Drugs That Make You Smarter by Beverly A. Potter, Ph.D., and Sebastian Orfali (Berkeley, Calif.: Ronin Publishing, 1993)

Eat Smart, Think Smart by Robert Haas (New York: HarperCollins, 1994)

Mind Food and Smart Pills by Ross Pelton, R.Ph., Ph.D., with Taffy Clarke Pelton (New York: Main Street Books/Doubleday, 1989)

Off-the-Shelf Natural Health: How to Use Herbs and Nutrients to Stay Well by Mark Mayell (New York: Bantam Books, 1995)

Smart Drugs II: The Next Generation by Ward Dean, M.D., John Morganthaler, and Steven W. Fowkes (Menlo Park, Calif.: Health Freedom Publications, 1993)

Smart Nutrients by Abram Hoffer, Ph.D., and Morton Walker, D.P.M. (Garden City Park, N.Y.: Avery Publishing Group, 1993)

Thorsons Guide to Amino Acids by Leon Chaitow, N.D., D.O. (London: Thorsons, 1991)

ESSENTIAL OILS

Aromatherapy for Common Ailments by Shirley Price (New York: Fireside, 1991)

Aromatherapy for Vibrant Health and Beauty by Roberta Wilson (Garden City Park, N.Y.: Avery Publishing Group, 1995)

Aromatherapy: The Complete Guide to Plant and Flower Essences for Health and Beauty by Danièle Ryman (New York: Bantam Books, 1993)

The Art of Aromatherapy by Robert Tisserand (Rochester, Vt.: Healing Arts Press, 1977)

Complete Aromatherapy Handbook by Susanne Fischer-Rizzi (New York: Sterling Publishing Company, 1990)

The Complete Book of Essential Oils and Aromatherapy by Valerie Ann Worwood (San Rafael, Calif.: New World Library, 1991)

The Complete Home Guide to Aromatherapy by Erich Keller (Tiburon, Calif.: H. J. Kramer, 1991)

The Encyclopaedia of Essential Oils by Julia Lawless (Rockport, Mass.: Element, 1992)

The Practice of Aromatherapy by Jean Valnet (Rochester, Vt.: Healing Arts Press, 1990)

Scentual Touch: A Personal Guide to Aromatherapy by Judith Jackson (New York: Henry Holt and Company, 1986)

Index

heart disease
    benefits of green tea, 30–31
    benefits of melatonin, 168
Henman, Anthony Richard, 72–73, 74
herbal ecstacy, 56, 62, 74
HerbalGram, 56, 62
Herb Research Foundation (HRF), 56
herbs
    California poppy, 160–162
    ephedra, 15, 49–65
    FDA list of unsafe, 216
    ginkgo, 135–140
    ginseng, 37–43
    green tea, 24, 28–34
    growing market for medicinal, 204
    guarana, 71–75
    kava, 191–205
    kola nut, 77–79
    licorice, 64, 153
    maté, 75–76, 77
    Siberian ginseng, 44–47
    St. John's wort, 89–93
    tonic, 35–37, 39, 44
    valerian, 147–157
    yohimbé, 207–220
heroin, 159
Hildegard of Bingen, 148
Hindmarch, Ian, 138
Hippocrates, 148
Hobbs, Christopher, 92
Hoffer, Abram, 200
Hofmann, Albert, 119–120
Holland, tea drinking, 26–27, 30
hormones
    vasopressin, 107–111
    See also melatonin
HRF. *See* Herb Research Foundation
HTP. *See* 5-HTP (5-hydroxytrypto-
    phan)
Huether, Gerald, 168
Hutchison, Michael, 109
Huxley, Aldous, 14
Hydergine, 107–108, 118
    antioxidant role, 121
    in combination with piracetam, 121

commercial products, 121–122
development, 119–120
dosages, 121, 122
effects, 107, 118, 120–121
research on, 120, 120–121
safety, 121
side effects, 121
uses, 120
hypericin, 91, 92
hypnotics. *See* relaxants
Hyssop oil, 100
    See also essential oils

*I*mmune system, effects of mela-
    tonin, 167
impotence remedies
    kola nut, 78
    yohimbine, 208, 211, 217–218
India, ephedra use, 50
Indian snakeroot, 213
inebriants, 11–12, 16
    controlled use of, 225
    kava, 191–205
    yohimbé, 209
insomnia remedies
    GABA, 187
    melatonin, 165, 166, 172
    over-the-counter, 172
    tryptophan, 177–178
    valerian, 149, 150, 155
    See also relaxants
insulin, 31, 181
intoxicants, 12
    See also inebriants
isoquinoline alkaloids, 161

*J*apan, tea drinking, 25, 31
jasmine (plant), 98
Jasmine oil
    absolute, 99
    cost, 97
    uses, 98–99
    See also essential oils
Jesuit's tea. *See* maté

jet lag, melatonin as remedy, 166, 172, 174
Johnson, Samuel, 32
Josta, 74
Joy, Dan, 13

*K*aempfer, Engelbert, 136
kava
    abuse of, 203
    beverage, 191–192, 193–194, 197–198, 204
    chemistry, 194–196, 199
    compared to alcohol, 200–202
    cultivation, 4–5, 192
    dosages, 199, 205
    effects, 195–196, 198–200, 202–203
    extracts, 198, 204, 205
    forms, 204–205
    medical applications, 202–203
    plant, 4–5, 192
    psychoactive compounds, 194–195, 199
    research on, 195–196, 199, 202
    safety, 203–204
    side effects, 203
    tea, 197, 205
    traditional preparation method, 193, 197–198
    use in Pacific region, 191, 193–194, 197, 200–202
kavalactones, 195–196, 199
    synthetic, 204
Kessler, David, 59
khat, 53
Kilham, Chris, 199
King, Penny, 62
kola nut
    caffeine content, 77
    effects on body, 78
    products containing, 78–79
    research on, 78
    theobromine content, 69, 77
    traditional preparation, 78
Krieglstein, J., 152

L-5-hydroxytryptophan, *see* 5-HTP
Lavender oil, 101
   See also essential oils
learning disorders, children with,
   116, 130–131
Lebot, Vincent, 193, 199
lecithin, 125–126
   dosages, 128
   safety, 127, 128
Lerner, Aaron, 173
Lewin, Louis, 7, 194, 199, 201
Lewis, Walter H., 37
licorice, 64, 153
Life Enhancement Products, 214
Lindstrom, Lamont, 193
lipofuscin, 117, 121, 173
Love, Lori A., 179
L-phenylalanine, 82, 83, 84
LSD-25, 119
L-tryptophan. *See* tryptophan
Lucidryl (centrophenoxine), 131
lypressin, 110
lysine-vasopressin, 110

*M*a huang, 50, 53, 64
   See also ephedra
Manders, Dean Wolfe, 180
MAO (monoamine oxidase)
      inhibitors
   antidepressants, 92, 173, 214
   California poppy as, 162
   deprenyl as, 112–113
   ginkgo as, 139
   hypericin as, 92
   side effects, 214
   yohimbé as, 213–214
MAO-A, 112
MAO-B, 112, 113
Mao Zedong, 31
Maradona, Diego, 63
marijuana, 109, 173
Martius, K. F. P. von, 72
massage, with essential oils, 102

maté
   caffeine content, 76
   dosages, 77
   plant, 75
   safety, 76
   side effects, 76
   teas containing, 77
   traditional preparation, 75–76
Maury, Marguerite, 98, 143
McCaleb, Robert, 62
McKenna, Terence, 69
MDMA. *See* ecstasy (drug)
melanin, 173
melanoma, 173
melatonin, 163
   antioxidant role, 167, 173
   combined with valerian, 156
   commercial products, 169, 174–175
   debate over taking supplements,
      168–172
   dosages, 171, 174, 175
   effects, 163, 165–166, 167–168,
      173, 227
   everyday use, 174–175
   interactions with other drugs, 173
   levels in body, 164 165
   popularity, 163–164
   prescription drugs based on, 169
   production in body, 164, 165,
      184–185
   research on, 163, 165–166,
      167–168, 171, 172, 173
   safety, 163, 168, 170–172, 173
   side effects, 169, 172–173
   storage, 175
   supplements, 166–167, 168–170,
      171
   synthetic vs. natural, 5, 175
   timed-release products, 175
   timing of doses, 174–175
   vasopressin levels and, 110
memory boosters
   choline, 125
   deprenyl, 112
   DMAE, 130
   5-HTP, 183

ginkgo, 135, 138–139
piracetam, 117
pyroglutamate, 132–133
Rosemary oil, 144
vasopressin, 108, 109
men
   effects of yohimbine on erections,
      209, 211, 212
   impotence remedies, 208, 211,
      217–218
menstrual tension and cramps
   use of melatonin, 168
   use of valerian, 153
mental illness
   safety of mind-alterants, 227
   See also depression
mental performance
   effects of caffeine, 70
   effects of ginseng, 40
   See also brain boosters; memory
      boosters; smart drugs
menthol, 142
Merlin, Mark, 193, 205
methylxanthines. *See* xanthines
Mexican gold, 160
migraine headaches, effects of
   5-HTP, 183
Mills, Simon, 53, 90
mind-alterants
   actions, 15–17
   advice from other users, 227
   allergic reactions, 18
   as alternatives to other
      substances, 14–15
   aphrodisiacs, 12–13, 16
   brain boosters, 9–10, 16
   categories, 7–13, 15, 16
   combining, 226
   compulsive use, 224, 226
   controlled use, 224, 225–228
   everyday use, 40, 174–175, 224
   individual relationships with,
      223–225, 226
   inebriants, 11–12, 16, 225
   information available, 17, 18–19,
      226–227

mind-alterants (*cont.*)
mood brighteners, 8–9, 16
pejorative context, 3, 4
potential adverse effects, 223
purchasing, 228
purposes, 6
relaxants, 10–11, 16
safety, 17–18, 226–228
set and setting of use, 224–225, 227
stimulants, 8, 16, 225
use across cultures, 13–14
use in United States, 14
mint, 142
See also Peppermint oil
Mintz, Sidney W., 27
monoamine oxidase (MAO) inhibitors. *See* MAO (monoamine oxidase) inhibitors
mood brighteners, 8–9, 16
5-HTP, 183–184
Jasmine oil, 97, 98–99
kava, 196
melatonin, 166
Neroli oil, 97, 99–100
phenylalanine, 82
Rose oil, 97–98, 99, 101
St. John's wort, 89–93
yohimbé, 208
mood disorders, 9
See also depression
Moore, Michael, 150, 161, 213
Morgenthaler, John, 13, 109, 211
Mormon tea, 49–50, 53
Morning Thunder tea, 77
morphine, 159, 160
Mucho Maté tea, 77
Murray, Michael, 63, 171, 216

*N*arcotics, 11
National Academy of Sciences, 126
National Collegiate Athletic Association (NCAA), 63
National Down Syndrome Congress, 116
National Institutes of Health, 91

National Nutritional Foods Association (NNFA), 60–61
natural high products, 54, 55–57, 58
FDA warning on, 59–60
guarana in, 74
opposition to, 61
natural products, definition, 4–5
NCAA (National College Athletic Association), 63
Neroli oil, 99–100
cost, 97
effects, 100
See also essential oils
nerve tonics, 90
nervous system. *See* central nervous system
neurasthenia, 98, 149
neurotransmitters
acetylcholine, 116–117, 123–124, 125, 133, 210
actions, 82–83
adrenaline, 50–51, 53, 68, 82–83, 123
dopamine, 82–83, 112, 184, 210
effects of deprenyl, 112
functions, 123
roles in sleep, 152
synthesized from phenylalanine, 82–83
synthesized from tyrosine, 84
See also noradrenaline; serotonin
Niaouli, 100
N-methylephedrine, 53
NNFA. *See* National Nutritional Foods Association
nootropic substances, 6–7
piracetam, 107–108, 115–118, 121
pyroglutamate, 132–133
Nootropil, 117
noradrenaline
actions in body, 82–83, 123, 164
effects of deprenyl, 112
effects of ephedrine, 53
effects of 5-HTP, 184
effects of yohimbine, 210
See also selective noradrenalin reuptake inhibitors (SNRIs)

norephedrine, 53
norpseudoephedrine, 53
NutraSweet, 82
nutritional supplements, regulation of, 18–19, 58–59, 169–170, 216–217

*O*ats, 79
Olympic Committee, U.S., 63
oolong tea, 24
opium, 14
opium poppy, 159–160
Orange Blossom oil. *See* Neroli oil
orange flower water, 100
Osmond, Humphry, 200
osteoporosis, 168
Ott, Jonathan, 12
oxiracetam, 117
oxitriptan. *See* 5-HTP (5-hydroxy-tryptophan)
oxygen, low levels of, 115–116, 153

*P*acific islands, kava use, 191, 193–194, 197, 200–202
PAF (platelet-activating factor), 135
pain relievers
caffeine, 29
California poppy, 161
for headaches, 29, 142, 183
kava, 196, 203
melatonin, 168
phenylalanine, 82, 83
valerian, 149, 153
Paraguay, maté consumption, 75–76
Paraguayan tea. *See* maté
Parkinson's disease, 112
use of ginkgo, 138
use of smart drugs, 107, 112
use of tyrosine, 85
PDIs. *See* peripheral decarboxylase inhibitors
PEA (phenylethylamine), 83, 111
Pelton, Ross, 110
Pendell, Dale, 7

women
    effects of melatonin on fertility,
        168, 171, 173
    effects of yohimbé, 214–215
    menstrual tension and cramps,
        153, 168
    nervous conditions, 149
    pregnant, 227
    premenstrual syndrome (PMS),
        32
    use of valerian, 153
Wurtman, Richard, 168–169

X anax. *See* benzodiazepines
xanthines, 67–68
    adverse health effects, 32–33
    effects on body, 70
    in guarana, 72
    in kola nut, 77
    in tea, 28

theobromine, 28, 67, 68, 69, 72, 77
theophylline, 28, 30, 67, 68–69, 72
See also caffeine

Y aupon, 76–77
yerba maté. *See* maté
Ylang Ylang, 97
yoco, 75
yohimbé
    commercial products, 217, 219
    compounds in, 208, 213
    controversies about, 207, 208
    dosages, 216, 217–220
    effects, 208–210, 213–214, 216
    regulators' views of, 216–217
    research on, 208, 210–211
    safety, 215–217
    side effects, 209, 216, 218
    standardized extracts, 213–214
    tea, 207, 210, 219–220

timing of doses, 219
    use in Africa, 207
    as weight loss aid, 208
yohimbine, 208
    actions in body, 210–213
    combined with other substances,
        56
    dosages, 214, 217–218
    effects on women, 214–215
    as impotence remedy, 208, 211,
        217–218
    prescription drugs containing,
        208
    research on, 210–211, 212–213,
        214–215, 217–218
Young, Anthony, 61

Z eisel, Steven, 126
Zinberg, Norman E., 224, 225,
    227

About the Author

⊚

Mark Mayell is the author of *Off-the-Shelf Natural Health: How to Use Herbs and Nutrients to Stay Well*. He is also coauthor, with the editors of *Natural Health* magazine, of *The Natural Health First-Aid Guide* and *52 Simple Steps to Natural Health*. His experience includes a seven-year stint as the editor of *Natural Health* and three years as the editor of the magazine's book publishing division. He has also served as the editor of *Nutrition Action,* the monthly newsletter of the Washington, D.C., nutrition advocacy group Center for Science in the Public Interest. Mark has written extensively on alternative approaches to health for *Natural Health, New Age Journal,* and other magazines. He serves on the advisory boards of the American Holistic Health Association and Food & Water, Inc. Mark has a master's degree in philosophy and social policy from George Washington University. He lives with his wife and two children in the Boston area.